Toxicity Testing
New Approaches and Applications in Human Risk Assessment

Toxicity Testing
New Approaches and Applications in Human Risk Assessment

Editor-In-Chief

A. P. Li, Ph.D.

Associate Editors

T. L. Blank, B.Sc.
D. K. Flaherty, Ph.D.
W. E. Ribelin, D.V.M., Ph.D.
A. G. E. Wilson, Ph.D.

Environmental Health Laboratory
Monsanto Company
St. Louis, Missouri

Raven Press ■ New York

Raven Press, 1140 Avenue of the Americas, New York, New York 10036

© 1985 by Raven Press Books, Ltd. All rights reserved. This book is protected by copyright. No part of it may be reproduced, stored in a retrieval system, or transmitted, in any form or by any means, electronic, mechanical, photocopying, recording, or otherwise, without the prior written permission of the publisher.

Made in the United States of America

Library of Congress Cataloging in Publication Data
Main entry under title:

Toxicity testing: New approaches and applications
in human risk assessment.

Based on a conference held Sept. 14–15, 1983, in the
World Headquarters of Monsanto Co., St. Louis, Mo.
Includes bibliographies and index.
1. Toxicity testing—Congresses. 2. Health risk
assessment—Congresses. I. Li, A. P. [DNLM:
1. Toxicology—methods—congresses. QV 602 N532 1983]
RA1199.N47 1985   615.9'07   84-27634
ISBN 0-88167-083-9

Papers or parts thereof have been used as camera-ready copy as submitted by the authors whenever possible; when retyped, they have been edited by the editorial staff only to the extent considered necessary for the assistance of an international readership. The views expressed and the general style adopted remain, however, the responsibility of the named authors. Great care has been taken to maintain the accuracy of the information contained in the volume. However, neither Raven Press nor the editors can be held responsible for errors or for any consequences arising from the use of information contained herein.

The use in this book of particular designations of countries or territories does not imply any judgment by the publisher or editors as to the legal status of such countries or territories, of their authorities or institutions, or of the delimitation of their boundaries.

Some of the names of products referred to in this book may be registered trademarks or proprietary names, although specific reference to this fact may not be made: however, the use of a name without designation is not to be construed as a representation by the publisher or editors that it is in the public domain. In addition, the mention of specific companies or of their products or proprietary names does not imply any endorsement or recommendation on the part of the publisher or editors.

Authors were themselves responsible for obtaining the necessary permission to reproduce copyright material from other sources. With respect to the publisher's copyright, material appearing in this book prepared by individuals as part of their official duties as government employees is only covered by this copyright to the extent permitted by the appropriate national regulations.

Materials appearing in this book prepared by individuals as part of their official duties as U.S. Government employees are not covered by the above-mentioned copyright.

Preface

For the past twenty years there has been a dramatic rise in both the manufacturing and application of chemicals in the work and home environments. While the benefits to the quality of life from the use of chemicals are readily apparent, there has been increasing concern in recent years about the potential health effects of such chemicals. This concern has led to a vigorous research effort in the establishment of promising approaches to evaluate the toxic potential of chemicals, as well as the validation and standardization of the established approaches. Regulatory policies, such as the Toxic Substances Control Act and the Federal Fungicide Insecticide Rodenticide Act, have been established.

Human health is the matter of concern in the regulation of the release of new chemicals in our environment; it is therefore of utmost importance to investigate experimental approaches that yield the most relevant scientific data upon which human risk assessment can be made. Such is the theme being addressed in this book.

The chapters in this book have been written by experts in various disciplines of toxicology—including genetic toxicology, xenobiotic metabolism, pharmacokinetics, immunology, reproduction biology, teratology, and epidemiology. This book is intended for the use of workers from academia, government, and industry who are interested in improving the sophistication of our toxicology testing procedures to reduce the uncertainty in the extrapolation of toxicity data to humans.

A. P. Li, Ph.D.
A. G. E. Wilson, Ph.D.

Acknowledgments

The conference on which this volume is based was held on September 14 and 15, 1983 in the World Headquarters of Monsanto Company, St. Louis, Missouri.

The following are acknowledged for their participation in the conference: Organizing Committee: Thomas L. Blank, Dennis K. Flaherty, Albert P. Li, William E. Ribelin, and Alan G. E. Wilson (Chairman); Public Relations: William H. Westendorf; World Headquarters Administration Meeting Planning: June Nienaber and Eugene F. McCoskey; Accounting and Administration: Jack G. Cooper, Dianne M. Olive, and Sharon A. Williams

The editors gratefully acknowledge the contribution of the Monsanto Graphics Department: Patricia Green, Shirley Hambee, Gary Kemper, Lynda Kraus, Khris Rice, and Jane Rupp.

Contents

Overview

Complexities of Evaluating the Toxicological Risk to Humans 3
Leon Golberg

Genetic Toxicology
Section Editor: A. P. Li

Use of Human Cells in Mutagenicity and Carcinogenicity
    Determination 17
J. Justin McCormick and Veronica M. Maher

Measurement of Chemically-Induced DNA Repair in Rodent
    and Human Cells 33
Byron E. Butterworth

Use of Cytogenetic Endpoints in Human Lymphocytes as
    Indicators of Exposure to Genotoxicants 41
R. Julian Preston

Use of Human T-Lymphocytes to Monitor Mutations in Human
    Populations 51
Richard J. Albertini

Identification of Environmental Carcinogens by Detecting the
    Induction of a Retrogenetic Expression 67
R. H. Stevens, P. A. Lindholm, D. A. Cole, P. T. Liu, and H. F. Cheng

Effects of Structurally Diverse Chemicals on Metabolic
    Cooperation *In Vitro* 79
A. Russell Malcolm and Lesley J. Mills

Use of Formalin-Treated Cells in the DNA-Cell Binding Assay for
    Genotoxic and Carcinogenetic Chemicals 93
H. Kubinski, Z. O. Kubinski, and J. Shahidi

Discussion 99

Metabolic and Pharmacokinetic Approaches
Section Editor: A. G. E. Wilson

Significance of Metabolism Studies in Toxicity Testing and Risk Assessment 105
Rick G. Schnellmann and I. Glenn Sipes

Drug Metabolizing Enzyme Systems and Their Relationship to Toxic Mechanisms 119
M. R. Boyd, V. Ravindranath, L. T. Burka, J. S. Dutcher, R. B. Franklin, C. N. Statham, W. M. Haschek, P. J. Hakkinen, C. C. Morse, and H. P. Witschi

Physiological Pharmacokinetics: Relevance to Human Risk Assessment 129
R. J. Lutz and R. L. Dedrick

Pharmacokinetics of Inhaled Chlorobenzene in the Rat 151
Timothy M. Sullivan, Gordon S. Born, Gary P. Carlson, and Wayne V. Kessler

Discussion 159

Toxicity to the Immune System and the Fetus
Section Editor: D. K. Flaherty

Assessment of the Effects of Chemicals on the Immune System 165
Peter H. Bick, Michael P. Holsapple, and Kimber L. White, Jr.

Risk Assessment for Transplacental Carcinogenesis 179
Lucy M. Anderson, Paul J. Donovan, and Jerry M. Rice

Validity of *In Vitro* Methods in Teratogenicity Testing 203
Allan R. Beaudoin

Development and Validation of a Panel of Host Resistance and Immune Function Assays Designed to Detect Chemical-Induced Immunomodulation 213
Peter T. Thomas, Ruth A. Fugmann, Catherine Aranyi, and James D. Fenters

Discussion 223

Dose-Response Models, Environment, and Epidemiology
Section Editor: W. E. Ribelin

Assessment of Various Dose-Response Models in the Determination of Risk 227
Tom Downs

Environmental Distribution and Fate: Its Role in Risk Assessment .. 235
W. Brock Neely

Use of Epidemiology in Risk Assessment 247
William R. Gaffey

Human Biologic Parameters as Epidemiologic Tools in Environmental Risk Assessment 253
Clark W. Heath, Jr.

Panel Discussion
Section Editor: T. L. Blank

Panel Discussion: New Approaches in Toxicity Testing and Their Application in Human Risk Assessment 263

Subject Index..273

Contributors

Richard J. Albertini
Department of Medicine
University of Vermont College of
  Medicine
Burlington, Vermont 05405

Lucy M. Anderson
Laboratory of Comparative
  Carcinogenesis
National Institutes of Health
National Cancer Institute
Frederick Cancer Research Facility
Building 538, Room 205E
Frederick, Maryland 21701

Catherine Aranyi
IIT Research Institute
Life Sciences Research
10 West 35th Street
Chicago, Illinois 60616

Allan R. Beaudoin
Department of Anatomy and Cell Biology
University of Michigan
Ann Arbor, Michigan 48109

Peter H. Bick
Department of Microbiology and
  Immunology
Virginia Commonwealth University
Richmond, Virginia 23298

Gordon S. Born
Schools of Pharmacy and Health Sciences
Purdue University
West Lafayette, Indiana 47907

M. R. Boyd
National Cancer Institute
Bethesda, Maryland 20205

L. T. Burka
Toxicology and Research Testing Program
NIEHS
Post Office Box 12233
Research Triangle Park, North Carolina
  27709

Byron E. Butterworth
Chemical Industry Institute of Toxicology
Research Triangle Park, North Carolina
  27709

Gary P. Carlson
Schools of Pharmacy and Health Sciences
Purdue University
West Lafayette, Indiana 47907

H. F. Cheng
Radiation Research Laboratory
Department of Radiology
University of Iowa
Iowa City, Iowa 52242

D. A. Cole
Radiation Research Laboratory
Department of Radiology
University of Iowa
Iowa City, Iowa 52242

R. L. Dedrick
Chemical Engineering Section
Biomedical Engineering and
  Instrumentation Branch
Division of Research Services
National Institutes of Health
Bethesda, Maryland 20205

Paul J. Donovan
Laboratory of Comparative
  Carcinogenesis
National Institutes of Health
National Cancer Institute
Frederick Cancer Research Facility
Building 538, Room 205E
Frederick, Maryland 21701

Tom Downs
The University of Texas School of Public
  Health
Houston, Texas 77025

J. S. Dutcher
Inhalation Toxicology Research Institute
Albuquerque, New Mexico 87105

CONTRIBUTORS

James D. Fenters
ITT Research Institute
Life Sciences Research
10 West 35th Street
Chicago, Illinois 60616

R. B. Franklin
National Cancer Institute
Bethesda, Maryland 20205

Ruth A. Fugmann
ITT Research Institute
Life Sciences Research
10 West 35th Street
Chicago, Illinois 60616

William R. Gaffey
Department of Epidemiology
Monsanto Company
800 North Lindbergh
St. Louis, Missouri 63167

Leon Golberg
Division of Community and Occupational
    Medicine
Duke University Medical Center
Durham, North Carolina 27710

P. J. Hakkinen
Proctor and Gamble Company
Sharon Woods Technical Center
Cincinnati, Ohio 45241

W. M. Haschek
Department of Veterinary Pathobiology
University of Illinois
2001 South Lincoln
Urbana, Illinois 60801

Clark W. Heath, Jr.
Masters of Public Health Program
Department of Community Health
Emory University School of Medicine
Atlanta, Georgia 30322

Michael P. Holsapple
Department of Microbiology and
    Immunology
Virginia Commonwealth University
Richmond, Virginia 23298

Wayne V. Kessler
Schools of Pharmacy and Health Sciences
Purdue University
West Lafayette, Indiana 47907

H. Kubinski
University of Wisconsin School of
    Medicine
Madison, Wisconsin 53706

Z. O. Kubinski
University of Wisconsin School of
    Medicine
Madison, Wisconsin 53706

P. A. Lindholm
Radiation Research Laboratory
Department of Radiology
University of Iowa
Iowa City, Iowa 52242

P. T. Liu
Radiation Research Laboratory
Department of Radiology
University of Iowa
Iowa City, Iowa 52242

R. J. Lutz
Chemical Engineering Section
Biomedical Engineering and
    Instrumentation Branch
Division of Research Services
National Institutes of Health
Bethesda, Maryland 20205

Veronica M. Maher
Carcinogenesis Laboratory—Fee Hall
Department of Biochemistry
Michigan State University
East Lansing, Michigan 48824

A. Russell Malcolm
United States Environmental Protection
    Agency
Narragansett, Rhode Island 02882

J. Justin McCormick
Carcinogenesis Laboratory—Fee Hall
Department of Microbiology
Michigan State University
East Lansing, Michigan 48824

Lesley J. Mills
Department of Microbiology
University of Rhode Island
Kingston, Rhode Island 02881

C. C. Morse
Biology Division
Oak Ridge National Laboratory
Oak Ridge, Tennessee 37830

CONTRIBUTORS

W. Brock Neely
Environmental Sciences Research
The Dow Chemical Company
Midland, Michigan 48640

R. Julian Preston
Biology Division
Oak Ridge National Laboratory
Oak Ridge, Tennessee 37831

V. Ravindranath
National Cancer Institute
Bethesda, Maryland 20205

Jerry M. Rice
Laboratory of Comparative
 Carcinogenesis
National Institutes of Health
National Cancer Institute
Frederick Cancer Research Facility
Building 538, Room 205E
Frederick, Maryland 21701

Rick G. Schnellmann
Department of Pharmacology and
 Toxicology
College of Pharmacy
University of Arizona
Tucson, Arizona 85721

J. Shahidi
University of Wisconsin School of
 Medicine
Madison, Wisconsin 53706

I. Glenn Sipes
Department of Pharmacology and
 Toxicology
College of Pharmacy
University of Arizona
Tucson, Arizona 85721

C. N. Statham
Toxicology Branch
10th Medical Laboratory
A.P.O., New York 09180

R. H. Stevens
Radiation Research Laboratory
Department of Radiology
University of Iowa
Iowa City, Iowa 52242

Timothy M. Sullivan
College of Medicine
University of South Florida
Saint Petersburg, Florida 33701

Peter T. Thomas
IIT Research Institute
Life Sciences Research
10 West 35th Street
Chicago, Illinois 60616

Kimber L. White, Jr.
Department of Microbiology and
 Immunology
Virginia Commonwealth University
Richmond, Virginia 23298

H. P. Witschi
Biology Division
Oak Ridge National Laboratory
Oak Ridge, Tennessee 37830

Foreword

Toxicology has experienced rapid growth over the past few years. What used to be defined as classical toxicology presently represents only a subset of the whole field. From the time of the first non-clinical experiment, toxicologists have been plagued with the problem of interpreting the data in a manner that has relevance to man. This has led to new techniques which explore more the "how" of toxicology than the "what" in anticipation that the resulting data will permit more accurate extrapolation to man.

The symposium speakers described new techniques and new approaches to old techniques, ranging from the use of human cells to computer modeling. Each of the techniques and study parameters presented added to our knowledge of mechanisms, our ability to predict human effects, as well as the complexity of the task. Progress can and will be made if consideration is given to eventual extrapolation to man during the experimental design.

Roger M. Folk, Ph.D.
Director, Environmental Health Laboratory
Monsanto Company

Toxicity Testing
New Approaches and Applications in Human Risk Assessment

Overview

New Approaches in Toxicity Testing and Their Application in Human Risk Assessment, edited by A. P. Li. Raven Press, New York © 1985.

Complexities of Evaluating the Toxicological Risk to Humans

Leon Golberg

Division of Community and Occupational Medicine, Duke University Medical Center, Durham, North Carolina 27710

In discussing the complexities of evaluating the toxicological risk to man, I am aware that one of the most important is the difficulty in communcation. This is illustrated by the wording "Washington Biological Survey", abbreviated to "WASH BIOL SURV" on the tags attached by the Department of the Interior in the course of their study of migratory birds. They had a letter from a farmer who said, "Dear Sirs, I shot one of your crows and I followed the instructions attached to it. I washed it, I boiled it and served it, and it was the most awful food we ever had."

People are our primary concern.

There has been a progressive subdivision of toxicology into specialties and subspecialties, a process which has created a multitude of scientists in this field, each of whom concentrates on one organism or type of chemical or particular organ or system, or a specific cell type, or even a subcellular organelle, enzyme system or other cellular component. Although this process of micronization is essential, unavoidable and even beneficial as far as progress is concerned, it is important not to lose sight of the big picture, the raison d'être of the whole enterprise, namely, safety for man. As William D. Ruckelshaus (1983) put it " . . . we must assume that life now takes place in a minefield of risks from hundreds, perhaps thousands of substances. We can no longer tell the public that they have an adequate margin of safety." I think he was referring to environmental contaminants, but that is a truth that applies on far wider scale, as we are realizing and as I shall attempt to elaborate. And so, since complete safety is unattainable, the process of evaluating risk becomes the practical approach, albeit fraught with daunting complexities. In thinking over what one might call the "Toxicologist's Progress", by analogy with the Pilgrim's Progress, in evaluating risk to man, I felt that only Greek mythology can adequately express what has been involved in the course of years. In Table 1 I have tried to summarize the different stages as they would be described. You will recall that Medusa had an infinite capacity to grow new heads as fast as the old ones were severed. That is reminiscent of the unending stream of objections that can be raised to any and all hazard assessments. In the context of the Toxicologist's Progress, Stage I represents the one-molecule theory, which began with carcinogenicity, was extended to mutagenicity and teratogencity and is still going strong. Disbelievers suffered dire penalties, including the one indicated in Table 1 or even worse, a cut-off of research funds.

TABLE I

Toxicologist's Progress in Evaluating Risk to Man

Stage	Nature of Obstacle				Penalty
	Name	Heads	Feet	Hair	
I	Medusa	1	2	Snakes	Turned to stone
II	Cerberus	Many	4	Snakes	Consigned to Hades
III	Scylla	6	12	?	Seized and devoured
IV	Sisyphus	1	2	Normal	Keep pushing heavy rock to top of steep hill

Stage II was a heretical belief in thresholds for any carcinogens. Cerberus, this many-headed dog with a mane and tail made up of snakes, waited at the door of Hades for those who had the temerity even to think in terms of thresholds.

In Stage III, Scylla was the siren who tempted men with the charms of epigenetic carcinogenesis. Once trapped, the penalty was frightful to behold. Those who survived the temptations of Scylla reached State IV, the mathematical models that have sought to quantify the relationship between dose and response as a basis for risk assessment. The fate that awaited them was that of Sisyphus who was condemned to roll a huge rock up to the top of the hill repeatedly, only to have it roll down again. In the field of mathematical modeling, the first time around, the models dealt with quantal responses and focused on $P(d)$ in expressions such as the probit, logit, Weibull and multi-stage models (Van Ryzin, 1980; Munro and Krewski, 1981). Before long, these approaches became passé because time to response had to be taken into account, in the absence of competing risks. The focus was now on $P(t,d)$ in expressions such as the log-linear, Cox regression, multi-hit, Hartley-Sielken and Krewski approximation. The third time around, we now have cause-specific models in those instances where carcinogenic response times are observable. These models utilize the time at which the event occurs, as well as taking into account competing risks and their effect on the probability of response at dose d (Sielken, 1983). Cause-specific probabilities can be estimated without untestable assumptions on competing risks.

Significant advances

So we have this repetitive struggling to push the rock up the hill and then have it come down and start all over again. However, there have been significant advances. Progress had been made in two directions, both involving greater depth of biological insight, as distinct from mathematical manipulation of end-results. The standard approach to the application of a mathematical model has traditionally involved reliance on Haber's law that the product of concentration and time, that is C x t is constant. On this basis a continuous exposure, 24 hours a day, 7 days week, over a lifetime or over a working lifetime has been calculated by simple proportion from the actual conditions of exposure, as the first step in determining dose. This approach has two serious flaws. First of all, in many cases C x t is not constant. An example is provided by the work of Swenberg et al. (1983) on inhalation of formaldehyde by rats, in which they studied the effect of concentration C, as opposed to cumulative dose Ct, on cell turnover in the nasal mucosa. They showed that the same product in terms of ppm-hours, 36 total ppm-hours of exposure, but with different concentrations for different times, gave rise to very different effects. At 12 ppm (for 3 hr) there was a 17-fold elevation in the proportion of ^{3}H-labeled cells, as compared with 3 ppm (for 12 hr). Similarly a 6-month exposure of rats at 15 ppm (6 hr/day, 5 days/week) yields 450 ppm-hr/week, with severe effects on the nasal mucosa, whereas 6 months at 3 ppm (22 hr/day, 7 days/week), a total of 462 ppm-hr/week (Rusch et al., 1983) produces much less toxicity to the nasal mucosa.

These results are simply a reflection of the fact that, at higher concentrations of formaldehyde, severe tissue damage occurs, with cell necrosis and death, followed by regeneration, compensatory proliferation and hyperplasia. Hence these pathological changes are concentration-dependent effects, rather than the overall product of cumulative exposure. The resulting carcinogenicity in this instance is dependent on long-continued and repeated production of cycles of severe, extensive tissue damage and repair. Where such exposure is intermittent, for example six hours a day, five days a week, important reparative changes occur overnight, and especially at week-ends. To ignore these restorative intervals by calculating a constant uniform exposure level is an unjustified exclusion of biological fact in order to achieve a hypothetical and false abstraction.

The second flaw in the application of Haber's law relates to the question of the "dose" administered. Calculating or measuring an ambient exposure level and representing this as "the dose" fails to take cognizance of the actual biologically effective or "delivered" dose to the target tissue or intracellular DNA, as well as the nature and time scale of repair of DNA damage. Calculation of the delivered dose in turn brings up the question of high dose to low dose extrapolation, in those instances, and there are many of them, where the activation and/or detoxication mechanisms become saturated as the dose is increased. Such saturation has consequences that have been described by Gehring and his colleagues (Gehring and Blau, 1977; Gehring et al., 1978) and have been summarized by Hoel et al. (1983), as well as by Starr (1983). As one example, Starr has taken the Maltoni and Lefemine (1975) results for hepatic hemangiosarcomas produced by vinyl chloride and plotted them in terms of the administered dose, but has shown that, by applying Michaelis-Menten kinetics, a vastly different dose response relationship, in terms of delivered dose, is obtained. Consideration is given below to other methods of arriving at the biologically effective dose.

Host susceptibility

The diversity of human susceptibility adds considerably to the complexity of evaluating risk. Each individual is of course unique. Ideally we should evaluate the toxicological risk for that particular individual, knowing the dose to which he or she is exposed, rather than the group as a whole. What many have been striving for is to develop appropriate methods for measuring individual exposure, by biological monitoring or other means. In seeking indices of effect, one needs to take into account the genetic, constitutional, dietary and lifestyle factors that, in addition to occupational and environmental exposures, determine host susceptibility. There is also another way of categorizing such host response factors, namely as congenital or acquired. The former includes familial susceptibility, immune deficiency disorders, important aspects of inborn errors of metabolism such as α_1-antitrypsin deficiency (Kidd et al., 1983). Among phenotypes predisposing to harm are metabolic characteristics such as slow acetylation in determining, for instance, response to benzidine exposure and producing bladder cancer (Cartwright et al., 1982; Lower, 1983; Weber et al., 1983). The work of Dr. R. L. Smith of St. Mary's Hospital, London, on individuals metabolizing debrisoquine has enabled him to classify them into two oxidation phenotypes: extensive metabolizers and poor metabolizers (Ritchie et al., 1980). Such means of differentiating genetic determinants of individual susceptibility are, of course, very valuable (Vesell, 1979).

Another aspect of metabolism is illustrated by the work of Bartsch et al. (1980), in which the enzymic capacities of individual human specimens of liver have been compared with rat liver, in regard to the production of electrophiles that are mutagenic to S. typhimurium strains TA1530 and TA100 in plate assays. A variety of nitrosamines and vinyl chloride served as substrates. The mean activity of up to 18 samples of human liver ranged from 43 to 754% of the rat liver activity. Even more noteworthy is the considerable variation which exists between different individual human specimens. This observation has been borne out time and again, starting from the work of Alexanderson et al. (1969). A substantial range of metabolic activities thus exists among people and this is bound to have an impact which is not always taken into account in risk assessment.

Atopy is one important factor predisposing to the development of human allergic reactions to drugs and other chemicals. Equally decisive may be the balance between metabolic production of antigenic determinants, on the one hand, and of degradation products, on the other. Despite recent advances in understanding of these effects (Winslow, 1981; Proceedings of the Immune System Symposium, 1982) much remains to be revealed concerning the intimate mechanisms involved. An illustration of this fact is provided by the so-called "quenching" phenomenon first reported by Opdyke (1976). This observation deals with the suppression of allergic contact sensitization elicited by such fragrance ingredient sensitizers as citral, cinnamic aldehyde or phenylacetaldehyde when they are applied to human skin in the form of the natural essential oils containing them, or as mixtures with various terpenes or other compounds.

In the occupational setting or in guinea pigs, the induction of pulmonary sensitivity and dermal reactivity (Karol et al., 1980, 1981; Karol, 1980, 1983) lends itself to detailed comparison of C x t effects. A striking example in the case of toluene diisocyanate (TDI) has been provided by Karol (1983). Guinea pig sensitization by exposure to 0.61 ppm TDI for 3 hr/day on 5 consecutive days (9.1 ppm-hr) elicited high IgE antibody titers, 25% responders for lung sensitivity and 100% for dermal reactivity to TDI challenge. Exposure at the current TLV, 0.02 ppm, 6 hr/day for 70 days (8.7 ppm-hr) elicited no antibody titers and no pulmonary or dermal response to TDI challenge.

Alkylation and repair of intracellular macromolecules

Pristine, unsubstituted DNA was at one time thought to be the normal form in eukaryotes, or at least to be attainable in the absence of xenobiotics and environmental pollutants. Contrary to this view, physiological DNA methylation is now assigned a significant regulatory role in gene expression (Boehm and Drahovsky, 1983). Vertebrate DNA contains only one naturally-occuring modified base, 5-methylcytosine (Ehrlich and Wang, 1981), and the proportion of this component is specific for both tissues and species (Gama-Sosa et al., 1983). Procedures like partial hepatectomy do not increase the level of 5-methylcytosine, but such a rise does take place in the course of normal development. Enzymatic methylation of DNA to produce 5-methylcytosine utilizies

S-adenosylmethionine as the source of the methyl group, and occurs as a follow-up to DNA replication in order to establish what has been termed "maintenance methylation" (Boehm and Drahovsky, 1983).

In recent years, evidence has accumulated that carcinogenesis can alter DNA methylation patterns, resulting in changes in gene expression, associated with expression of a tumor cell phenotype (Nyce et al., 1983; Boehm and Drahovsky, 1983; Riggs, 1983). Diala et al. (1983) have reported that total genomic DNA methylation (i.e. the percentage of methylated cytosines) is reduced in human tumor cell lines, in comparison with normal cells and tissues. This work lends emphasis to efforts being made to elucidate the mechanism(s) responsible for hypomethylation of specific genes in the DNA of tumor cells. The aberrant methylation theory of carcinogenesis has also focused on hypomethylation of tRNA and rRNA, with decreased levels of 2'-O-methylated uridylic acid residues (Sitz et al., 1983). As Nyce et al. (1983) have pointed out, the hypomethylation model provides a potential link between mutational and epigenetic mechanisms of carcinogenesis.

Chemical alkylation of DNA bases by carcinogens, and the speed, extent and fidelity of DNA repair, are topics that call for more adequate treatment than is possible here. The basic principles, as they relate to nitrosamines and similar carcinogens, have been presented with admirable clarity by Pegg (1983) and apply to such diverse systems as E. coli and animal (including human) cells (Myrnes et al., 1982). The key enzymes involved in the repair of resulting DNA lesions are glycosylases that excise N-alkylpurines, and the inducible enzyme O^6-methylguanine-DNA methyltransferase (OMDM). With respect to OMDM activity, the mouse is apparently not susceptible to induction in the same way as the rat is (Maru et al., 1982). According to Pegg (1983), human liver possesses 4-10 times the OMDM activity of rat liver. Fotte et al. (1983) reported two strains of HeLa cells: methylation-repair proficient (Mer$^+$) and repair deficient (Mer$^-$). The Mer$^+$ strain contains 10^5 molecules of OMDM/cell whereas Mer$^-$ displays no activity. These results are in line with earlier findings (Waldstein et al., 1982), and illustrate yet again the wide variation and OMDM activity in human and animal tissues.

The observations referred to above apply to simple products of alkylation; with more complex adducts, the mechanisms involved may be very different. Even with simple derivatives, complexities abound. Thus, with diethylnitrosamine, rat hepatocytes form O^6-ethyldeoxyguanosine, which is efficiently repaired and does not accumulate, and O^4-ethyldeoxythymidine, which does accumulate in hepatocyte DNA (Dyroff et al., 1983). According to Scicchitano and Pegg (1982), the rate at which OMDM demethylates O^6-methylguanine in DNA is dependent on the extent of methylation of the DNA. In rat liver at 37°C, 2 minutes suffices for 90% demethylation of DNA containing a proportion of 1:2000 alkylated guanines, but a ratio of 1:500,000 requires 27 minutes. Montesano et al. (1983) studied the effect of pretreatment with dimethylnitrosamine (DMN) on the speed and capacity of DNA repair with respect to O^6-methylguanine. At a large enough dose of DMN, even the induced increased capacity of OMDM had little impact on the O^6-methylguanine generated in liver DNA. Increased cell proliferation did not appear to be necessarily coupled to enhanced OMDM activity. However, the excision repair was characteristic of the cell type (Lee et al., 1983).

Human biological monitoring

Evaluation of toxicological risk to man is greatly facilitated if measurements are carried out in people rather than rats. Biological monitoring has the added advantage that it provides, not only indices of chemical exposure, but also measures of effect, if any. A fascinating example is the current effort to measure individual capacity for endogenous N-nitrosamine formation, a far more important source of these potential human carcinogens than those nitrosamines derived exogenously from food, drinking water and air.

Bartsch and his colleagues (Ohshima and Bartsch, 1981; Ohshima *et al.*, 1982; Bartsch *et al.*, 1983; Ohshima *et al.*, 1983a) applied a procedure using beetroot juice as a source of nitrate and L-proline as an amino acid whose N-nitroso derivative is excreted unchanged, virtually quantitatively in the urine and feces. A similar approach has been used in cigarette smokers (Hoffmann and Brunnemann, 1983). As might have been expected, the results of measurements of endogenous N-nitrosation are affected by a host of factors such as amines ingested, catalysts and inhibitors (vitamins A and C, plant phenols) in the diet, the presence of bacteria to reduce nitrate to nitrite, and gastric pH in relation to the pH optimum for nitrosation of the particular amines. It is now realized that, in future, compounds formed in the human stomach will have to be characterized and measured individually (Craddock, 1983).

In the course of this work, major hitherto unknown N-nitroso compounds have been identified in human urine; they were dervied from L-thiazolidine 4-carboxylic acid (Ohshima *et al.*, 1983b), and its 2-methyl derivatives (*cis*- and *trans*-) (Tsuda *et al.*, 1983). These compounds are thought to arise by interaction of L-cysteine with formaldehyde and acetaldehyde in the body.

An attractive approach to dose monitoring has been based on the claim by Ehrenberg and his coworkers (Osterman-Golkar *et al.*, 1976) that alkylation of the amino acids cysteine and histidine of hemoglobin can act as indirect indicators of the level of alkylation of DNA in various cells of the body. The concept has been applied to ethylene, ethylene oxide, propylene oxide and several other compounds (Calleman, 1982; Segerbäck, 1983; Ehrenberg *et al.*, 1983; Osterman-Golkar *et al.*, 1983; Pereira and Chang, 1982). Farmer and his colleagues (1980, 1982) have employed combined gas chromatography-mass spectrometry for direct analysis of the alkylated amino acids in globin hydrolysates. This work has led to the discovery of normal background levels of derivatives such as S-methylcysteine in hemoglobin, the amount varying with the species (Bailey *et al.*, 1981; Farmer, 1982). S-ethylcysteine was undetectable at a limit of sensitivity of 5 nmol/g globin. Background levels (0-3 nmol/g globin) of N-3'-(2-hydroxyethyl) histidine have also been observed (Table 2).

TABLE 2

Background of Alkylated Derivatives in Hemoglobin and Urine

Derivative	Amounts
S-Methylcysteine	High and variable
N-3'Methylhistidine	Very high
N-3'(2-Hydroxyethyl)histidine	Considerable amounts
N-3'(2-Hydroxypropyl)histidine	Lower amounts
N-7-Methylguanine	

Finally, mention should be made of the exciting developments in the use of immunological and other techniques to detect DNA adducts as a measure of individual exposure in human populations known to be subjected to the action of specific mutagens and carcinogens (IARC Report of Working Group, 1982). The ultimate objective is to quantify the excised alkylated bases that are excreted unchanged in urine. Thus Bennett et al. (1981) measured the dose-dependent urinary output of the aflatoxin B_1-guanine adduct 2,3-dihydro-2-(N^7-guanyl)-3-hydroxyaflatoxin B_1 in rats given the mycotoxin. A further example along these lines was provided by Gombar et al. (1983) in rats to whom radiolabeled aminopyrine was administered together with nitrite as a source of endogenously formed dimethylnitrosamine. Alkylation of liver DNA and RNA to yield 7-methylguaine led to the excretion of about 95% of this excised base in urine, the amount recovered increasing linearly with dose. Even after doses of aminopyrine as low as 0.3 mg/kg, the 7-methylguanine in urine was readily detectable. The application of these techniques to patients who had undergone the aminopyrine breath test or to other exposed populations holds great promise for the future.

Envoi

The proper study of mankind is man. For obvious reasons, laboratory animals serve as surrogates for man. But the complexities of evaluating the toxicological risk to man can be substantially reduced by doing as much as possible with material derived from human sources and by making the maximum use of the opportunities provided by existing human exposure to substances of interest. The presentations that follow will illustrate what new approaches can accomplish in this direction.

REFERENCES

Alexanderson, B.; Evans, D. A. P., and Sjöqvist, F.: Steady-state plasma levels of nortriptyline in twins: Influence of genetic factors and drug therapy. *Brit. Med. J.*, 4:764, 1969.

Bailey, E.; Connors, T. A., Farmer, P. B., Gorf, S. M., and Rickard, J.: Methylation of cysteine in hemoglobin following exposure to methylating agents. *Cancer Res.*, 41:2514, 1981.

Bartsch, H.; Malaveille, C., Camus, A. M., Martel-Planche, G., Brun, G., Hautefeuille, A., Sabadie, N., Barbin, A., Kuroki, T., Drevon, C., Piccoli, C., and Montesano, R.: Validation and comparative studies on 180 chemicals with S. typhimurium strains and V79 chinese hamster cells in the presence of various metabolizing systems. *Mutation Res.*, 76:1, 1980.

Bartsch, H.; Ohshima, H., Muñoz, N., Crespi, M., and Lu, S. H.: Measurement of endogenous nitrosation in humans: potential applications of a new method and initial results.

In Human Carcinogenesis. Eds. C. C. Harris and H. N. Autrup, Academic Press, New York, 1983, pp. 833-856.

Bennett, R. A.; Essigman, J. M., and Wogan, G. N.: Excretion of an aflatoxin-guanine adduct in the urine of aflatoxin B_1-treated rats. *Cancer Res.*, 41:650, 1981.

Boehm, T. L. J.; and Drahovsky, D.: Alteration of enzymatic methylation of DNA cytosines by chemical carcinogens: A mechanism involved in the initiation of carcinogenesis. *J. Nat. Cancer Inst.*, 71:429, 1983.

Calleman, C. J.: In vivo dosimetry by means of alkylated hemoglobin-a tool in the design of tests for genotoxic effects. In *Banbury Report 13. Indicators of Genotoxic Exposure*, B. A. Bridges, B. E. Butterworth and I. B. Weinstein (eds.). Cold Spring Harbor Laboratory, 1982 pp. 157-168.

Cartwright, R. A.; Glashan, R. W., Rogers, H. J., Ahmad, R. A., Barham-Hall, D., Higgins, E., and Kahn, M. A.: Role of N-acetyltransferase phenotypes in bladder carcinogenesis: a pharmacogenetic epidemiological approach to bladder cancer. *Lancet, ii*:842, 1982.

Craddock, V. M.: Nitrosamines and human cancer: proof of an association? *Nature, 306*:638, 1983.

Diala, E. S.; Cheah, M. S. C., Rowitch, D., and Hoffman, R. M.: Extent of DNA methylation in human tumor cells. *J. Nat. Cancer Inst., 71*:755, 1983.

Dyroff, M. C.; Bedell, M. A., Popp, J. A., and Swenberg, J. A.: Initiation of hepatic GGT-positive foci by continuous oral diethylnitrosamine (DEN) administration for one to ten weeks. *The Pharmacologist, 25*:185, 1983.

Ehrenberg, L.; Moustacchi, E., Osterman-Golkar, S., and Ekman, G.: Dosimetry of genotoxic agents and dose-response relationships of their effects. *Mutation Res., 123*:121, 1983.

Ehrlich, M.; and Wang, R. Y.: 5-Methylcytosine in eukaryotic DNA. *Science, 212*:1350, 1981.

Farmer, P. B.: The occurrence of S-methylcysteine in the hemoglobin of normal untreated animals. In *Banbury Report 13. Idicators of Genotoxic Exposure*, B. A. Bridges, B. E. Butterworth and I. B. Weinstein (eds.). Cold Spring Harbor Laboratory, 1982 pp. 169-175.

Farmer, P. B.; Bailey, E., Lamb, J. H., and Connors, T. A.: Approach to the quantitation of alkylated amino acids in haemoglobin by gas chromatography mass spectrometry. *Biomed. Mass Spectrom., 7*:41, 1980.

Farmer, P. B.; Gorf, S. M., and Bailey, E.: Determination of hydroxypropylhistidine in haemoglobin as a measure of exposure to propylene oxide using high resolution gas chromatography mass spectrometry. *Biomed Mass Spectrom., 9*:69, 1982.

Foote, R. S.; Pal, B. C., and Mitra, S.: Quantitation of O^6-methylguanine-DNA methyltransferase in HeLa cells. *Mutation Res., 119*:221, 1983.

Gama-Sosa, M.A.; Midgett, R. M., Slagel, V. A. Githens, S., Kuo, K. C., Gehrke, C. W., and Ehrlich, M.: Tissue-specific differences in DNA methylation in various mammals. *Biochim. Biophys. Acta, 740*:212, 1983.

Gehring, P. J., and Blau, G. E.: Mechanisms of carcinogenesis; dose response. *J. Environ. Path. Toxicol. 1*:163, 1977.

Gehring, P. J.; Watanabe, P. G., and Park, C. N.: Resolution of dose-response toxicity data for chemicals requiring metabolic activation: example vinyl chloride. *Toxicol. Appl. Pharmacol. 44*:581, 1978.

Gombar, C. T.; Zubroff, J., Strahan, G. D., and Magee, P. N.: Measurement of 7-methylguanine as an estimate of the amount of dimethylnitrosamine formed following administration of aminopyrine and nitrite to rats. *Cancer Res., 43*:5077, 1983.

Hoel, D. G.; Kaplan, N. L., and Anderson, M. W.: Implication of nonlinear kinetics on risk estimation in carcinogenesis. *Science, 219*:1032, 1983.

Hoffmann, D.; and Brunnemann, K. D.: Endogenous formation of N-nitrosoproline in cigarette smokers. *Cancer Res., 43*:5570, 1983.

IARC Report of Working Group: Development and possible use of immunological techniques to detect individual exposure to carcinogens. International Agency for Research on Cancer, Lyon, 1982.

Karol, M. H.: Study of guinea pig and human antibodies to toluene diisocyanate. *Amer. Rev. Resp. Dis., 122*:965, 1980.

Karol, M. H.: Concentration-dependent immunologic response to toluene diisocyanate (TDI) following inhalation exposure. *Toxicol. Appl. Pharmacol., 68*:229, 1983.

Karol, M. H.; Dixon, C., Bradie, M., and Alarie, Y.: Immunologic sensitization and pulmonary hypersensitivity by repeated inhalation of aromatic isocyanates. *Toxicol. Appl. Pharmacol., 53*:260, 1980.

Karol, M. H.; Hauth, B. A., Riley, E. J., and Magreni, C.M.: Dermal contact with toluene diisocyanate (TDI) produces respiratory tract hypersensitivity in guinea pigs. *Toxicol. Appl. Pharmacol., 58*: 221, 1981.

Kidd, V. J.; Wallace, R. B. Itakura, K., and Woo, S. L. C.: α-Antitrypsin deficiency detection by direct analysis of the mutation in the gene. *Nature, 304*:230, 1983.

Lee, K. A.; Vollberg, T. M., and Sirover, M. A.: The regulation of base excision repair during cell proliferation. *The Pharmacologist, 25*:190, 1983.

Lower, G. M., Jr.: Arylamines and bladder cancer causality: Application of conceptual and operational criteria. *Clin. Pharmacol. Therap., 34*:129, 1983.

Maltoni, C.; and Lefemine, G.: Carcinogenicity assays of vinyl chloride: current results. *Ann. N. Y. Acad. Sci., 246*:195, 1975.

Maru, G. B.; Margison, G. P., Chu, Y., H., and O'Connor, P. J.: Effects of carcinogens and partial hepatectomy upon the hepatic O^6-methylguanine repair system in mice. *Carcinogenesis, 3*:1247, 1982.

Montesano, R.; Brésil, H., Planche-Martel, G., Margison, G. P., and Pegg, A. H.: Stability and capacity of dimethylnitrosamine-induced O^6-methylguanine repair system in rat liver. *Cancer Res., 43*:5805, 1983.

Munro, I. C.; and Krewski, D. R.: Risk assessment and regulatory decision making. *Food Cosmet. Toxicol, 19*:549, 1981.

Myrnes, B.; Giercksky, K. E., and Krokan, H.: Repair of O^6-methylguanine residues in DNA takes place by a similar mechanism in extracts from HeLa cells, human liver, and rat liver. *J. Cell. Biochem., 20:381, 1982.*

Nyce, J.; Weinhouse, S., and Magee, P. N.: 5-Methylcytosine depletion during tumour development: An extension of the miscoding conept. *Brit. J. Cancer, 48*:463, 1983.

Ohshima, H.; and Bartsch, H.: Quantitative estimation of endogenous nitrosation in humans by monitoring N-nitrosoproline excreted in the urine. *Cancer Res., 41*:3658, 1981.

Ohshima, H.; Bereziat, J. C., and Bartsch, H.: Monitoring N-nitrosamino acids excreted in the urine and feces of rats as an index for endogenous nitrosation. *Carcinogenesis, 3*:115, 1982.

Ohshima, H.; Mahon, G. A. T., Wahrendorf, J., and Bartsch, H.: Dose-response study of N-nitrosoproline formation in rats and a deduced kinetic model for predicting carcinogenic effects caused by endogenous nitrosation. *Cancer Res., 43*:5072, 1983a.

Ohshima, H.; Friesen, M., O'Neill, I., and Bartsch, H.: Presence in human urine of a new N-nitroso compound, N-nitrosothiazolidine 4-carboxylic acid. *Cancer Letters, 20*:183, 1983b.

Opdyke, D. L. J.: Inhibition of sensitization reactions induced by certain aldehydes. *Food Cosmet. Toxicol., 14*:197, 1976.

Osterman-Golkar, S.; Ehrenberg, L., Segerbäck, D., and Hällström, I.: Evaluation of genetic risks of alkylating agents. II. Haemoglobin as a dose monitor. *Mutation Res., 34*:1, 1976.

Osterman-Golkar, S.; Farmer, P. B., Segerbäck, D., Bailey, E., Calleman, C. J., Svensson, K., and Ehrenberg, L.: Dosimetry of ethylene oxide in the rat by quantitation of alkylated histidine in hemoglobin. *Teratog Carcinog Mutagen, 3*:395, 1983.

Peg, A. E.: Alkylation and subsequent repair of DNA after exposure to dimethylnitrosamine and related carcinogens. In *Reviews in Biochemical Toxicology*, Vol. 5 Eds. E. Hodgson, J. R. Bend and R. M. Philpot. Elsevier, New York, 1983 pp. 83-133.

Pereira, M. A.; and Chang, L. W.: Hemoglobin binding as a dose monitor for chemical carcinogens. In *Banbury Report 13. Indicators of Genotoxic Exposure*, B. A. Bridges. B. E. Butterworth and I. B. Weinstein (eds.);. Cold Spring Harbor Laboratory, 1982 pp. 177-187.

Proceedings of the Immune System Symposium. Environ. Health Persp., 43:1, 1982.

Riggs, A. D.: 5-Methylcytosine, gene regulation, and cancer. *Adv. Cancer Res., 40*:1, 1983.

Ritchie, J. C.; Sloan, T. P. Idle, J. R. and Smith, R. L.: Toxicological implications of polymorphic drug metabolism. In *Environmental Chemicals, Enzyme Function and Human Disease. Ciba Foundation Symposium No. 76*, 219. Amsterdam, Excerpta Medica, 1980.

Ruckelshaus, W. D.: Science, risk and public policy. *Science, 221*:1026, 1983.

Rusch, G. M.; Clary, J. J., Rinehart, W. E., and Bolte, H. F.: A 26-week inhalation toxicity study with formaldehyde in the monkey, rat and hamster. *Toxicol. Appl. Pharmacol., 68*:329, 1983.

Scicchitano, D.; and Pegg, A. E.: Kinetics of repair of O^6-methylguanine in DNA by O^6-methylguanine-DNA methyltransferase *in vitro* and *in vivo*. *Biochem. Biophys. Res. Commun., 109*:995, 1982.

Segerbäck, D.: Alkylation of DNA and hemoglobin in the mouse following exposure to ethene and ethene oxide. *Chem.-Biol. Interactions, 45*:139, 1983.

Sielken, R. L.: Cancer dose-response models. In *Proc. Third Internat. Congress on Toxicol.* In press, 1983.

Sitz, T. O.; Godburn, K. E., Somers, K. D., and Nazar, R. N.: Significance of S-adenoxylmethionine pools in the hypomethylation of ribosomal RNA during the propagation of tissue culture cells and oncogenesis. *Cancer Res., 43*:5681, 1983.

Starr, T. B.: Mechanisms of formaldehyde toxicity and risk evaluation. In *Formaldehyde: Toxicology, Epidemiology, Mechanisms*, J. J. Clary, J. E. Gibson and R. S. Waritz (eds.). New York, Marcel Dekker, 1983, p. 237.

Swenberg, J. A.; Gross, E. A., Randall, H. A., and Barrow, C. S.: The effect of formaldehyde exposure on cytotoxicty and cell proliferation. In *Formaldehyde: Toxicology, Epidemiology, Mechanisms*, J. J. Clary, J. E. Gibson and R. S. Waritz (eds.);. New York, Marcel Dekker, 1983, p. 225.

Tsuda, M.; Hirayama, T., and Sugimura, T.: Presence of N-nitroso-L-thioproline and N-nitroso-L-methylthioprolines in human urine as major N-nitroso compounds. *Gann, 74*:331, 1983.

Van Ryzin, J.: Quantitative risk assessment. *J. Occup. Med., 22*:321, 1980.

Vesell, E.: Pharmacogenetics: Multiple interactions between genes and environment as determinants of drug response. *Amer. J. Med., 66*:183, 1979.

Waldstein, E. A.; Cao, E. H., and Setlow, R. B.: Adaptive increase of O^6-methylguanine-acceptor protein in HeLa cells following N'-methyl-N-nitro-N-nitrosoguanidine treatment. *Nucleic Acid Res., 10*:4595, 1982.

Weber, W. W.; Hein, D. W., Litwin, A., and Lower, G.M., Jr.: Relationship of acetylator status to isoniazid toxicity, lupus erythematosus, and bladder cancer. *Fed. Proc. 43*:3086, 1983.

Winslow, S. G.: The effects of environmental chemicals on the immune system. A selected bibliography with abstracts, 1969-1980. F.A.S.E.B., Special Publications, 1981.

Genetic Toxicology

Section Editor: A. P. Li

…

Use of Human Cells in Mutagenicity and Carcinogenicity Determination

J. Justin McCormick and Veronica M. Maher

Carcinogenesis Laboratory—Fee Hall, Departments of Microbiology and Biochemistry, Michigan State University, East Lansing, Michigan 48824

A great deal of evidence, drawn from experimental studies with animals and from epidemiologic studies of the incidence of human cancer, indicates strongly that tumors arise as the result of a multi-stepped process. The requirement that a normal cell acquire a series of discrete changes before emerging as a fully transformed tumor cell and the fact that a tumor cell can be identified only much later after it has given rise to a tumor makes it extremely difficult to elucidate the nature of the steps involved. One approach to this problem, an approach that we are taking, is to make use of cells in culture rather than intact animals or humans in an effort to dissect the individual steps involved. Although studies with intact animals are indispensable in analyzing many aspects of carcinogenesis, the use of cells in culture permits a more direct experimental manipulation and quantitation of the individual steps and can yield information on their nature. An added advantage in using cells in culture instead of whole animals is that it allows one to experimentally manipulate human cells in ways that cannot ethically be done with human beings and permits direct comparisons between animal cells and human cells.

Our initial studies with diploid cells in culture were directed at developing quantitative assays for the induction of mutations by carcinogens (Maher and McCormick, 1976; Maher et al., 1976a, b, 1977, 1979; McCormick and Maher, 1981). Our working hypothesis for these experiments was that carcinogenic agents, such as chemicals and radiation, cause cancer by acting as mutagens and that an essential event leading ultimately to the transformation of a normal cell into a tumor-forming cell results from damage to DNA that gets converted into a mutation. At the time, there were no quantitative assays for measuring the frequency of neoplastic transformation of normal diploid human cells. More recently several groups, including our own, have developed such systems (Kakunaga, 1977, 1978; Milo and DiPaolo, 1978; Maher et al., 1982; McCormick et al., 1980; Silinskas et al., 1981; Sutherland et al., 1980, 1981; and Zimmerman and Little, 1983.)

Indirect support for the involvement of mutations in neoplastic transformation came from the finding (Cleaver, 1968) that cells derived from xeroderma pigmentosum (XP) patients, persons genetically predisposed to sunlight-induced skin cancer (Robbins et al,

1974), are deficient in the rate of excision of ultraviolet (UV)-induced DNA damage. This finding predicted that such cells would be extremely sensitive to the mutagenic action of UV radiation and of any other agent causing DNA damage that XP cells cannot excise as rapidly as normal human cells. This is because the XP cells would be expected to have more of the initial damage remaining in their DNA at the time such lesions are translated into permanent changes in DNA (mutations). If genetic changes resulting from the presence of unrepaired lesions are causally involved in the neoplastic transformation process, XP cells should also be more sensitive than normal, repair-proficient cells to transformation by UV radiation or these other agents. Our studies over the past several years have been directed toward testing these predictions, and determining the effect of DNA repair on the cytotoxic, mutagenic, and transforming action in diploid human fibroblasts of a variety of chemical carcinogens and of ultraviolet and ionizing radiation (Aust *et al.*, 1980, 1984; Drinkwater *et al*, 1982; Heflich *et al.*, 1980; Howell *et al.*, 1984; Konze-Thomas *et al.*, 1982; Maher *et al.*, 1982; McCormick *et al.*, 1980; Patton *et al.*, 1984; Silinskas *et al.*, 1981; Simon *et al.*, 1981; and Yang *et al.*, 1980, 1982). The results of our studies indicate that DNA excision repair by human cells can eliminate potentially cytotoxic, mutagenic, and transforming damage before these lesions can be translated into permanent cellular effects. They further suggest that at least one step on the path to full neoplastic transformation, viz., loss of anchorage dependence, results from a mutagenic event (Maher *et al.*, 1982; and Silinskas *et al.*, 1981).

COMPARATIVE STUDIES OF THE CYTOTOXIC EFFECT OF CARCINOGENS IN HUMAN CELLS

Studies have shown that the best method for determining the cytotoxic effect of an agent on cells in culture is to compare treated and untreated populations for their ability to form colonies when plated at low density (survival of reproductive capacity). For such studies to be reliable, care must be taken to insure that the cloning efficiency of the untreated cells is as high as possible and that the cell densities used for the treated populations with expected low survivals do not affect the cloning efficiency. We now routinely achieve cloning efficiencies of greater than 50% with fibroblasts derived from normal persons and 20 to 45% with cells derived from persons with various genetic predispositions to cancer. The techniques we use to achieve these high cloning efficiencies have been described (McCormick and Maher, 1981).

We have used two approaches to determine the effect of DNA excision repair on the cytotoxic action of carcinogens in human fibroblasts. One is to expose a series of cell strains (i.e., cell lines with limited lifespan in culture) that differ in their rate of excision repair of DNA lesions to increasing doses of the DNA damaging agent and compare their survival curves, as shown in Figure 1 and 2. A second method is to prevent cells from replicating by growing them to confluence (density inhibition) and then treating a series of such confluent cultures with carcinogens. One set of treated cells is assayed immediately for the initial number of DNA adducts and for survival by releasing the cells from confluence and plating them at cloning density. The cells in the other sets of cultures are maintained in the density-inhibited state for various periods to allow time for excision repair. They are subsequently assayed for the number of DNA adducts remaining unexcised and plated for survival of colony-forming ability. Examples of the results of these kinds of studies are shown in Figures 3 and 4A and B.

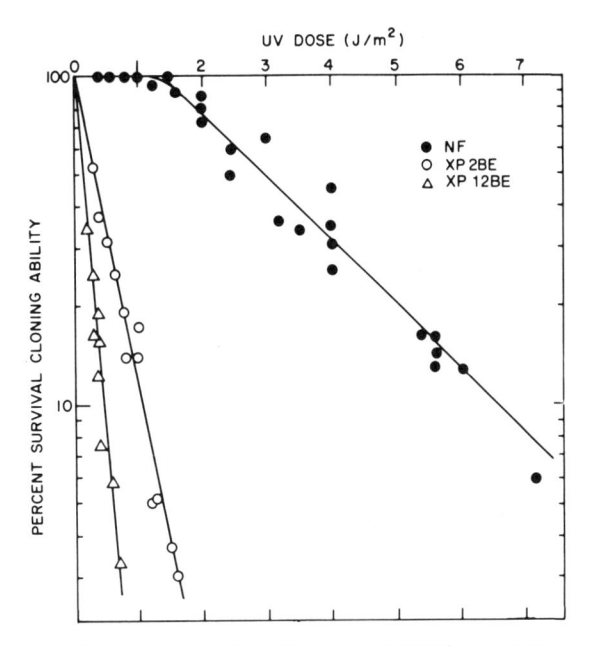

FIGURE 1: Comparing the cytotoxic effect of low doses of UV 254 nm radiation in diploid human fibroblasts with different rates of DNA excision repair of pyrimidine dimers. Cells from exponentially-growing cultures were plated into 60 mm-diameter dishes at appropriate densities to yield a countable number of colonies (cloning densities), allowed 12 hr for attachment, irradiated *in situ* in a film of buffer, fed with Ham's F10 medium supplemented with fetal bovine serum, and allowed to develop colonies. (●) normal cells; (○) XP2BE cells from complementation group C (Robbins *et al.*, 1974); (△) XP12BE from group A. (Figure adapted from similar figure in Maher *et al.*, 1979). Recent data using an improved dosimeter suggest that the doses shown are half of the actual doses used for the study in 1979).

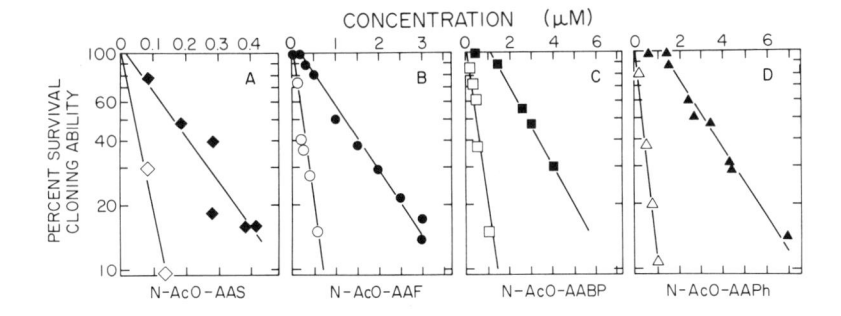

FIGURE 2. Comparing the cytotoxic effect of reactive derivatives of four aromatic amide carcinogens, N-acetoxy-4-acetylaminostilbene (N-AcO-AAS); N-acetoxy-2-acetylaminofluorene (N-AcO-AAF); N-acetoxy-4-acetylaminobiphenyl (N-AcO-AABP); and N-acetoxy-2-acetylaminophenanthrene (N-AcO-AAPh) in normal fibroblasts and XP12BE cells. Cells were plated at cloning densities and allowed 12 hr to attach. The growth medium was replaced with serum-free medium and the carcinogen introduced by micropipette. The cells were then allowed to form colonies *in situ*. (Taken from Maher *et al.*, 1981).

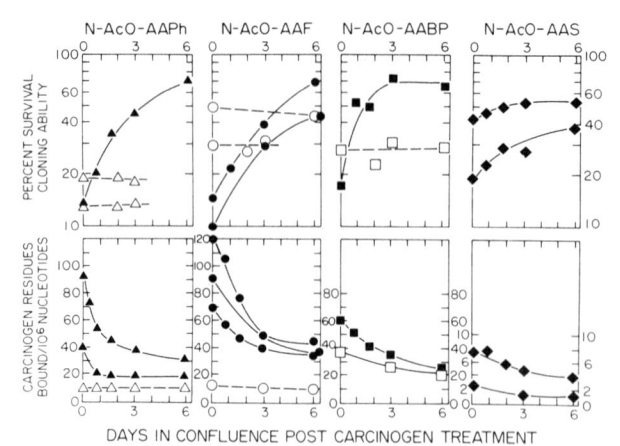

FIGURE 3: Comparison of the rates of recovery from the potentially lethal effects of four aromatic amine derivatives with the rate of removal of radioactive labeled residues from the DNA of normal (closed symbols) or XP12BE cells (open symbols). Cells were treated at confluence as described and then assayed after the designated period of time in the G_0 state. (Taken from Maher et al., 1981).

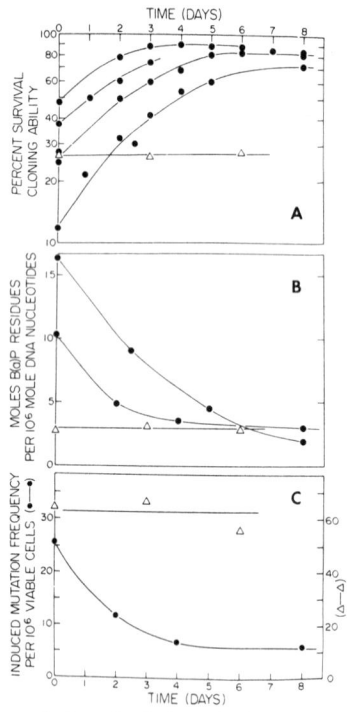

FIGURE 4: Kinetics of removal of covalently bound adducts (B) and recovery of normal (circles) or XP12BE cells (triangles) from the potentially cytotoxic (A) or mutagenic (C) effects of anti BPDE. The cells were treated in the G_0 state, released on the designated days, and assayed for survival of colony-forming ability, for the number of residues bound to DNA, and after a suitable expression period, for the frequency of induced mutations to TG resistance. (Taken from Yang, et al., 1980) with permission.)

We have found in diploid human fibroblasts that there is a direct correlation between the cells' ability to repair DNA lesions (rate of excision) and their ability to exhibit high survival after exposure to a potentially cytotoxic dose of an agent (Maher et al., 1977, 1979, 1982). For example, in Figure 1 the XP12BE cells are virtually incapable of excising UV-induced DNA damage and after a dose of 1 J/m^2, their survival is less than 1%. XP2BE cells excise UV-induced damage slowly and after such a dose, exhibit 15% survival. Normal cells excise UV-induced damage very rapidly and exhibit 100% survival, even after a dose that reduces the survival of XP12BE cells below 1%. In contrast, we have found that normal human cells excise DNA adducts produced by N-acetoxy-4-acetylaminostilbene or N-acetoxy-2-acetylaminofluorene (N-AcO-AAF) very slowly compared to their rate of pyrimidine dimer excision, and when exposed to doses of these agents large enough to reduce the survival of XP12BE cells to 1%, the normal cells cannot attain 100% survival. Instead they show a survival of 20 to 35% (Figure 2).

As shown in Figure 3 and 4A and B, XP12BE cells are unable to excise DNA adducts formed by a series of reactive derivatives of polycyclic aromatic amides or hydrocarbons. Neither can these cells remove potentially cytotoxic lesions. In contrast, normal cells held in confluence gradually remove these DNA adducts and when released and assayed for survival, they show the higher survival levels expected for cells with correspondingly lower numbers of DNA adducts.

COMPARATIVE STUDIES OF THE MUTAGENIC EFFECT OF CARCINOGENS IN HUMAN CELLS

We have carried out similar comparative studies with normal and XP cells to determine the effect of excision repair on the mutagenic action of carcinogens. For the majority of our studies of mutagenesis in diploid human cells, resistance to 6-thioguanine (TG) was the genetic marker. Our procedures for obtaining reproducible, concentration-dependent results with this marker have been described (Konze-Thomas et al., 1982; Maher et al., 1979; and McCormick and Maher, 1981). We and our colleagues have also worked out quantitative assays for using resistance to diphtheria toxin (DT) as a genetic marker (Aust et al., 1984; Drinkwater et al., 1982). Recently we simultaneously assayed human cells for the frequency of DT resistant cells and TG resistant cells induced by exposure of the population to carcinogens in order to gain insight into the kinds of mutations induced by a series of carcinogens including X-rays, ethylnitrosourea (ENU), the anti isomer of the 7,8-diol-9,10-epoxide of benzo(a)pyrene (BPDE), N-AcO-AAF and the classic frameshift mutagen ICR-191 (Aust et al., 1984). Recovery of DT resistant colonies requires that the mutation in the elongation factor EF-2 render the protein resistant to DT, but still capable of carrying on protein synthesis. Therefore, the mutation responsible for DT resistance cannot involve major changes in the gene. In contrast, cells can acquire TG resistance by any mechanism that eliminates hypoxanthine (guanine) phosphoribosyltransferase activity, e.g., base substitutions, frameshifts, deletions, chromosome loss, etc. As expected, X-rays which cause breaks in DNA and the frameshift mutagen ICR-191 yielded little or no increase in frequency of DT resistant mutants, but a great increase in TG resistant cells (data not shown, cf. Aust et al., 1984). ENU, a classic base substitution mutagen, as expected, gave a large increase in DT resistant cells and a similarly large increase in the frequency of TG resistant cells (DT to TG ratio ~1.5) (Figure 5). BPDE and N-AcO-AAF also gave a DT to TG ratio of ~1.5, suggesting that in diploid human fibroblasts these chemicals yield predominantly base substitutions, rather than frameshifts. This result for N-AcO-AAF is in contrast to its mutagenic action in Salmonella (Aust et al., 1984).

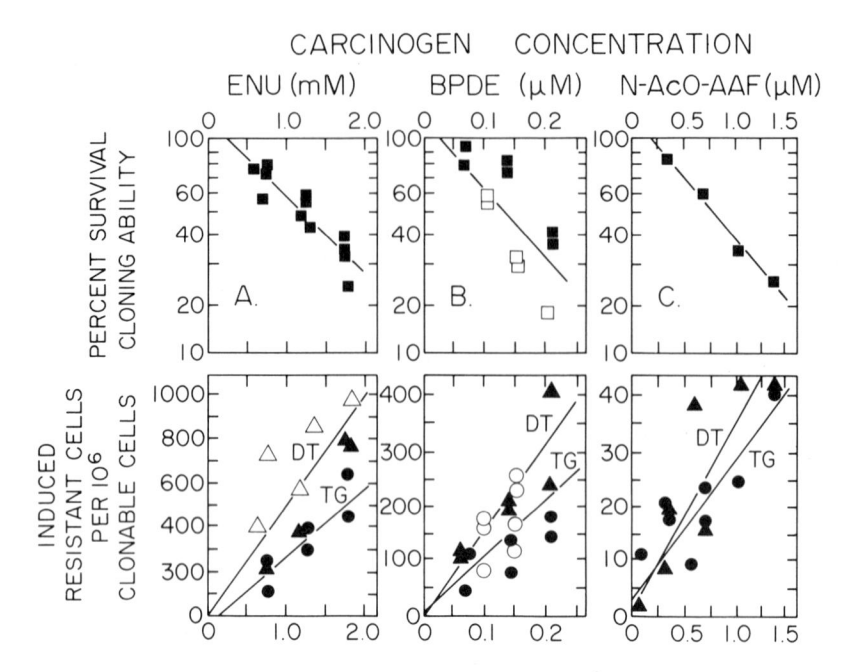

FIGURE 5. Cytotoxicity and frequency of diphtheria toxin (DT) resistant or 6-thioguanine resistant cells induced in a population of normal diploid human fibroblasts by increasing concentrations of ENU; BPDE; and N-AcO-AAF. (Data taken from Aust et al., 1984 with permission.)

We also examined the effect of DNA excision repair on the mutagenic action of carcinogens, using the same two approaches described above for our studies on cytotoxicity. Cell strains that differed in excision repair capacity were compared for the frequency of TG resistant cells induced by increasing doses of UV radiation (Konze-Thomas et al., 1982; Maher et al., 1979, 1982) or chemical carcinogens, such as BPDE and benzo(a)pyrene 4, 5-oxide (Maher et al., 1977; Yang et al., 1980, 1982); ENU (Simon et al., 1981); and N-AcO-AAF (Maher et al., 1980). Alternatively, cells were treated in the non-replicating (confluent) state and then assayed immediately or after various times posttreatment for the number of photolesions or adducts in DNA and, after a suitable expression period, for the frequency of TG resistant cells induced.

An example of results using the first approach, i.e., comparing cells that differ in rate of repair, is shown in Figure 6B. Clearly, for a given exposure of UV 254 nm, the XP7BE cells, which excise at a rate ~16% that of normal cells, or XP12BE cells which are unable to excise pyrimidine dimers, exhibit a significantly higher frequency of mutants than do normal cells. This is to be expected since, in a given period of time, the excision-proficient normal cells can remove many more of the potentially mutagenic lesions than either XP cell strain can. We found similar results with human cells treated with chemical carcinogens that produce bulky DNA adducts which these XP cells are unable to excise or excise only very slowly (Maher et al., 1977). In contrast, XP12BE cells give a normal response to the potentially mutagenic effects of N-methyl-N'-nitro-N-nitrosoguanidine (MNNG) and have a normal rate of repair of MNNG-induced lesions (Domoradzki et al., 1984).

USE OF HUMAN CELLS 23

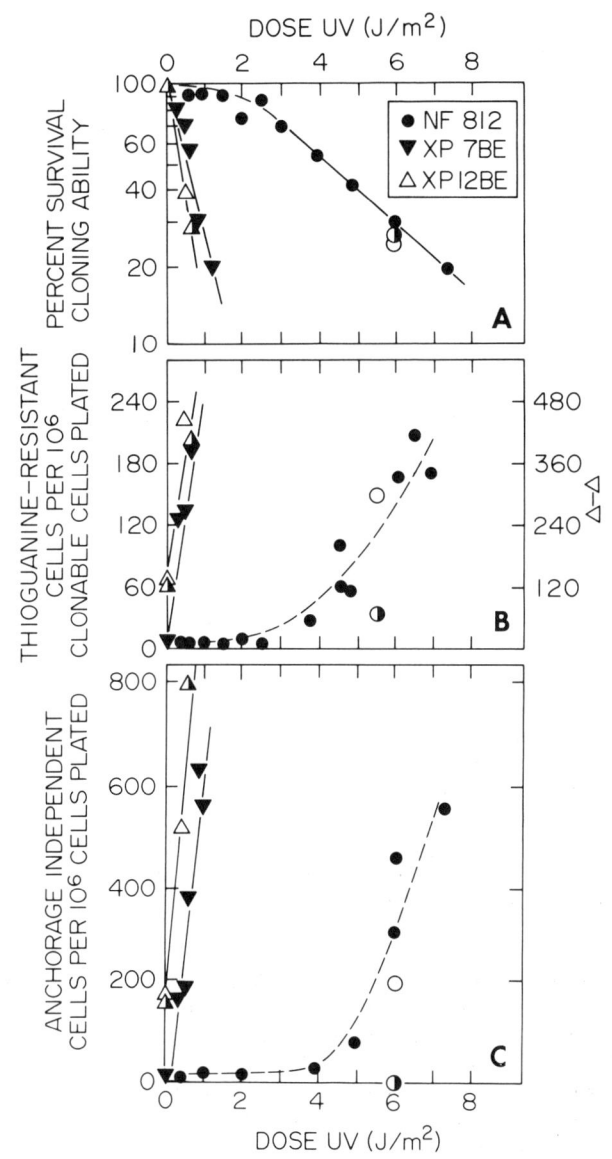

FIGURE 6: Cytotoxicity, mutagenicity, and transforming ability of UV radiation in normal (circles) and XP cells (XP12BE, triangles; XP7BE, inverted triangles). The frequency of thioguanine resistant cells was assayed after 6 doublings; that of anchorage-independent cells after 9 to 11 doublings. The former were corrected for cloning efficiency on plastic. Solid symbols, populations irradiated in exponential growth; open symbols, cells synchronized by release from confluence and irradiated shortly before onset of S phase; half-solid symbols, cell irradiated 18-20 hrs prior to S. See text for details. The background frequencies have not been subtracted from the induced values. The open and half-solid circules in the middle panel represent data from a separate mutagenesis experiment, not identical to the one represented by the same symbols in the bottom panel. Otherwise, all data are from experiments in which cells were assayed for all three parameters. (After a Figure in Maher *et al.*, 1982).

Figure 4C gives an example of the results obtained using the second approach, i.e., holding cells in confluence before assaying the effect of the treatment. There is a direct correlation between the cells' ability to excise BPDE adducts from DNA and their ability to decrease the potentially mutagenic effects of this carcinogen (Yang et al., 1980).

EFFECT ON MUTATIONS AND SURVIVAL OF ALLOWING TIME FOR EXCISION BEFORE DNA SYNTHESIS

Since the essential difference between XP cells and normal cells is their respective rates of excision repair of UV-induced damage, the data in Figure 1 and 6A and B are consistent with the hypothesis that there is a limited amount of time for excision repair between the initial radiation and the onset of the critical cellular events responsible for cell killing and/or mutation induction in these cells. We suggested that such an event could be semiconservative DNA synthesis on a damaged template (Maher et al., 1977, 1979). We tested this hypothesis by synchronizing normal cells and excision repair-deficient XP12BE cells by release from density-inhibition (Konze-Thomas et al., 1982), and irradiating them just prior to the onset of DNA synthesis (S-phase); in early G_1, ~ 18 hr prior to S-phase; or in the density-inhibited G_0 state so that upon release from confluence there would be ~ 24 hrs before onset of DNA synthesis. We knew from previous studies that human fibroblasts capable of repair were able to carry out excision while in the confluent state; during the interval between release from confluence and onset of DNA synthesis (G_1); as well as during S-phase (Heflich et al., 1980; Konze-Thomas et al., 1979; McCormick and Maher, unpublished studies; Yang et al., 1980, 1982).

Figure 7 shows the results of this study (Konze-Thomas et al., 1982). As expected for cells that are unable to excise the DNA damage induced by UV 254 nm radiation, the frequency of mutations induced in XP12BE cells was the same whether they were irradiated just before S, 18 hrs prior to S, or 24 hrs before DNA synthesis began. In contrast, the slope of the dose response for TG resistance induced in the normal cells irradiated just prior to S was about 10-fold steeper than that of cells irradiated 18 hrs earlier. The frequencies induced in cells treated in confluence and then released, so as to have at least 24 hrs prior to the onset of S phase, were still lower. (Part of this decrease reflects the fact that $\sim 10\%$ of the cells in confluence are shielded by the crowding and do not receive the same effective dose as the other cells. The cells to be irradiated in early G_1 or at the beginning of S-phase are already plated at lower density ($3\text{-}8 \times 10^3$ cells/cm^2) and can continue to traverse the cell cycle following irradiation without a need for trypsinization. Those in G_0 have to be replated from confluence immediately following irradiation and then allowed to proceed to S phase.) These results in the bottom panel of Figure 7 support the idea that mutations are "fixed" (i.e., made permanent) by DNA replication and that the frequency is determined by the number of unexcised lesions remaining during DNA replication.

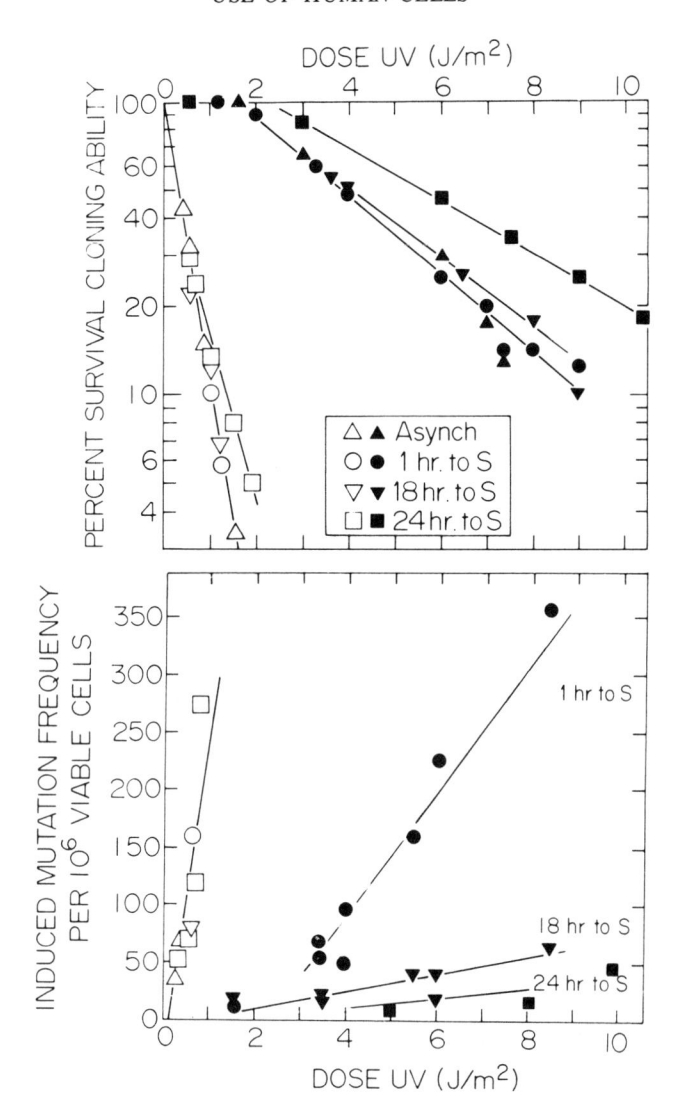

FIGURE 7: Cytotoxicity and mutagenicity of UV in normal (closed symbols) or XP12BE cells (open symbols) irradiated under conditions designed to allow various lengths of time for excision repair to take place prior to the onset of S phase. Cells irradiated in confluence (G_0) and then released and plated at lower densities (■, □); cells released from G_0 and irradiated 6 hrs later (∇,▼); cells released and irradiated 24 hrs later (○,●); cells replated from asynchronously growing cultures, and irradiated ~16 hrs later (△,▲). (Taken from Konze-Thomas *et al.*, 1982) with permission).

The effect of time for excision repair between irradiation and the onset of S was much less pronounced for cell survival (top panel of Figure 7). The XP12BE cells, of course, were not expected to exhibit any real difference in survival when irradiated at various times prior to the onset of S, but the repair-proficient normal cells were. In contrast to the corresponding mutagenicity data, the data for normal cells show little difference in survival between the cells irradiated at the onset of S; and in G_1, 18 hrs prior to S-phase; or in G_0. Again, we showed that part of the increase in survival of the cells irradiated in G_0 is caused by the shielding that occurs when cells become tightly packed by the protocol used to prepare the G_0 population (cf. Konze-Thomas et al., 1982). The fact that XP12BE cells irradiated with low doses of UV, e.g., 1 J/m^2, are far more sensitive than repair-proficient normal cells indicates that excision repair following irradiation can eliminate potentially cytotoxic lesions. This fact was also demonstrated using the method illustrated by Figure 3 and 4A, but with UV 254 nm as the DNA damaging agent (Konze-Thomas et al., 1979; Maher et al., 1979). In fact, normal cells exhibiting a survival of 20% if released from confluence immediately, showed a survival of 90 to 100% if held in the G_0 state for 18 hrs. Therefore, we interpret the data in Figure 7 (top panel) to suggest that the time available for repair of potentially lethal lesions is determined, not by the onset of S-phase, but by the cell's need for critical cellular proteins and their respective mRNA's. If the DNA template for transcription of these mRNA's is still blocked by lesions at the time the cell has need of them, reproductive death (i.e., inability to form a colony), is the result. This would explain why holding cells in a resting state (G_0) following exposure to DNA damaging agents, before releasing them into the cycling state, results in a higher survival than does immediate release. Cells held in confluence have a lower metabolic state than cells in exponential growth and therefore fewer critical proteins are needed before the cell has time to remove the blocking DNA damage. We suggest that reproductive death from exposure to UV-radiation or the agents shown in Figures 3 and 4 results from the failure of cells to synthesize needed proteins because transcription is blocked by DNA photoproducts or adducts (Konze-Thomas et al., 1982, Yang et al., 1982). This conclusion is consistent with the fact that the XP12BE cells, which do not remove such lesions from their DNA, show no dose modifying effect on being held in the resting state.

STUDIES ON NEOPLASTIC TRANSFORMATION OF DIPLOID HUMAN FIBROBLASTS

As indicated in the Introduction, the underlying purpose of our research is to determine the number and nature of the steps involved in the transformation of cells in culture in order to understand the mechanisms of human carcinogenesis. Because of our previous experience with carcinogen-induced mutagenesis of human cells, we approached the problem of carcinogen-induced transformation from the point of view of it being the result of a mutation. In the past, many workers developing transformation assays assumed either explicitly or implicitly that mutations or genetic changes were not responsible. This explains why most transformation assays were not designed to simultaneously yield information on transformation frequencies and mutations frequencies using the same treated cell populations. Furthermore, the protocols used, as well as the type of cell line used (aneuploid), often precluded recognition of whether mutation(s) were involved in transformation. This problem was enhanced by the fact that, even when early passage diploid cells derived from Syrian hamster embryos were used (Berwald and Sachs, 1965; DiPaolo et al., 1972; Barrett and Ts'o, 1978), the earliest end point, morphological transformation, developed at such a high frequency (0.1 to 1%) that genetic mutations were considered an unlikely cause. Furthermore, it was clear that these morphologically transformed colonies were not tumorigenic *per se* (Barrett and et al., 1980). Rather, cells able to cause tumors arose randomly in progeny of the carcinogen-treated cultures but only after 35 to 70 population doublings posttreatment, long after the control cells from nontreated cultures had senesced and the progeny of the treated cell population had become aneuploid. This delay made it difficult to associate the ultimate tumorigenicity with the original carcinogen treatment.

For many years, workers had tried without success to induce the transformation of human fibroblasts with carcinogens. Finally in 1977, Kakunaga demonstrated that human fibroblasts treated with a carcinogen could give rise to cells which formed foci (small areas, apparently clonal in origin, where cells grow in a three dimensional array) on the top of confluent monolayers. The progeny of these cells were tumorigenic when injected subcutaneously into athymic mice.

Therefore, we began our studies by repeating the protocol of Kakunaga (1977, 1978), and were able to confirm his results. However, we realized that this method of assaying transformants (i.e., from the formation of foci in confluent cultures of progeny cells that had been allowed to undergo ~13 doublings since carcinogen treatment) would not be suitable for quantitative comparative studies. Although we can routinely recognize such foci, the focus assay for transformed human fibroblasts is further complicated by the fact that the foci are far less distinct than SV40 virus-induced foci in these cells (McCormick *et al.*, 1980). Therefore, we tried the assay of Milo and DiPaolo (1978) who reported detecting anchorage independent (AI) transformed human fibroblasts by their ability to form colonies in semi-solid medium. Cells derived from pooled AI colonies, upon injection into sub-lethally irradiated athymic mice, form tumors (nodules) within 2-3 weeks. This system offered the obvious advantage that transformed cells could more easily be identified, and their frequency quantitated. We, therefore, repeated their protocol using MNNG and propane sultone and confirmed their results (McCormick *et al.*, 1980, and Silinskas *et al.*, 1981). More recently we have found that the nodules formed after injection of AI human cells eventually regress.

EVIDENCE THAT NEOPLASTIC TRANSFORMATION INVOLVES GENETIC CHANGES FROM DNA DAMAGE

Because of our conviction that the transformation process was likely to involve one or more mutagenic events, we then proceeded to design a human cell transformation assay involving induction of anchorage independence and modeled after our human cell mutagenesis assays. For example, we expected the process of transformation to have in common with the process of mutagenesis: a) an expression period, i.e., a period of time between carcinogen damage of cells and their ability to express the new (i.e., transformed) phenotype: b) a linear increase in the frequency of transformants with increase in carcinogen dose; c) a concentration dependence for the carcinogenic agent which resembled that required for induction of mutations, so that strong mutagens would usually be strong transforming agents; d) a low, but measurable frequency of transformed cells in non-carcinogen treated cell populations just as one finds low, but measurable, frequency of mutant cells in such populations; e) a higher frequency of transformation per dose in DNA repair-deficient cells than in normal cells, as we had shown for the induction of mutants in XP cells; f) a cell cycle dependence similar to that which occurs for mutation induction, so that populations of cells treated just before S phase would show a higher frequency of transformation than cell populations treated with the same dose of the agent far from S-phase. We tested each of these predictions and found them to be true.

Although our transformation assay is based on selection of AI cells by their ability to form colonies in soft agar, our protocol differs substantially from that of Milo and his associates (Milo and DiPaolo, 1978; Milo et al., 1981). Most important, perhaps, is our finding that to bring about the induction of anchorage independence it is *not* necessary to synchronize the cells and treat them at the beginning of S-phase. The data on the frequency of UV-induced anchorage independence in normal cells and XP7BE cells in Figure 6C are derived from cells irradiated in exponential growth. Secondly, we have determined that waiting for 20 population doublings posttreatment is not an optimal expression period. An increase in frequency of AI cells is detected after an expression period of ~7 doublings and if cultures are maintained in exponential growth during expression, the frequency of AI cells begins to decrease after ~12 population doublings so that, in our hands, after 20 doublings it is only 10% of maximum. A third difference is that we now grow our cells in Ham's F10 medium supplemented with 10% fetal bovine serum during the entire period before selection in soft agar and use this same medium for selection in agar. (Our Ham's F10 medium lacks hypoxanthine, but only because we also use this medium for selecting cells resistant to thioguanine. In addition, we add additional bicarbonate to bring the total to 2.2 g/l for additional buffering capacity.) A fourth significant difference between our protocol and Milo's is that we can obtain a linear dose-response for induction of AI cells using doses of UV radiation (and other carcinogens, such as propane sultone) at doses that bring the survival of colony-forming ability down to 20%. (Maher et al., 1982; Silinskas et al., 1981).

If genetic changes resulting from the presence of unrepaired DNA photoproducts or adducts are causally involved in the transformation of human cells to anchorage independence, DNA excision repair-deficient XP cells should be more sensitive to transformation by UV radiation than normal cells are. We tested this hypothesis by irradiating the two kinds of cells and assaying the population simultaneously for the frequency of TG resistant cells and AI cells. The results are included in Figure 6. As shown in Figure 6C, the frequency of anchorage independent cells induced by low doses of UV radiation is significantly higher in XP cells than in normal cells. *(Note that these XP cells are not malignant; the biopsies from which they are derived are always obtained from non-sunlight exposed areas of the skin. This is confirmed by the fact that injection of >2 x 10⁷ unirradiated cells into athymic mice did not produce tumors (Maher et al., 1982).* The data designated by solid symbols were derived from cells irradiated in exponential growth and assayed for colony-formation in soft agar after an expression period of about nine population doublings. Taken all together the data in Figure 6 indicate that to achieve a particular degree of cell killing, mutagenesis, and transformation, normal (NF) cells have to be exposed to 8- to 10-fold higher doses of UV radiation than XP cells. As discussed above, this is the result expected if induction of anchorage independence as well as TG resistance results ultimately from DNA damage remaining unexcised in the cell at some critical time after irradiation and if, because of the difference in their respective rates of excision repair, the average number of lesions remaining at this critical time is approximately equal in the three populations.

We tested the hypothesis that semiconservative DNA synthesis on a template containing unexcised lesions was responsible for the induction of anchorage independence by techniques similar to those described in Figure 7. Synchronized populations of normal and XP12BE cells were irradiated in early and late G_1 and their progeny assayed for frequency of AI cells. The results are included in Figure 6 as open and half-solid symbols. The tranformation frequencies of the normal cells irradiated with $6 J/m^2$ ~3 hours prior to onset of S phase yielded 200 anchorage-independent cells per 10^6 cells plated, whereas cells irradiated in early G_1 (20 hours prior to onset of S) showed no colonies out of 2 x 10^6 cells plated. The untreated control cells in this particular experiment also gave no colonies out of 2 x 10⁶. In contrast, the frequency of anchorage independent cells in XP12BE population irradiated in early G_1 was not lower than those irradiated just before the S phase. In fact it was somewhat higher. In the corresponding mutation experiment (Figure 6B), the frequencies were equal. In the mutagenesis experiments with normal cells from which the data in the middle panel were taken, the frequency of mutant cells did not decrease completely to the background level. However, in this mutagenesis experiment, the cells irradiated in G_1 had somewhat less time for excision repair before onset of S than was available in the transformation experiments. The fact that allowing substantial time for excision before DNA synthesis eliminated the potentially mutagenic and transforming effect of UV radiation in normal cells, but not in XP12BE cells, suggests that DNA synthesis on a template still containing unexcised lesions is the cellular event responsible for "fixing" the mutations and transformation.

If one assumes that anchorage independence, like TG resistance, results from a simple mutation, it is tempting to speculate about the size of the DNA target involved. The difficulties inherent in making a direct comparison between the data in Figure 6B and 6C have been discussed in detail (Maher *et al.,* 1982). It seems to us that the more important conclusion to be drawn from the three panels in Figure 6 is that there is obvious similarity in the dose-response curves for the two phenotypes and there is a close relationship between the ability of a cell population to remove photoproducts from DNA and its degree of sensitivity to the transforming (and mutagenic) effect of this carcinogenic agent. Taken all together, these data support the hypothesis that mutations are involved in transformation.

Progeny cells derived from AI colonies of XP7BE or normal cells were injected into sub-lethally irradiated athymic mice (~10⁷ cells/injection, 5 mice/assay). The cells gave rise to nodules about 1 cm in diameter within 10 days. No tumors arose in animals injected with 2 x 10⁷ anchorage dependent cells. These nodules were excised and diagnosed as fibrosarcomas by pathologists studying coded slides. At that time, it was our experience that the majority of such nodules did not progress to kill the animal but remained at that size. Our present experience with our closed colony of athymic Balb/hc(nu/nu) mice is that they do regress and, therefore, anchorage independent human cells are only partially transformed. One or more additional steps are required before they can escape the residual immune surveillance of these animals.

CONCLUSION

In summary, our studies indicate that, although the transformation of diploid human fibroblasts into tumor-forming cells is a multi-stepped process, an initial step to anchorage independence resembles a mutagenic event. The data indicate that excision repair in these fibroblasts is essentially an error-free process and that the ability to excise potentially cytotoxic, mutagenic, or transforming lesions induced in DNA by UV radiation or by several classes of chemical carcinogens determines their ultimate biological consequences. The data presented here suggest that there is a certain limited amount of time available between the initial exposure and the onset of the cellular events responsible for mutation induction, for cell transformation, and for cell killing, and that the critical event for the mutation and transformation to anchorage independence is DNA replication on a template containing unexcised lesions. This explains the abnormal sensitivity of excision repair-deficient XP cells. The accompanying cytotoxicity studies indicate that although a population's survival is determined by the extent of excision repair of potentially lethal damage from DNA before some critical cellular event, no single cell cycle-related event such as DNA synthesis on a damaged template is responsible for cell death.

ACKNOWLEDGEMENTS

We wish to express our indebtedness to our colleagues, A. E. Aust, J. C. Ball, J. Domaradzki, N. R. Drinkwater, R. H. Heflich, J. N. Howell, B. Konze-Thomas, J. W. Levinson, J. D. Patton, K. C. Silinskas, and L. L. Yang for their invaluable contributions to the research summarized here. The excellent technical assistance of M. Antczak, R. C. Corner, K. D. Debien, D. J. Dorney, K. J. Falahee, R. M. Hazard, S. A. Kately, T. E. Kinney, L. Lommel, L. D. Milam, A. L. Mendrala, M. M. Moon, T. G. O'Callaghan, D. Richmond, L. A. Rowan, J. E. Tower and T. VanNoord is gratefully acknowledged. The labeled anti BPDE was provided by the Cancer Research Program of the National Cancer Institute and the labeled aromatic amines by Dr. John Scribner of the Pacific Northwest Research Foundation. The research summarized in this report was supported in part by Contract ES-78-4659 from the Department of Energy and by Grant CA 21253, CA 21289 and ES 07076 from the Department of Health and Human Services, NIH. Additional financial assistance was provided by the Michigan Osteopathic College Foundation.

REFERENCES

Aust, A. E., Falahee, K. J. Maher, V. M., and McCormick, J. J.: Human cell-mediated benzo(a)pyrene cytotoxicity and mutagenicity in human diploid fibroblasts. *Cancer Res.* 40:4070-4075, 1980.

Aust, A. E., Drinkwater, N. R., Debien, K. D., Maher, V. M. and McCormick, J. J.: Comparison of the frequency of diphtheria toxin and thioguanine resistance induced by a series of carcinogens to analyze their mutational specificities in diploid human fibroblasts. *Mutation Res.* 125, 95-104, 1984.

Barrett, J. C. and Ts'o, P.O.P.; Evidence for the progressive nature of neoplastic transformation in vitro. *Proc. Natl. Acad. Sci. (U.S.A.).* 75:3761-3765, 1978.

Barrett, J. C., Crawford, B. D., and Ts'o, P.O.P.: The role of somatic mutation in a multistage model of carcinogenesis. In *Mammalian Cell Transformation by Chemical Carcinogens* (N. Mishra, V. Dunkel, and M. Mehlman, eds.) pp. 467-501, Princeton, Senate Press Inc., 1980.

Berwald, Y. and Sachs, L.: In Vitro transformation of normal cells to tumor cells by carcinogenic hydrocarbons. *J. Natl. Cancer Inst.* 35:641-661, 1965.

Cleaver, J. E.: Defective repair replication of DNA in xeroderma pigmentosum. *Nature (London)* 218:652-656, 1968.

DiPaolo, J. A., Nelson, R. L., and Donovan, P. J.: In vitro transformation of Syrian hamster embryo cells by diverse chemical carcinogens. *Nature (London)* 235:270-280, 1972.

Domoradzki, J., Pegg, A. E., Dolan, M. E., Maher, V. M., and McCormick, J. J.: Correlation between O6-methylguanine-DNA methyltransferase activity and resistance of human cells to the cytotoxic and mutagenic effect of N-methyl-N'-nitro-N-Nitrosoguanidine. *Carcinogenesis* in press, 1984.

Drinkwater, N. R., Corner, R. C., McCormick, J. J., and Maher, V. M.: An in situ assay for induced diphtheria toxin resistant mutants of diploid human fibroblasts. *Mutation Res.* 106:277-289, 1982.

Heflich, R. H., Hazard, R. M., Lommel L., Scribner, J. D., Maher, V. M., and McCormick, J. J.: A comparison of the DNA binding, cytotoxicity and repair synthesis induced in human fibroblasts by reactive derivatives of aromatic amide carcinogens.
Chem. Biol. Interactions, 29:43-56, 1980.

Howell, J. N., Greene, M. H., Corner, R. C., Maher, V. M., and McCormick, J. J.: Fibroblasts from patients with hereditary cutaneous malignant melanoma are abnormally sensitive to the mutagenic effect of simulated sunlight and 4-nitroquinoline 1-oxide.
Proc. Natl. Acad. Sci. (USA), 81,1179-1183, 1984.

Kakunaga, T.: The transformation of human diploid cells by chemical carcinogens. In *Origins of Human Cancer,* (H. H. Hiatt, J. D. Watson, J. A. Winsten, eds.) Vol. C, pp. 1537-1548, Cold Spring Harbor, New York, Cold Spring Harbor Laboratory Press, 1977.

Kakunaga, T.: Neoplastic transformation of human diploid fibroblast cells by chemical carcinogens. *Proc. Natl. Acad. Sci. (U.S.A.),* 75:1334-1338, 1978.

Konze-Thomas, B., Levinson, J. W., Maher, V. M., and McCormick, J. J.: Correlation among the rates of dimer excision, DNA repair replication, and recovery of human cells from potentially lethal damage induced by ultraviolet radiation. *Biophys. J.* 28:315-326, 1979.

Konze-Thomas, B., Hazard, R. M., Maher, V. M., and McCormick, J. J.: Extent of excision repair before DNA synthesis determines the mutagenic but not the lethal effect of UV radiation. *Mutation Res.* 94:421-434, 1982.

Maher, V. M., and McCormick, J. J.: Effect of DNA repair on the cytotoxicity and mutagenicity of UV irradiation and of chemical carcinogens in normal and xeroderma pigmentosum cells. In *Biology of Radiation Carcinogenesis* (J. M. Yuhas, R. W. Tennant, and J. D. Regan, eds.) pp. 129-145, 1976.

Maher, V. M., Curren, R. D., Ouellette, L. M., and McCormick, J. J.: Role of DNA repair in the cytotoxic and mutagenic action of physical and chemical carcinogens. In *In Vitro Metabolic Activation in Mutagenesis Testing.* (F. J. deSerres, J. R. Fouts, J. R. Bend, and R. M. Philpot, eds.) pp. 313-336, Elsevier Scient. Publ. Co., Amsterdam, 1976a.

Maher, V. M., Ouellette, L. M., Curren, R. D., and McCormick, J. J.: Frequency of ultraviolet light-induced mutations is higher in xeroderma pigmentosum variant cells than in normal human cells. *Nature* 261:593-595, 1976b.

Maher, V. M., McCormick, J. J., Grover, P. L., and Sims, P.: Effect of DNA repair on the cytotoxicity and mutagenicity of polycyclic hydrocarbon derivatives in normal and xeroderma pigmentosum human fibroblasts. *Mutation Res.* 43:117-138, 1977.

Maher, V. M., Dorney, D. J., Mendrala, A. L., Konze-Thomas, B., and McCormick, J. J.: DNA excision repair processes in human cells can eliminate the cytotoxic and mutagenic consequences of ultraviolet irradiation. *Mutation Res.* 62:311-323, 1979.

Maher, V. M., Hazard, R. M., Beland, F. J., Corner, R., Mendrala, A. L., Levinson, J. W., Heflich, R. H., and McCormick, J. J.: Excision of the deacetylated C-8-guanine DNA adduct by human fibroblasts correlates with decreased cytotoxicity and mutagenicity. *Proc. Amer. Assoc. Cancer Res.* 21:71, 1980.

Maher, V. M., Heflich, R. H., and McCormick, J. J.: Repair of DNA damage induced in human fibroblasts by N-substituted aryl compounds. In *Carcinogenic and Mutagenic N-Substituted Aryl Compounds* (S. S. Thorgeirsson, E. K. Weisberger, C. W. King, and J. D. Scribner) Monograph 58, p. 217-222, National Cancer Institute, 1981.

Maher, V. M., Rowan, L. A., Silinskas, K. C., Kately, S. A., and McCormick, J. J.: Frequency of UV-induced neoplastic transformation of diploid human fibroblasts is higher in xeroderma pigmentosum cells than in normal cells. *Proc. Natl. Acad. Sci. (U.S.A.), 79*:2613-2617, 1982.

McCormick, J. J. and Maher, V. M.: Measurement of colony-forming ability and mutagenesis in diploid human cells. In *DNA Repair: A Laboratory Manual of Research Procedures* (E. C. Friedberg and P. C. Hanawalt, eds.), Vol. 1, Part B, pp. 501-521, New York, Marcel Dekker, Inc., 1981.

McCormick, J. J., Silinskas, K. C., and Maher, V. M.: Transformation of diploid human fibroblasts by chemical carcinogens. In *Carcinogenesis, Fundamental Mechanisms and Environmental Effects* (B. Pullman, P.O.P. Ts'o, and H. Gelboin, eds.) pp. 491-498, Dordrecht, D. Reidel Publ. Co., 1980.

Milo, G. E., Jr., and DiPaolo, J. A.: Neoplastic transformation of human diploid cells in vitro after chemical carcinogen treatment. *Nature 275*:130-132, 1978.

Milo, G. E., Oldham, J. W., Zimmerman, R., Hatch, G. G., and Weisbrode, S. A.: Characterization of human cells transformed by chemical and physical carcinogens in vitro. *In Vitro 17*:719-729, 1981.

Patton, J. D., Rowan, L. A., Mendrala, A. L., Howell, J. N., Maher, V. M. and McCormick, J. J.: Xeroderma pigmentosum (XP) fibroblasts including cells from XP variants are abnormally sensitive to the mutagenic and cytotoxic action of broad spectrum simulated sunlight. *Photochem. Photobiol., 39*:37-42 1984.

Robbins, J. H., Kraemer, K. H., Lutzner, M. A., Festoff, B. W., and Coon, H. G.: Xeroderma pigmentosum an inherited disease with sun sensitivity, multiple cutaneous neoplasms, and abnormal DNA repair. *Annals of Internal Medicine. 80*:221-248, 1974.

Silinskas, K. C., Kateley, S. A., Tower, J. E., Maher, V. M., and McCormick, J. J.: Induction of anchorage independent growth in human fibroblasts by propane sultone. *Cancer Res. 41*, 1620-1627, 1981.

Simon, L., Hazard, R. M., Maher, V. M., and McCormick, J. J.: Enhanced cell killing and mutagenesis by ethylnitrosourea in xeroderma pigmentosum cells. *Carcinogenesis 2*:567-570, 1981.

Sutherland, B. M., Cemino, J. S., Delihas, N., Shih, A., and Oliver, R.: Ultraviolet light-induced transformation of human cells to anchorage-independent growth. *Cancer Res. 40*:1934-1939, 1980.

Sutherland, B. M., Delihas, N. C., Oliver, R. O., and Sutherland, J.C.: Action spectra for ultra-violet light-induced transformation of human cells to anchorage-indepdent growth. *Cancer Res. 41*:2211-2214, 1981.

Yang, L. L., Maher, V. M., and McCormick, J. J.: Error-free excision of the cytotoxic, mutagenic N2-deoxyguanosine DNA adduct formed in human fibroblasts by ($\pm$)-7β, 8α-dihydroxy-9α, 10α-epoxy-7, 8, 9, 10-tetrahydrobenzo(a)pyrene. *Proc. Natl. Acad. Sci. (U.S.A), 77*,5933-5937, 1980.

Yang, L. L., Maher, V.M., McCormick, J. J.: Relationship between excision repair and the cytotoxic and mutagenic effect of the "anti" 7,8-diol-9,10-epoxide of benzo(a)pyrene in human cells. *Mutation Res. 94*:435-447, 1982.

Zimmerman, R. J. and Little, J. B.: Characterization of a quantitative assay for the in vitro transformation of normal human diploid fibroblasts to anchorage independence by chemical carcinogens. *Cancer Res. 43*:2176-2182, 1983.

Measurement of Chemically-Induced DNA Repair in Rodent and Human Cells

Byron E. Butterworth

Chemical Industry Institute of Toxicology, Research Triangle Park, North Carolina 27709

COMING OF AGE OF THE SCIENCE OF GENETIC TOXICOLOGY

The information that controls the structure, function, and reproduction of the cell is encoded ultimately in the DNA. Thus, both theoretical considerations and experimental evidence indicate that alternation of the DNA is involved in carcinogenesis. Dr. Bruce Ames of the University of California at Berkeley was the first to examine a large number of chemicals and demonstrate that, in general, mutagens were carcinogens (McCann et al., 1975). The key elements to the assay were strains of *Salmonella* in which mutants could easily be identified under selective conditions and which were engineered to be exquisitely sensitive to mutagens. The incorporation of a rat liver homogenate in the assay facilitated the production of potential genotoxic metabolites. The concept of a short-term test for potential carcinogens was embraced by many regulatory agencies and toxicology laboratories and genetic toxicology now has become a factor that is always considered in human risk assessment.

Extent of Application of Short-Term Tests

There is a reluctance on the part of many to accept the predictive value of cell culture assays because of examples where the Ames test has failed to predict the carcinogenicity of a specific chemical. Indeed, genetic toxicology assays are often forced to accept the unrealistic challenge of perfect correlation with cancer studies. In such an exercise, if a compound has produced a tumor in any species, in any organ, at any dose, it becomes a "plus". The only correct result for the short-term test is then defined as a plus. Cell culture assays cannot be expected to reflect the species, strain, sex, and organ specificities that are common in chemical carcinogenesis. If the same criterion were applied to rodent bioassays, the rat is, indeed, a poor predictor of carcinogenicity in the mouse.

Genetic toxicology has made tremendous progress since the Ames test. Numerous assays are available that can be applied to obtain a meaningful profile of a chemical's genotoxic potential (Hollstein et al., 1979; Butterworth, 1979). Yet, if anything, the results from an Ames test is commonly the only information ever generated on the genotoxic potential of a chemical.

By eliminating flagrant and massive exposures to chemicals in the workplace and practicing reasonable industrial hygiene, the level of occupationally related disease usually drops below the background produced by environmental factors such as cigarette smoking. Thus, by eliminating the obvious problem there is no resulting demand to examine the genotoxic activity of chemicals in the workplace. There is little incentive to generate sometimes difficult to explain data that could precipitate expensive further testing or retrospective litigation.

In a voluntary testing program a negative result in the Ames test usually brings a sigh of relief and satisfies immediate concerns. In most instances no demands are made for more elegant test methods. The more assays that are run, the greater the chance of a spurious positive result. In a program to develop new products, if a marginal compound is positive in the Ames test, it is often dropped without further testing. It is the perception of many that no amount of experimentation in other assays will be sufficient to override a positive Ames test. If industry were allowed to refute bacterial data with more meaningful assays, this would provide the incentive to do more thorough testing, and science and the public interest would be better served.

Scope of Genotoxicity Assays

In point of fact there has been significant advances in genetic toxicology since the advent of the Ames test. Assays are available that measure genotoxicity in mammalian cells (Hsie *et al.,* 1979), metabolically competent cells (Williams, 1976), specific target organs in the whole animal, primary human cell cultures, and samples from exposed individuals (Bridges *et al.,* 1982). Often, the key to understanding the mechanism of action of a chemical is found by contrasting the activity in several genotoxicity assays. Compounds that are uniformly positive in a battery of short-term tests are invariably carcinogenic. Mutagens are, in fact, carcinogens. More farsighted laboratories find that an accurate assessment of the profile of genotoxic activity of a compound is essential in human risk assessment. It must be remembered that rodent bioassays are only models for human toxicity. Genetic toxicology provides the means to evaluate the relevance of these rodent models in predicting human health effects. An entire conference was held that dealt only with genotoxicity assays in the whole animal or people (Bridges *et al.,* 1982). For example, one can measure chemically induced DNA repair in primary cultures of human hepatocytes (Butterworth *et al.,* 1983a) and human bronchial epithelium (Doolittle *et al.,* 1983a). Mutagenic activity suggests not only carcinogenic potential but also warns of potential genetic damage to germ cells. Germ cell assays are available
(Sega, 1982) including DNA repair in pachytene spermatocytes (Working and Butterworth, 1984).

Genetic Toxicology in the Regulatory Arena

Genetic toxicology has reached the point that results could be applied in the regulatory process. One such recommendation for testing relating to product registration would be to substitute a well-chosen battery of genetic toxicology assays to replace a second species in long-term cancer risk evaluation. Such a program would allow a wiser use of resources and, if anything, provide better data. For example, let us assume that compound X is negative in a 2-year rat feeding study. If the compound were also negative in bacterial and mammalian cell mutagenesis assays, did not induce DNA repair *in vitro* or *in vivo* in rat or human hepatocytes, produced no chromosomal aberrations in treated animals, and was negative in the C3H/10T½ cell transformation/promotion assay, it is doubtful that spending $500,000 and two years for a mouse study would provide any useful new information.

Genotoxicity assays also provide the basis of distinguishing between genotoxic and nongenotoxic carcinogens. Initiating agents exhibit cumulative, nonreversible effects while the effects of promoters appear to be reversible. Other compounds appear to be carcinogenic because they are toxic to a specific tissue, and prolonged high doses result in tissue damage followed by continual, compensating cell turnover. Such basic information should be considered in risk assessment decisions. A nongenotoxic compound that is a weak carcinogen at high doses in one tissue of one species might well be regulated less stringently than a genotoxic chemical that produces tumors in multiple tissues in several species. Sometimes other relevant information is available such as hormonal effects, the ability to activate specific genes, or immunosuppressive activity. To lump all carcinogens together for regulatory purposes is to deny that any progress has been made in the science of carcinogenesis or genetic toxicology.

CHEMICALLY INDUCED DNA REPAIR

The determination of chemically induced DNA repair as measured by unscheduled DNA syntheses (UDS) is a valuable tool that lends itself to assessment of organ-specific genotoxic activity. Cells can be exposed to the compound of interest either in culture or in the intact animal. If the compound or its active metabolites bind to the DNA, the damage may be repaired by a process in which cellular enzymes excise the altered region of the DNA and resynthesize the missing DNA sequence according to the template on the opposite strand. If this excision repair process occurs in the presence of ^{3}H-thymidine, the radiolabelled base will be incorporated and can be measured by quantitative autoradiography. DNA repair is a natural response to chemical insult to the genetic material, occurs in most cells, is readily detected, does not require proliferating cells, and can be measured in various cell types in culture or in the whole animal. If one is interested in predicting the ability of a chemical to cause liver tumors in rats, one should examine the genotoxic effects in liver cells from exposed rats.

Rat Hepatocytes

One advance in this area was the development in this laboratory of an *in vivo - in vitro* hepatocyte DNA repair assay (Mirsalis and Butterworth, 1980). Following treatment of the animal by an appropriate route of exposure, primary hepatocyte cultures are prepared and incubated with ^{3}H-thymidine. If the DNA has been damaged in the intact animal such that the cells are undergoing excision repair, ^{3}H-thymidine will be incorporated into the DNA of the freshly isolated cells in culture. This assay detects genotoxic hepatocarcinogens from a variety of chemical classes including nitroaromatics, aromatic amines, direct acting agents, mycotoxins, nitrosamines, and azo compounds. The assay also detects cells in S-phase and can help distinguish between true genotoxic carcinogens and those which are only cytotoxic and induce cell turnover such as carbon tetrachloride and chloroform (Mirsalis *et al.*, 1982b).

One advantage of the *in vivo* approach is that factors such as uptake, distribution, metabolism, detoxification, and excretion are inherently taken into account. Most genotoxic hepatocarcinogens such as dimethylnitrosamine (DMN) and 2-acetylaminofluorene (AAF) induce UDS in hepatocytes both *in vitro* (Williams, 1976; Probst *et al.*, 1981), and *in vivo* (Mirsalis *et al.*, 1982b). There are, however, interesting exceptions. Some polycyclic aromatic hydrocarbons that are not hepatocarcinogens such as benzo(a)pyrene (B(a)P), induce DNA repair in the *in vitro* hepatocyte assay but not in the *in vivo* hepatocyte system. The reasons for this dichotomy are not presently understood, but may relate simply to delivery of the compound to the cells. In contrast, the potent hepatocarcinogen technical grade dinitrotoluene (tech-DNT) induces a response in the *in vivo* assay but not in the *in vitro* system because gut flora are obligatory in its metabolism to genotoxic products (Bermudez et al., 1979; Mirsalis et al., 1982a). Tech-DNT consists of approximately 80% 2,4-DNT and 20% 2,6-DNT. 2,6-DNT was shown to be at least an order of magnitude more potent than 2,4-DNT in inducing hepatocyte DNA repair (Mirsalis and Butterworth, 1982). Long-term feeding studies have confirmed 2,6-DNT to be the carcinogenic component in the mixture (Leonard and Popp, 1983). These studies have been extended to the mononitrotoluenes (NT) (Doolittle et al., 1983b). 2-NT produces a dose-related increase in hepatic UDS while the 3-NT and 4-NT isomers do not. As with DNT, gut flora are obligatory for the genotoxic activity of 2-NT. These experiments illustrate the value of the *in vivo* - *in vitro* hepatocyte DNA repair assay in predictive and mechanistic studies.

Not all nitroaromatic compounds require gut flora for metabolic activation. Nitropyrenes are extraordinarily mutagenic environmental pollutants found in diesel exhaust, coal-fired power plants, and cigarette smoke (Mermelstein et al., 1981). 1,6-Dinitropyrene (DNP) is the most potent compound thus far observed in inducing DNA repair in primary cultures of rat or human hepatocytes. Therefore, 1,6-DNP does not require gut glora for metabolic activiation (Butterworth et al., 1983b). No DNA repair was observed in hepatocytes isolated from rats treated with 1,6-DNP by gavage 2, 12, or 24 hours previously. The reason for the lack of response *in vivo* is not known, but may relate to detoxification or distribution of the compound in the animal.

Human Hepatocytes

It is important to know the extent to which rodent models are relevant in predicting human health effects. The *in vitro* hepatocyte DNA repair assay is directly applicable to freshly isolated human hepatocytes obtained from surgical samples normally discarded during prescribed surgery (Butterworth et al., 1983a). In experiments with primary cultures of human hepatocytes, a positive dose-related response up to the concentration indicated was observed with the genotoxicants aflatoxin B_1 (AFB_1) (0.01 mM), 2-acetylaminofluorene (0.01 mM), benzo(a)pyrene (0.01 mM), dimethylnitrosamine (1 mM), 2,4-diaminotoluene (1 mM) and 2,6-diaminotoluene (1 mM). No response was observed with 2-napthylamine (2NA) (1 mM), aniline (1 mM), or nitrobenzene (1 mM). 2,4-Dinitrotoluene (1 mM), 2,6-dinitrotoluene (1 mM), and 2-nitrotoluene (1 mM) were also negative, which is consistent with the observation in rat hepatocytes that these compounds require gut flora for metabolic activation. Thus, the response in human hepatocytes is qualitatively similar to rodent hepatocyte DNA repair models (Williams, 1976; Probst et al., 1981). AFB_1 has been implicated in human liver cancer and these results confirm it to be a potent genotoxicant in human hepatocytes. 2NA is a human bladder carcinogen but did not induce DNA repair in human hepatocytes, indicating that organ specificity is a key factor to be considered in predictive toxicology.

Rat Tracheal Epithelium

Lung cancer is currently the leading cause of mortality from cancer in men in the United States, and the incidence in women is increasing dramatically. Carcinoma of the lung is usually bronchogenic with the most common site being the large bronchi at or near the lung hilus. Rodent tracheas have been used extensively as model systems for studying human bronchogenic carcinoma. Accordingly, an assay has been developed for measuring chemically induced DNA repair as unscheduled DNA synthesis in primary cultures of rat tracheal epithelial (TE) cells (Doolittle and Butterworth, 1984). The cells may be exposed in culture or in the whole animal. Dimethylnitrosamine (DMN) produced a positive response *in vitro* and *in vivo* following administration by inhalation. Of the chemicals tested *in vitro* methyl methanesulfonate (0.01 - 1.0 mM), N-methyl-N'-nitro-N-nitrosoguanidine (0.5 - 5.0 µg/ml), dimethylnitrosamine (0.1 - 10 mM), and 1,6-dinitropyrene (0.05 - 5 µM) induced UDS in TE cells in a concentration-dependent manner, whereas N-acetylaminofluorene (0.001 - 0.1 mM), benzo(a)pyrene (0.001 - 0.1 mM) and 1-nitropyrene (0.001 - 0.1 mM) did not. These data indiciate that the TE UDS assay is capable of detecting genotoxic agents, some of which require metabolic activation. The observation of selective activation of some compounds demands that the response be compared to human bronchial epithelial cells to assess the appropriateness of the animal model.

Human Bronchial Epithelium

Because 90% of human lung cancers originate in the bronchial epithelium, methodology was developed to prepare primary culture of human bronchial epithelial cells as a means of measuring chemically induced DNA repair in these target cells (Doolittle *et al.*, 1983a). Bronchi were obtained as fresh autopsy material or as material normally discarded during prescribed surgery. The epithelial layer was selectively released by digestion with a protease solution. Cultures were judged as viable by actively beating cilia and trypan blue dye exclusion. DNA repair was measured in basal cells. The direct acting agent MMS induced UDS in all cultures and indicated that the cells were viable and capable of DNA repair. DNA repair was induced in all cultures with B(a)P while no DNA repair was observed with DMN. 1,6-DNP induced DNA repair only in the cultures obtained from autopsy material. Thus, the patterns of metabolic activation and genotoxic activity in rat tracheal epithelium were not the same as those in the human bronchial epithelium, indicating that in this case the rat model is inappropriate for assessing activity in human cells. Similar studies will be conducted with hamster tracheal epithelial cells which have been shown to metabolize B(a)P differently than the analogous cells in the rat (Mass and Kaufman, 1983).

Rat Nasal Epithelium

Many chemicals such as formaldehyde and hexamethylphosphoramide, when administered by inhalation, specifically induce squamous cell carcinomas of the nasal epithelium, and yet, no assay exists to assess genotoxicity in this tissue. The conditions necessary to initiate organ and primary cultures of the rat nasal epithelium have been characterized as a means of measuring chemically induced DNA damage and repair in these cells (Bermudez and Allen, 1983). Primary cultures of the epithelium were obtained by protease digestion. Explanted tissues could be maintained for two weeks with vigorous ciliary movement and little desquamation. DNA repair in these cells was induced in primary cultures treated with DMN or in cells isolated from animals treated with 1000 ppm DMN for 4 hours by inhalation. Therefore, the culture of rat nasal epithelium as an intact tissue or single cells provides the means to determine the genotoxic effects of *in vivo* or *in vitro* exposure, by the quantitation of DNA damage and repair to those chemicals that are specific for the nasal epithelium.

Rat Alveolar Macrophages

Because rat alveolar macrophages (RAM) are phagocytic, a genotoxicity assay in these cells would be useful for the study of inhaled environmental toxicants bound to particulates and could provide an index for assessing genotoxic activity in the lung. A DNA repair assay for RAM has been developed (Cheng et al., 1983). RAM were isolated by pulmonary lavage and incubated with ^{3}H-thymidine and the compound of interest. The direct acting agent MMS produced a strong positive response. Compounds such as B(a)P, AAF, and DMN failed to respond indicating the lack of metabolic activity in these cells and, thus, limiting the use of this system.

Rat Spermatocytes

Mutagens are of concern in human risk assessment not only because they are potential carcinogens but because they may induce heritable mutations in the germ cells with the serious consequence of altering the genetic information in the human gene pool. Several means have been developed to measure DNA repair in mouse spermatocytes (Sega, 1982).

A quantitative assay to measure DNA repair as unscheduled DNA synthesis in rat pachytene spermatocytes (PS) has been developed to assess chemically induced DNA damage in germ cells (Working and Butterworth, 1984). PS were isolated at various times following treatment and incubated *in vitro* in the presence of ^{3}H-thymidine for 24 hr. Incorporation was quantitated by autoradiography. Spermatocytes isolated from animals treated at 1 hour post exposure (PE) with MMS (25 mg/kg) or cyclophosphamide (200 mg/kg) exhibited DNA repair. This is consistent with the observations that these chemicals also induce dominant lethal mutations. No UDS was observed at 2 hr PE with 10 mg/kg dimethylnitrosamine, 50 mg/kg 1,6-DNP, 2 mg/kg aflatoxin B$_1$ or at 12 hr PE with 50 mg/kg 2-acetylaminofluorene, 20 mg/kg 2,6-dinitrotoluene, 50 mg/kg 1,6-DNP or at 24 hr PE with 50 mg/kg 1,6-DNP. The lack of UDS response in PS to many known genotoxicants probably reflects the relative inaccessibility of the germ cells to these compounds or their active forms *in vivo*.

CONCLUSION

The results from genetic toxicology studies are used increasingly by industry, academia, and regulatory agencies to support conclusions relating to human risk assessment. It is imperative that more meaningful assays be developed and employed that relate to the whole animal and people. Measurement of chemically induced DNA repair in target tissues from exposed animals and in primary human cell cultures should prove to be among the most valuable tools of the genetic toxicologist.

REFERENCES

Bermudez, E., and Allen, P. F.: Assessment of the genotoxicity of airborne chemicals: Isolation and culture of rat nasal epithelium. *Environ. Mutagen.* 5, 413, 1983.

Bermudez, E., Butterworth, B. E., and Tillery, D.: The effect of 2,4-diaminotoluene and isomers of dinitrotoluene on unscheduled DNA synthesis in primary rat hepatocytes. *Environ. Mutagen.* 1, 391-398, 1979.

Bridges, B. A. Butterworth, B. E., and Weinstein, I. B., eds.: *Indicators of Genotoxic Exposure, Banbury Report 13,* Cold Spring Harbor Laboratory, Cold Spring Harbor, NY, 1982.

Butterworth, B. E.: Strategies for Short-Term Testing for Mutagens/Carcinogens, CRC Press, Inc., West Palm Beach, FL, 1979.

Butterworth, B. E., Earle, L. L., Strom, S., Jirtle, R., and Michalopoulos, G.: Measurement of chemically induced DNA repair in human hepatocytes.
Proc. Am. Assoc. Cancer Res. 24, 69, 1983a.

Butterworth, B. E., Earle, L. L., Strom, S., Jirtle, R., and Michalopoulos, G.: Induction of DNA repair in human and rat hepatocytes by 1,6-dinitropyrene.
Mutat. Res., 122, 73-80, 1983b.

Cheng, M., Kligerman, A. D., and Butterworth, B. E.: Chemical induction of unscheduled DNA synthesis in rat alveolar macrophages. *The Pharmacologist 25,* 190, 1983.

Doolittle, D. J., and Butterworth, B. E.: Assessment of chemically-induced DNA repair in isolated rat tracheal epithelial cells. *Carcinogenesis 5,* 773-779, 1984.

Doolittle, D. J., Furlong, J. W., Earle, L. L., and Butterworth, B. E.: Measurement of chemically-induced DNA repair in human bronchial epithelial cells.
The Pharmacologist 25, 174, 1983a.

Doolittle, D. J., Sherrill, J. M., and Butterworth, B. E.: The influence of intestinal bacteria, sex of the animal, and position of the nitro group on the hepatic genotoxicity of nitrotoluene isomers *in vivo. Cancer Res. 43,* 2836-2842, 1983b.

Hollstein, M., McCann, J., Angelosanto, F. A., and Nichols, W. W.: Short-term tests for carcinogens and mutagens. *Mutat. Res. 65,* 133, 1979.

Hsie, A. W., O'Neill, J. P., McElheny, V. K, eds.: *Mammalian Cell Mutagenesis: The Maturation of Test Systems. Banbury Report 2,* Cold Spring Harbor Laboratory, Cold Spring Harbor, NY, 1979.

Leonard, T. L., and Popp, J.: Hepatocarcinogenicity of 2,6-dinitrotoluene.
Proc. Am. Soc. Cancer Res 24, 91, 1983.

McCann, J., Choi, E., Yamasaki, E., and Ames, B. N.: Detection of carcinogens as mutagens in the *Salmonella*/microsome test: Assay of 300 chemicals.
Proc. Nat. Acad. Sci USA 72, 5135-5139, 1975.

Mass, M. J., and Kaufman, D. G.: A comparison between the activiation of benzo(a)pyrene in organ cultures and microsomes from the tracheal epithelium of rats and hamsters. *Carcinogenesis 4,* 297-303, 1983.

Mermelstein, R., Kiriazides, D. K, Butler, M., McCoy, E. C., and Rosenkranz, H. S.: The extraordinary mutagenicity of nitropyrenes in bacteria. *Mutat. Res. 89,* 187-196, 1981.

Mirsalis, J. C., and Butterworth, B. E.: Detection of unscheduled DNA synthesis in hepaocytes isolated from rats treated with genotoxic agents; An *in vivo - in vitro* assay for potential mutagens and carcinogens. *Carcinogenesis 1,* 621-625, 1980.

Mirsalis, J. C., and Butterworth, B. E.: Induction of unscheduled DNA synthesis in rat hepatocytes following *in vivo* treatment with dinitrotoluene.
Carcinogenesis 3, 241-245, 1982.

Mirsalis, J. C., Hamm, T. E., Jr., Sherrill, M., and Butterworth, B. E.: Role of gut flora in the genotoxicity of dinitrotoluene. *Nature 295,* 322-323, 1982a.

Mirsalis, J. C., Tyson, K. C., and Butterworth, B. E.: Detection of genotoxic carcinogens in the *in vivo - in vitro* hepatocyte DNa repair assay.
Environ. Mutagen. 4, 533-562, 1982b.

Probst, G. S., McMahon, R. E., Hill, L. E., Thompson, C. Z., Epp, J. K., and Neal, S. B.: Chemically-induced unscheduled DNA synthesis in primary rat hepatocyte cultures: A comparison with bacterial mutagenicity using 218 compounds.
Environ. Mutagen. 3, 11-32, 1981.

Sega, G. A.: DNA repair in spermatocytes. *In Indicators of Genotoxic Exposure,* B. A. Bridges, B. E. Butterworth, and I. B. Weinstein, eds. *Banbury Reports, 13,* Cold Spring Harbor, NY, pp. 503-514, 1982.

Williams, G. M.: Carcinogen induced DNA repair in primary rat liver cell cultures: A possible screen for chemical carcinogens. *Cancer Lett. 1,* 231-236, 1976.

Working, P. K., and Butterworth, B. E.: An assay to detect chemically-induced DNA repair in rat spermatocytes. *Environ. Mutagen. 6,* 273-286, 1984.

New Approaches in Toxicity Testing and Their Application in Human Risk Assessment, edited by A. P. Li. Raven Press, New York © 1985.

Use of Cytogenetic Endpoints in Human Lymphocytes as Indicators of Exposure to Genotoxicants

R. Julian Preston

Biology Division, Oak Ridge National Laboratory, Oak Ridge, Tennessee 37831

Since the observation by Moorhead *et al* (1960) hat peripheral lymphocytes could be stimulated by phytohemagglutinin (pha) to enter the cell cycle and observed at metaphase, there has been an enormous amount of data obtained on the induction of chromosome alternations by radiation and chemical agents with this lymphocyte assay system. It has generally been regarded as a simple and informative assay for human population monitoring, as an aid to providing information on potential clastogenic (or mutagenic) exposures. As will be suggested below this view should be regarded with great caution with regard to chemical exposures, particularly in contrast to radiation exposures. It is premature to assume that information on the level of exposure or subsequent adverse health effects can be ascertained or determined from measures of chromosome alteration frequencies or sister chromatid exchange frequency in mitogenically stimulated human peripheral lymphocytes.

This chapter will address the issue of the utility of the lymphocyte assay, with reference to the underlying mechanisms of induction of chromosome alterations, and also will discuss possible ways of increasing the sensitivity of the assay in order to make it more useful for population monitoring. The application of the lymphocyte assay for detecting gene mutations is discussed by Dr. R. J. Albertini in a chapter in this volume.

It will be apparent that there has not been an attempt to provide a complete review of the available literature, citing the many studies on the analysis of lymphocytes from a few to many individuals presumed to have been exposed to clastogenic and/or mutagenic agents. Examples are only given to indicate the potential utility and the associated pitfalls and problems of the lymphocyte assay.

LYMPHOCYTE ASSAY
Methods of Culture

The techniques for culturing peripheral lymphocytes have been described many times, and in general it is reasonable to state that any culture conditions that provide adequate analysable metaphases are acceptable (Bloom, 1981). However, it is important to add that each laboratory using the assay should determine the rate of progression of mitogenically stimulated cells through the first and subsequent cell cycles with their specific culture conditions, using blood samples from several individuals. This can be done by growing the cells in the presence of bromodeoxyuridine (BrdU), sampling cells over a range of times (for example, every 2 h. from 46 h. to 60 h. after mitogenic stimulation), and staining the fixed preparations by a technique for obtaining differentially stained chromatids (for example, Goto et al., 1978). In this way the cells that had replicated their DNA once in the presence of BrdU will contain evenly stained chromatids; those that had replicated twice in BrdU will contain differentially stained chromatids, one light blue and one dark blue when Giemsa stain is used; cells that progress through three or more cell cycles in BrdU will contain some differentially stained chromosomes and some evenly, but lightly stained, chromosomes. For studies of chromosome aberrations, it is important to analyse cells in their first metaphase after mitogenic stimulation, and so a fixation time should be chosen when a high proportion of analysable cells are in this first division. It is generally not feasible to use a fixation time when all the cells are in their first division because this requires a very early fixation (approximately 42 h. after stimulation, when the number of mitotic cells is too low), and so a compromise time is selected when about 90% of the cells are in their first division (usually 48 h.). Of course, there is a considerable variation from individual to individual in the percentage of cells in their first or subsequent division event at 48 h., and so it is good practice to check the proportions in parallel cultures containing BrdU, such that the possible effects of analysing different proportions of first division cells from different samples upon aberration frequencies can be ascertained. It is also possible to *analyse* chromosome aberrations from cultures grown with BrdU, where the preparations have been differentially stained - cells showing no differentiation, and clearly M1 cells can then be analysed. However, there is still some disagreement about the possible confounding effects of BrdU upon aberration frequency, and so no consensus has been reached on the appropriateness of this method.

For the analysis of sister chromatid exchanges (SCE) it is necessary to analyse cells in their second mitotic division (M2) after stimulation and growth in BrdU, so that differentially stained chromatids can be obtained. Since only clearly identified M2 cells will be analysed, the fixation time chosen should simply be one at which a high proportion of M2 cells are obtained (usually from 56-72 h. depending upon culture conditions). Each laboratory should establish a fixation time for their own particular set of culture conditions.

The only other technical feature of the lymphocyte assay that bears comment here is on the use of tissue culture media containing a low concentration of folic acid. It has been noted that growth of human lymphocytes in such media (notably TC199) can result in the appearance of specific chromosome breaks at so-called fragile sites (Jacky et al., 1983) or in an increase in aberrations at possible fragile sites (Reidy et al., 1983). It is recommended for population monitoring studies that low folate medium be avoided, although, it is clear that additional cultures with low folate medium could provide additional or different types of information.

Chromosome aberrations

It is not necessary to provide a complete classification of chromosome aberration types in this chapter as these are readily available (for example Bloom, 1981; Savage, 1975). The only point of emphasis is the relationship between the aberration type and the cell cycle stage at the time of formation. Chromosome-type aberrations are formed in G_1, *ie* prior to DNA replication, and chromatid-type aberrations are formed during or after DNA replication, in the S or G_2 stages. Thus, the specific types of aberrations can indicate the stage of their formation, although not necessarily the time of exposure. The different aberration types also have different consequences with regard to the induction of cell lethality, and transmission to subsequent cell generations. Such considerations will be of great importance when considering the possible adverse health effects from exposure to chemical and physical clastogens. For these reasons, the types of chromosome aberrations observed should be recorded as completely as possible, and not included in a general category of "aberrant metaphases".

Radiation induced aberrations and estimates of exposure

For a variety of reasons, it is sensible to discuss the utility of the lymphocyte assay for estimating exposure to ionizing radiation separately from cases of chemical exposure. It was in some ways fortunate, but in retrospect perhaps also unfortunate, that all the original studies of the analysis of chromosome aberrations in the lymphocytes of exposed or possible exposed persons were for situations where exposure was to radiation. The fact that in these cases estimates of exposure could be made with some accuracy has often led to the assumption that similar exposure-estimating procedures could be applied to persons, groups or populations exposed environmentally or occupationally to chemical agents. A clear note of caution in accepting this assumption is made here, and will be discussed further.

Radiation and a small number of chemical agents (egs., streptonigrin, bleomycin, neocarzinostatin, cytosine arabinoside, and 8-methoxycaffeine) are able to *produce* aberrations in all stages of the cell cycle; chromosome-type aberrations in G_1 and chromatid-type aberrations in S and G_2.

The peripheral lymphocytes, a subpopulation of which is mitogenically stimulated when blood samples are placed in culture, are essentially noncycling, and are in the G_0 stage of the cell cycle, the term usually applied to a noncycling G_1 cell. Thus, following radiation exposure, chromosome-type aberrations will be induced in these noncycling, G_0 lymphocytes, and can be observed at the first metaphase following mitogenic stimulation in culture. The fact that the aberration can be produced in G_0 cells means that their frequency can be directly related to the dose received (*ie* aberration frequency is proportional to dose). In addition, it has been shown for many species that the frequency of aberrations induced *in vitro* is the same as the frequency induced by the same dose delivered *in vivo* (Brewen and Gengozian, 1971; Preston et al., 1972; Clemenger and

Scott, 1973). This means that a standard dose response curve, for any particular radiation type, can be obtained for *in vitro* exposures, and can then be used for estimating doses received by individuals as a result of radiation accidents, and medical or environmental exposures. The frequency of aberrations (usually dicentrics) is measured in cultured blood samples from exposed individuals, and then converted into a dose estimate from the standard dose response curve. There is an extensive literature on the use of the lymphocyte assay as a biological dosimeter for many different radiations (Bender and Gooch, 1966; Lloyd *et al.,* 1976). Of course, there are still some limitations to the utility of the assay. These include time of blood sampling after exposure, partial body exposures, nonhomogeneous exposures. There are way to partially circumvent these problems, but these will not be discussed here.

It will also be apparent that the lymphocyte assay is amenable to estimating doses following chronic radiation exposures (Evans, *et al.,* 1979)). This again is possible because the aberrations are induced in G_0 cells, and their frequency will be directly related to exposure. Cells containing radiation induced aberrations will gradually be lost from the peripheral lymphocyte pool, as will normal cells, as a result of lymphocyte turnover. However, the cells repopulating the peripheral pool will be derived largely from normal precursor cells, and not from those containing aberrations. The majority of chromosome-type aberrations are cell lethal as the result of loss of acentric fragments at division, or because of a mechanical interference of the aberration with division. Thus, during long chronic exposures (months or years) the aberration frequency will not be additive with time (or dose), but will reach some equilibrium where new aberrations are formed and some existing ones are lost from the sampled population.

A similar argument holds for determining the maximum sampling time after acute exposures that can be used in order to measure the maximum aberration frequency or true induced frequency. The lymphocyte turnover will result in loss of cells from the peripheral pool, both normal and abnormal, and repopulation largely by normal precursor cells. It appears that the aberration frequency stays constant for about 6 weeks after exposure (Brewen *et al.,* 1972)

Samples have been taken many years after exposure, for example with radiation-treated ankylosing spondylitis patients (Buckton *et al.,* 1978) and persons exposed to the atomic bomb in Hiroshima and Nagasaki (Awa *et al.,* 1978). The fact that some portion of lymphocytes are very long-lived (in excess of 20 years) means that radiation-induced aberrations can still be observed in cells present as peripheral lymphocytes at the time of exposure. If it is assumed that the aberration frequency declines exponentially with time an approximate estimate of the dose received can be made. However, emphasis is made on the word *approximate.*

The lymphocyte assay is clearly very applicable to the estimation of radiation exposures, and has been used extensively. The aberration frequency is directly proportional to dose, making this possible.

Chemical-induced aberrations and estimates of exposure

Based upon the success of the lymphocyte assay for estimating radiation exposures, it seemed appropriate to many to analyse chromosome aberrations in blood samples from individuals occupationally exposed to chemical agents or mixtures (many examples can be found in Office of Technology Assessment, 1983), and attempt to determine whether there had been an exposure to a clastogen, and to relate aberration frequencies to the possible exposure level. At this point in time this is an overly-optimistic approach. However, current and future research can realistically improve the assay to make it more reliable and applicable, and make the results more readily interpretable.

The present low sensitivity of the assay for measuring the frequency of chromosome aberrations following chemical exposure is due to the mechanism of induction of aberrations by chemical agents. This mechanism of induction will also result in induced aberration frequencies being only indirectly related to exposure dose, in contrast to radiation-induced aberrations.

Chromosome aberrations induced by chemical treatments are produced during the S-phase irrespective of the cell cycle stage treated. Thus, all aberrations will be of the chromatid-type. It has been assumed that aberrations induced by most chemicals are the result of an S-phase dependent mechanism - either DNA replication itself or a post-replication phenomenon. However, this is an oversimplification. It has been shown from experiments in this and other laboratories (Preston and Gooch, 1981; Evans and Vijayalaxmi, 1980) that under specific conditions chromosome-type aberrations can be induced in G_1 and G_0 cells by what are usually considered to be S-phase dependent chemicals. It is, therefore, more appropriate to consider that the probability of producing aberrations in G_1 or G_2 cells following chemical treatments is normally low, and that the probability is considerably increased when treated cells pass through the S-phase, giving the apparent S-phase dependence.

As discussed above, peripheral lymphocytes are in a non-cycling G_1 stage of the cell cycle, and so chemically-induced DNA damage will not generally be converted into chromosome aberrations until the cells are stimulated to re-enter the cell cycle *in vitro*, and undergo DNA replication. Since repair of DNA damage can take place in G_0 cells and during the long first *in vitro* G_1 stage, the aberration frequency will not necessarily be porportional to the amount of induced DNA damage but rather to the amount of DNA damage remaining at the time of DNA replication. It is clear that the amount of DNA damage present at the time of replication that has the potential to be converted into chromosome aberrations will be dependent upon several factors including: 1) the dose received 2) the induced amounts of those particular DNA damages that can result in chromosome aberrations (a value that can vary from agent to agent) 3) the amount of DNA repair in G_0 cells before sampling (*ie* time between exposure and sampling) 4) the amount of repair in G_1 cells from mitogenic stimulation to the first *in vitro* S-phase. Many of these will, of course, be further subject to individual to individual variation. The outcome is that for most chemical agents only some proportion of induced DNA damage can be converted into aberrations at the time of replication. These DNA repair factors all work to reduce the sensitivity of the lymphocyte assay for measuring exposure, and also clearly will result in the aberration frequency being at best indirectly proportional to exposure.

This reduced sensitivity and indirect relationship between aberration frequency and exposure allow for the following conclusions when the lymphocyte assay is used for population monitoring. If an increase in chromosome aberrations is observed in the potentially exposed group when compared to a "matched" control, and the only suspected variable is exposure or non-exposure to the agent under investigation, it is reasonable to conclude that there had been an exposure to a clastogenic agent, but no exposure level can be estimated. In addition, at this time no estimate of subsequent adverse health effects (genetic or somatic) can be made. If there is no difference in aberration frequency between the possibly exposed group and "matched" control it is not possible to rule out an exposure, although from some previous experiences it might be feasible to provide a maximum likely exposure.

There are many other facets of population monitoring in cases of chemical exposures, particularly regarding population selection, chronic exposures and risk estimation, and these are discussed further in a review by Preston (1984).

The situation is certainly not an impossible one to overcome, at least in theory, and future research will, I think, prove optimists correct. In later sections of this chapter some approaches we are taking to improve the sensitivity of the assay and interpretation of the data are described.

Sister chromatid exchanges (SCE)

If cells are grown for two rounds of replication in the presence of a thymidine analog, usually bromodeoxyuridine (BrdU), it is possible using specific staining procedures to obtain chromosomes with differentially stained chromatids. In such differentially stained preparations it is also possible to observe exchanges between the sister chromatids (SCE). SCE are induced as a consequence of the technique itself, due to the misreplication of the thymidine analog (O'Neill *et al.,* 1983), and their frequency is consequently influenced by analog concentration (or % incorporation) into DNA; in general, the higher the concentration in the medium the higher the SCE frequency over a range giving 0 to 100% incorporation in DNA (Heartlein et al., 1983). The SCE frequency can also be increased over background levels by a wide range of chemical agents (eg. Perry and Evans, 1975; Evans, 1983). In many cases a significant increase in SCE can be shown at concentrations of chemicals about two orders of magnitude less than those required to induce significant increases in chromosome aberrations. This does not necessarily imply a different mechanism of induction of the two events, although one has often been suggested, but perhaps rather the probability of producing an SCE as the result of an error of replication is higher than the same misreplication event resulting in an aberration.

SCE are not induced to any great extent by radiation treatment of cells in any stage of the cell cycle. There is no increase in SCE in lymphocytes irradiated in G_0 because the rapid repair of radiation-induced DNA damage means that little or no unrepaired damage is present when cells reach the S-phase - the stage when SCE are formed. Thus the analysis of chromosome aberrations in lymphocytes is considerably preferable to analysis of SCE in cases of radiation exposure.

In the case of chemical exposures it appears that the analysis of SCE provides a more sensitive assay for attempting to determine if persons have been exposed to an agent capable of producing chromosomal changes. However, it should be added that at this time no adverse health effects have been associated with increases in SCE. Therefore, it is preferable to analyse both chromosome aberrations and SCE from each blood sample.

This greater sensitivity of the SCE assay is possibly due to the fact that DNA damage induced in G_0 cells and remaining unrepaired until replication has a higher probability of resulting in an SCE than a chromosome aberration. However, the SCE assay with human lymphocytes exposed in vivo is still subject to most of the problems discussed for chromosomal aberrations above. Since SCE are produced at the time of DNA replication, and the exposures will be to non-cycling G_0 cells, the frequency of SCE will be influenced by the repair of induced DNA damage between exposure and sampling G_0 cells, and repair during the first *in vitro* G_1 phase. For chronic exposures there will be an equilibrium between repair of induced DNA damage and the induction of damage, thus allowing the assay to be utilised for cases of chronic exposure, with the condition that the sensitivity of the assay will be fairly low. There are many reports of increases in SCE in the lymphocytes of persons exposed to clastogenic or mutagenic agents (Latt *et al.,* 1981), indicating that there are situations where the assay can be applied to provide information on whether or not a particular group has been exposed. The absence of an increase in SCE cannot be interpreted as indicating an absence of exposure. The same requirements hold for including "matched" control samples in parallel with those from possibly exposed persons, as described for chromosome aberration analysis. There are many extrinsic and intrinsic factors that can influence SCE frequency, and so control matching becomes difficult. There are also likely to be as yet unidentified factors that can perhaps increase or decrease the SCE frequency, and so analysis and interpretation of the results from population monitoring studies have to be very carefully considered, and conclusions should necessarily be cautious.

There is little information available to indiciate whether or not the increases in SCE frequency can be associated with exposure level. Of course, because of the confounding factors, such as repair of induced DNA damage, the frequency of SCE will only be indirectly proportional to exposure. One of the major problems to obtaining such relationships is that the information on *in vivo* exposure itself is very limited. In two cases, where some reasonable estimate of exposure can be determined there is some semblance of a linear relationship between increases in SCE and increases in exposure: these cases are cigarette smoking and ethylene oxide exposure (Evans, 1983; Jones, 1982). More information on exposure levels and frequency of SCE is needed before it can be determined just how reliable the SCE assay is for determining exposure, even in a relative way.

Studies related to increasing the sensitivity of the lymphocyte assay

Two studies carried out recently in this laboratory as part of our attempts to determine the mechanism of induction of chromosome aberrations and SCE have some potential for producing an increased sensitivity of the lymphocyte assay.

In a series of experiments it has been shown that cytosine arabinoside (ara-C) can inhibit DN repair resynthesis, and on reversing this inhibition with deoxycytidine, the ara-C inhibited repairing regions are able to interact to produce chromosome aberrations (Preston and Gooch, 1981; Preston, 1980; Preston, 1982). Very large increases in chromosome aberration frequency can be obtained by incubating lymphocytes with ara-C after X-irradiation or chemical treatment. These studies have led to several conclusions concerning the mechanism of induction of chromosome aberrations, but these will not be discussed here, because they are perhaps incidental. The important point is the increased sensitivity to aberration induction when cells are incubated with ara-C after radiation or chemical treatments. With X-rays, the increases in aberrations in G_0- or G_1- treated cells are for chromosome-type aberrations, the type of aberrations normally induced by X-rays in cells treated at these cycle stages. It is possible to enhance the sensitivity, *ie* produce more aberrations at any particular dose, by incubating radiation exposed blood samples with ara-C. This would allow for less cells having to be analysed in the case of low doses or chronic exposures. However, the rapid repair of radiation-induced DNA damage makes this approach somewhat impractical.

In the case of chemical exposures, ara-C incubation of lymphocytes treated with, for example, methyl methanesulfonate or 4-nitroquinoline-N-oxide in G_1, results in a significant frequency of chromosome-type (dicentric) aberrations. These agents, as discussed above (d), normally only induce chromatid-type aberrations, and then only at very low frequencies in G_1-treated cells. By incubating blood samples, from possibly exposed persons, with ara-C, it is possible that the repair of DNA damage unrepaired at the time of sampling can be inhibited by ara-C, and subsequently converted into chromosome-type aberrations. This will not only increase the sensitivity of the assay, but will result in the production of chromosome-type aberrations that are more easily and accurately analysed than chromatid-type aberrations, are present at low background frequencies, and their frequencies appear to be less influenced by extrinsic factors. This approach is currently being studied.

The second series of studies that might be adapted to improve the sensitivity of the lymphocyte assay involve the induction of SCE. It has been shown that differential staining of chromatids can be obtained by growing cells for two rounds of replication in chlorodeoxyuridine (CldU) instead of the more usual BrdU (Pal *et al.,* 1981). However, the frequency of SCE is about 5 times as high with CldU compared to BrdU, for equivalent substitution in the DNA. SCE are, in the absence of any additional treatment, induced by the misreplication of analog-containing DNA, such that more errors in replication resulting in SCE occur for DNA containing CldU than BrdU. Following chemical treatments, it is possible that SCE are formed from misreplication of damaged DNA bases or from misreplication of BrdU incorporated during repair resynthesis, prior to DNA replication. The thymidine analog is normal added immediately after treatment, or, in the case of *in vivo* exposure, at the time the lymphocyte cultures are set up. The approach proposed is to incubate cells in CldU through the first *in vitro* G_1, during the time when DNA damage remaining in sampled lymphocytes is being repaired, and then allow them to replicate in BrdU, so that the "background" SCE frequency will be kept low. The intention is to enhance the SCE frequency induced by a chemical exposure and not the "background" frequency, thus making the assay more sensitive for detecting chemical exposures. Along the same lines, there are ways of further enhancing the sensitivity, but preliminary results do not yet indicate their feasibility.

There are certainly many other ways of improving or changing the lymphocyte assay such that it is of greater utility for detecting genotoxic exposures. In the future it should be possible to use the analysis of chromosome aberrations and SCE as one of a set of assays that could be used to estimate the level of exposure. It is too premature to predict the usefulness or application of the lymphocyte assay for determining estimates of sugsequent genetic and/or somatic risks to exposed persons and their offspring, in the case of chemical exposures.

ACKNOWLEDGEMENTS

Authors are indebted to Susan Barnett for her excellent secretarial assistance. Financial support was received by grants PHS CA30967 awarded by NCI, NIOSH grants RO3-OHO-1705 and RO3-OHO-1672. Drs. P. A. Lindholm and P. T. Liu received support from training grant T32-CA-09125.

Research sponsored by the Office of Health and Environmental Research, U. S. Department of Energy, under contract W-7405-eng-26 with the Union Carbide Corporation.

REFERENCES

Awa, A. A., T. Sofumi, T. Honda, M. Iton, S. Nerishi, and M. Otake: Relationship between the radiation dose and chromosome aberrations in atomic bomb survivors of Hiromshima and Nagasaki, *J. Radiat. Res. (Tokyo) 19*:126-140, 1978.

Bender, M. A., P. C. Gooch: Somatic chromosome aberrations induced by human whole-body irradiation: The "Recuplex" criticality accident, *Radiation Res. 29*:568-582, 1966.

Bloom, Arthur D. Ed.: Guidelines for Studies of Human Populations Exposed to Mutagenic and Reproductive Hazards, March of Dimes Birth Defects Foundation, New York, pp. 1-35, 1981.

Brewen, J. G. and N. Gengozian: Radiation-induced human chromosome aberrations. II. Human *in vitro* irradiation compared to *in vitro* and *in vivo* irradiation of marmoset leukocytes, *Mutation Res. 13*:383-391, 1971.

Brewen, J. G., R. J. Preston and L. G. Littlefield: Radiation-induced human chromosome aberration yields following an accidental whole-body exposure to 60_{Co} γ-rays, *Radiation Res. 49*:647-656, 1972.

Buckton, K. E., G. E. Hamilton, L. Paton, and A. D. Langlands: Chromosome aberrations in ankylosing spondylitis patients, In *Mutagen-Induced Chromosome Damage in Man* (H. J. Evans and D. C. Lloyd, eds.) Edinburgh University Press, Edinburgh, pp. 142-150, 1978.

Clemenger, J. F. P. and D. Scott: A comparison of chromosome aberrations yields in rabbit blood lymphocytes irradiated *in vitro,* and *in vivo, Int. J. Radiat. Biol. 24*:487-496, 1973.

Evans, H. J.: Effect on chromosomes of carcinogenic rays and chemicals. In *Chromosome Mutation and Neoplasia (J. German, ed.) Alan R. Liss, Inc., New York, pp. 253-279, 1983.*

Evans, H. J., K. E. Buckton, G. E. Hamilton and A. Carothers: Radiation-induced chromosome aberrations in nuclear dockyard workers, *Nature 277*:531-534, 1979.

Evans, H. J. and Vijayalaxmi: Storage enhances chromosome damage after exposure of human leukocytes to mitomycin C, *Nature 284*:370-372, 1980.

Goto, K., S. Madea, Y. Kano, and T. Sugeyama: Factors involved in differential Giemsa staining of sister chromatids, *Chromosoma 66*:351-359, 1978.

Heartlein, M. W., J. P. O'Neill, and R. J. Preston: SCE induction is proportional to substitution in DNA for thymidine by CldU and BrdU, Mutation Res. 107 :103-109, 1983.

Jacky, P. B., B. Beck, and G. R. Sutherland: Fragile sites in chromosomes: Possible model for the study of spontaneous chromosome breakage, *Science 220*:69-70, 1983.

Jones, J. P.: Chromosome changes in employers exposed to ethylene oxide, In *Ethylene Oxide Worker Safety Issues* (J. F. Jorkasky, ed.) HIMA Report No. 82-2, Health Industry Manufacturers Association, Washington, D.C., pp. 5-25, 1982.

Latt, S. A., J. W. Allen, S. E. Bloom, A. V. Carrano, E. Falke, D. Kram, E. Schneider, R. R. Schreck, R. Tice, B. Whitfield, and S. Wolff: Sister chromatid exchanges, *Mutation Res.* 87:17-62, 1981.

Lloyd, D. C., R. J. Purrott, J. S. Prosser, G. W. Dolphin, P. A. Tipper, E. J. Reeder, C. M. White, S. J. Cooper, and B. D. Stephenson: The study of chromosome aberration yield in human lymphocytes as an indicator of radiation dose. VI. A review of cases investigated, 1975, *NRPG-R41,* National Radiological Protection Board, Harwell, 1976.

Moorehead, P. S., P. C. Nowell, W. J. Mellman, D. M. Battips, and D. A. Hungerford: Chromosome preparations of leukocytes from human peripheral blood, *Exptl. Cell Research* 20:613-616, 1960.

Office of Technology Assessment, U.S. Congress: *The Role of Genetic Testing in the Prevention of Occupational Disease OTA-BA-194,* U.S. Government Printing Office, Washington, D. C., April 1983.

O'Neill, J. P., M. W. Heartlein, and R. J. Preston: Sister-chromatid exchanges and gene mutations are induced by the replication of 5-bromo- and 5-chloro-deoxyuridine substituted DNA, *Mutation Res.* 109:259-270, 1983.

Pal, B. C., R. B. Cumming, M. F. Walton, and R. J. Preston: Environmental pollutant 5-chlorouracil is incorporated in mouse liver and testis DNA, *Mutation Res.* 91:395-401, 1981.

Perry, P. and H. J. Evans: Cytological detection of mutagen-carcinogen exposure by sister-chromtid exchange, *Nature* 258:121-125, 1975.

Preston, R. J.: Cytogenetic abnormalities as an indicator of mutagenic exposure, In *Single-Cell Mutation Monitoring Systems (A. Ansari and F. J. de Serres, eds.) Plenum Publishing Corporation, New York, 127-143, 1984.*

Preston, R. J.: The effect of cytosine arabinoside on the frequency of x-ray-induced chromosome aberrations in normal human lymphocytes, *Mutation Res.* 69:71-79, 1980.

Preston, R. J.: The use of inhibitors of DNA repair in the study of the mechanisms of induction of chromosome aberrations, *Cytogenet. Cell Genet.* 33:20-26, 1982.

Preston, R. J., J. G. Brewen and K. P. Jones: Radiation-induced chromosome aberrations in Chinese hamster leukocytes. A comparison of *in vivo* and *in vitro* exposures, *Int. J. Radiat. Biol.* 21:397-450, 1972.

Preston, R. J. and P. C. Gooch: The induction of chromosome-type aberrations in G_1 by methyl methanesulfonate and 4-nitroquinoline-N-oxide, and the non-requirement of an S-phase for their production, *Mutation Res.* 83:395-402, 1981.

Reidy, J. A., X. Zhou and A. T. L. Chen: Folic acid and chromosome breakage. I. Implications for genotoxicity studies, *Mutation Res.* 122:217-221, 1983.

Savage, J. R. K.: Classification and relationship of induced chromosome structural changes, *J. Med. Genet.* 13:103-122, 1975.

New Approaches in Toxicity Testing and Their Application in Human Risk Assessment, edited by A. P. Li. Raven Press, New York © 1985.

Use of Human T-Lymphocytes to Monitor Mutations in Human Populations

Richard J. Albertini

Department of Medicine, University of Vermont, Burlington, Vermont 05405

The most direct way to monitor human populations for genotoxicity, at either the germinal or somatic level, would be to study large numbers of individuals and to record incidences of genetic diseases in the population over a given time interval. Birth defects would be enumerated to define frequencies of germinal genotoxicities while cancer frequencies would estimate some harmful genetic events at the somatic level. It must be admitted that such a scheme has the advantage of relevance to the problem at hand-*i.e.* that of human health risk assessment. However, the scheme also has the disadvantage of impracticality to the point of impossibility. Furthermore, it is "after the fact". The diseases in humans that you wish to prevent must occur in order to allow monitoring to operate.

Direct mutagenicity testing may be defined as mutagenicity testing that quantifies genetic events occuring *in vivo* in either germinal or somatic cells (DeMars, 1979). Human direct mutagenicity testing defines such events in human cells immediately after the cells are removed from the body. Standard cytogenetic tests using human lymphocytes are the "classical" direct mutagenicity tests (Evans and O'Riordan, 1977; Brogger, 1979); measurements of sister chromatid exchanges (SCE) also score genetic events occuring *in vivo* (Perry and Evans, 1975; Stetka and Wolff, 1976; Latt et al., 1977; Wolff, 1977). Novel systems such as the detection of sperm head abnormalities (Wyrobek and Bruce, 1978) or the recognition of double Y bodies in sperm (Kapp et al., 1979) have been described for the detection of presumed genetic events occurring *in vivo* in germ cells.

The "classic" direct mutagenicity tests, and those mentioned for sperm, either score for chromosomal genetic events, or the bases for the abnormalities are unknown. There clearly is need for tests that detect specific locus somatic cell mutations occurring *in vivo.*

Two human direct mutagenicity tests purporting to detect specific locus somatic cell mutations ocurring *in vivo* are currently under development. The mutant hemoglobin system is based on detecting and quantifying rare, mature RBC's circulating *in vivo* that

51

contain one or another mutant hemoglobin (Papayannopoulou, et al., 1976; Stamatoyannopoulos and Nute, 1983; Bigbee et al., 1983). Over 250 mutant human hemoglobins are known; many of them can be detected immunologically, thus opening the way to score for cells bearing altered molecules. Variant RBC's containing mutant hemoglobin are presumed to be descendants of mutant stem cells arising in the bone marrow. Thus, quantification of these variant RBC's is a measure of somatic cell mutation occurring *in vivo*. Initial determinations have shown that mutant hemoglobin S containing human RBC's occur spontaneously at a frequency of approximately 10^{-7} (Stamatoyannopoulos and Nute, 1983).

An alternative system for human direct mutagenicity testing quantifies 6-thioguanine resistant (TG^r) T-lymphocytes arising *in vivo* in humans. This test is described here in detail.

Ideally, human direct mutagenicity tests should be interposed between environmental exposures and disease occurrences. Test results should serve as early warnings concerning the latter. However, in order to so use these tests with any confidence, the tests themselves must be "validated" in terms of their performance as predictors of human disease. Such "validation" may be possible if direct mutagenicity test results in individuals can be compared with the health outcomes of the same individuals.

6-THIOGUANINE RESISTANT (TG^r) T-LYMPHOCYTE SYSTEM
Rationale For The Method

The TG^r T-lymphocyte system is based on detecting inactivation of the X-chromosomal gene (hpt locus) that specifies the enzyme hypoxanthine-guanine phosphoribosyltransferase (HPRT). This enzyme is constitutive but dispensable in mammalian cells. It is operative in the purine salvage pathway where it phosphorylates its normal substrates hypoxanthine and guanine (Kelley, 1968; Caskey and Kruh, 1979). HPRT also phosphorylates purine analogues such as 6-thioguanine and 8-azaguanine (Elion and Hitchings, 1965; Elion, 1967). Because the cytotoxicity of these analogues requires their phosphorylation, lack of HPRT activity renders HPRT deficient cells resistant to killing by these agents (DeMars, 1974; DeMars and Held, 1972).

In man, the rare, naturally occuring Lesch-Nylan (LN) mutation results in inactivation of the gene for HPRT (Kelley, 1968; Balis, 1968; Seegmiller et al., 1967). Males with the LN syndrome have a well-recognized clinical phenotype (Lesch and Nyhan, 1964; Seegmiller et al., 1967). Furthermore, the LN mutation results in a clear and unambiguous phenotype at the single cell level (DeMars, 1971; Albertini and DeMars, 1973). Somatic cells from LN patients: (i) are deficient in HPRT activity (ii) are resistant to killing by purine analogues, and (iii) fail to incorporate hypoxanthine or guanine into DNA. These cells may thus serve as prototypes for mutation ocurring at the somatic level at the hpt locus.

Because of random X-chromosomal inactivation, females who are heterozygous for the LN mutation are somatic mosaics as regards normal and LN mutant cells. The relative frequencies of these two cell types is as expected for skin fibroblasts but is not for peripheral blood T-lymphocytes (Albertini and DeMars, 1974; Strauss et al., 1980)). Rather, there is a relative paucity of LN T-lymphocytes in heterozygotes which is presumed to be due to adverse selection *in vivo* of HPRT deficient cells. Nonetheless, LN heterozygotes serve as prototypes for one type of naturally occurring low frequency mosaicism-*i.e.* infrequent HPRT deficient T-lymphocytes in a majority population of HPRT sufficient cells.

HPRT deficiency with resulting purine analogue resistance is the basis for several mammalian cell *in vitro* mutagenicity test systems, including the human diploid fibroblast (Albertini and DeMars, 1973; Jacobs and DeMars, 1977) and the human diploid lymphoblast systems (Thilly *et al.,* 1978; 1976). Clearly, spontaneous and induced somatic cell mutations occur at the hpt locus in human cells *in vitro* with sufficient frequency to be detected. It is assumed that such mutations occur also *in vivo* at comparable frequencies. Thus the TG^r T-lymphocyte system depends on detecting the *in vivo* occurrences of somatic cell mutations in man by quantitating the frequency of mutant TG^r T-lymphocytes in blood.

Autoradiographic Assay For TG^r T-Lymphocytes

Method

The autoradiographic assay for TG^r T-lymphocytes depends on detecting rare cells that are resistant to 6-thioguanine inhibition of phytohemagglutinin (PHA) induced tritiated thymidine incorporation *in vitro* in short-term culture. The culture interval is sufficiently brief so that cell division and mutation does not occur *in vitro*. The method, described in detail elsewhere (Albertini *et al.,* 1982), is briefly summarized here.

Mononuclear cells (MNC's) are separated from whole heparinized blood by the Ficoll-Hypaque method (Boyum, 1968). Cells are initially suspended in medium (RPMI 1640), human serum and 7.5% dimethylsulfoxide (DMSO) and frozen in a Union Carbide biological freezer. The cells are stored in the vapor phase of liquid nitrogen until used. Cryopreservation is important for removing "phenocopies" as will be discussed below.

After thawing, the MNC's are put into short-term culture and stimulated with PHA. Replicate flask cultures, with or without 2×10^{-4} M 6-thioguanine, are established and incubated for 30 hours under standard conditions at 37°C in a 5% CO_2 in air humidified atmosphere. Cultures then are labelled with tritiated thymidine and again incubated for 12 hours. Cultures are terminated by adding cold 0.1 M citric acid so as to prepare free nuclei. The nuclei are fixed in seven parts methanol: 1.5 parts glacial acetic acid fixative and finally suspended in small volumes of fixative. The number of nuclei in the fixative suspension is determined electronically (Coulter Counter). Nuclei are added in measured volumes to coverslips affixed to microscope slides which are then stained and autoradiographed according to standard procedures.

The scoring of autoradiographs is by light microscopy. Coverslips made with nuclei from control, non-6-thioguanine containing cultures, are used to determine the control labelling index (LI_C). Five thousand nuclei are counted on these coverslips under high-power oil immersion microscopy (1000 X) and the labelled nuclei scored. The LI_C is calculated as:

$$LI_C = \frac{\text{number of labelled nuclei in 5000 scored}}{5000}$$

All coverslips made with nuceli from test, 6-thioguanine containing cultures are scanned in their entirety under low-power light microscopy (160 X). The total number of labelled nuclei on all coverslips is determined. The total number of nuclei on these coverslips is known from the Coulter counts. The labelling index of test cultures (LI_t) is calculated as:

$$LI_t = \frac{\text{total number of labelled nuclei on all test culture coverslips}}{\text{total number of nuclei on all test culture coverslips}}$$

The variant frequency (V_f), or frequeny of TG^r T-lymphocytes, is calculated as the ratio of test to related control labelling indices:

$$V_f = \frac{LI_t}{LIC_c}$$

Confidence intervals for V_f values may be determined as discussed elsewhere (Albertini et al., 1982).

Phenocopies

We initially reported TG^r T-lymphocyte V_f values as determined autoradiographically to be 10^{-4} or greater for normal non-mutagen exposed adults (Strauss and Albertini, 1979; Albertini, 1979; 1980). Cancer patients knowingly exposed to mutagenic chemotherapeutic agents showed even higher values. These frequencies did not seem compatible with somatic cell mutation rates at the hpt locus as determined for human cells *in vitro* (DeMars and Held, 1972). Subsequently, we found that V_f values determined with T-lymphocytes that had been cryopreserved were much lower-e.g. approximately $2\text{-}3 \times 10^{-6}$ for normal individuals (Albertini et al., 1981). These lower values are much more in accord with expectations. We feel that these V_f values determined with cryopreserved cells more closely approximate "true" TG^r T-lymphocyte mutant frequencies. Our reasoning is as follows.

The vast majority of T-lymphocytes in human peripheral blood are non-dividing and in an arrested G_0 stage of the cell cycle *in vivo*. However, rare cells are "in cycle". This small "cycling" T-lymphocyte population probably arises *in vivo* in response to antigenic or other stimuli. Although infrequent, the precise fraction of cycling T-lymphocytes at a given time *in vivo* in an individual is probably variable and the result of physiological or pathological conditions.

When we began our studies, our concept of PHA (or other mitogen) induced T-lymphocyte simulation *in vitro* was that the PHA effect was direct-i.e. the mitogen itself was thought to directly induce T-lymphocytes into DNA synthesis (Figure 1a). We supposed that this effect was inhibitable by 6-thioguanine at several points. Whether or not a cell was in cell cycle at the onset of culture was not thought of to be of consequence.

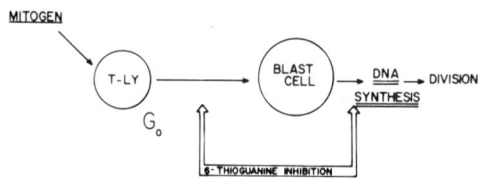

FIGURE 1a: Scheme depicting a concept of the sequence of events in a mitogen stimulated T-lymphocyte culture where the mitogen directly induced target T-lymphocytes into DNA synthesis. 6-Thioguanine could inhibit all cells at a variety of points proximal to their initial DNA synthetic period.

More recently, it has been shown by others that *in vitro* T-lymphocyte stimulation by mitogens is much more complex (Figure 1b) (Maizel *et al.*, 1981). The direct effect of mitogen on the "target" T-lymphocyte is simply to "transform" the cell to an activated cell in early G_1. This activation process is accompanied by profound metabolic alterations (Allison *et al.*, 1977; Hovi *et al.*, 1977) and results in the acquisition of surface receptors for T-cell growth factor (TCGF or interleukin-2) on the transformed cells (Maizel *et al.*, 1981). An unknown stimulus in these lymphocyte cultures affects monocytes resulting in their production of the growth factor interleukin-1. Interleukin-1, in turn, stimulates other T-lymphocytes to produce interleukin-2. It is the interleukin-2 that stimulates "activated" T-lymphocytes to DNA synthesis.

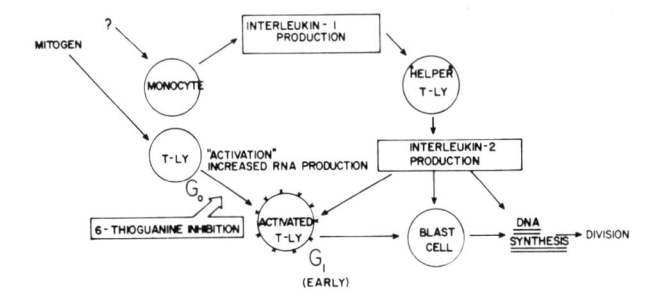

FIGURE 1b: Scheme depicting a concept of the sequence of events in mitogen stimulated T-lymphocyte cultures wherre the mitogen only "transforms" resting G_0 T-lymphocytes to their activated state in early G_1. The activated cells have acquired receptors for T-cell growth factor. Interleukin 1 and 2 are involved in ultimate DNA synthesis by the activated cells. 6-Thioguanine probably inhibits T-lymphocyts from their first round of DNA synthesis *in vitro* by inhibiting the "activation" step.

According to this scheme, resting G_0 T-lymphocytes of peripheral blood proceed to DNA synthesis *in vitro* by a route that is quite different from that used by "cycling" T-lymphocytes. The former require an "activation" step that the latter do not. We feel that it is this activation step that is inhibited by the short interval high dose (2×10^{-4}M) 6-thioguanine present in the test cultures. We do not feel that cycling cells can be inhibited from their first round of DNA synthesis *in vitro* by such a short exposure to 6-thioguanine, even though cycling cells are inhibited following one or more rounds of replication even at 6-thioguanine concentrations less than 10^{-4}M (Albertini and Borcherding, 1982; Albertini *et al.*, 1982). Thus, some non-mutant cycling cells may synthesize DNA, even in the presence of 6-thioguanine. They then become labelled with tritiated thymidine and are scored in the assay as "mutants". This occurs when fresh MNC's are tested, but not when cryopreserved MNC's are tested.

Elsewhere we show that cryopreservation moves cycling cells that incorporate label in 6-thioguanine through their initial in vitro DNA synthetic period earlier during the culture interval than is the case with fresh MNC preparations (Albertini *et al.*, 1981; Albertini, 1982). These cycling cells then are not in DNA synthesis during the 30 to 42 hour labelling "window" used for the assay. The frequency of labelled cells determined with cryopreserved samples therefore more nearly approximates the frequency of G_0 cells that are truly resistant to 6-thioguanine inhibition of their transformation to G_1-*i.e.* the mutant TG^r T-lymphocytes.

Recent Results

TG^r T-lymphocytes V$_f$ values determined with cryopreserved MNC samples from normal, non-mutagenized adults are routinely of the order of 10^{-6}. Similar values are found when T-lymphocytes from placental blood samples from newborns are studied. Cancer patients receiving mutagenic therapies often show values considerably above the normal range-e.g. 10 to 50 fold increases over normal individuals. (Albertini, 1982)

Clonal Assay For Mutant TG^r T-Lymphocytes

Using T-cell growth factors, it is now possible to clone peripheral blood T-lymphocytes directly *in vitro*, and establish long-term cultures (Paul *et al.*, 1981). Cloning can be accomplished directly in 6-thioguanine, thereby selecting for pre-existing TG^r cells present in blood (Albertini and Borcherdin, 1982; Albertini *et al.*, 1982). The method can be made quantitative, allowing another method for determining TG^r T-lymphocyte mutant frequencies (M$_f$'s.) Furthermore, with cloning, the mutants themselves are available for characterization.

Method

Peripheral blood lymphocytes are initially pre-incubated or "primed" with PHA for approximately 24 hours in order to activate them as outlined above. They then are resuspended, diluted, and inoculated in limiting dilutions into the wells of microtiter plates. In order to establish cloning efficiencies (CE's), cell suspensions containing, on average, one cell per well, are inoculated into wells without 6-thioguanine. Because only rare cells are expected to be TG^r and grow in thioguanine containing medium, a larger number of cells, usually 10^5, is inoculated into wells containing 6-thioguanine. All wells contain, in addition to T-lymphocytes, human serum and medium (RPMI 1640) with or without 6-thioguanine, an appropriate concentration of TCGF and feeder cells. X-irradiated (9000 Rads) HPRT deficient B-lymphoblasts (cell line TK-6), present at approximately 10^4 cells per well, serve as feeders. Selection is with 6-thioguanine at 10^{-5}M.

Microtiter plates are incubated at 37°C under standard conditions for approximately two weeks. Wells may be fed at 10 to 12 days by removing 0.1 ml volumes and adding the appropriate medium containing TCGF. Wells may be scored visually at two weeks when growing colonies are readily apparent. Alternatively, wells may be labelled with tritiated thymidine for scintillation counting, which distinguishes negative wells containing only "background counts" from positive wells which show incorporation of label into the DNA of growing cells. Growing clones may be "picked" and passaged in order to obtain populations for study.

It is assumed that single cells are distributed among the 96 wells of microtiter plates according to Poisson expectations. Similarly, it is assumed that the rare TG^r cells also are distributed among the 96 wells of selection microtiter plates according to Poisson expectations. Therefore, CE's are calculated from the P$_0$ classes of the distributions of positive and negative wells as observed in plates receiving, on average, one cell per well-*i.e.* P$_0$ = e^{-x}, where x is the average number of clonable cells per well. Similarly, the incidence of TG^r T-lymphocytes in selective wells is calculated from the P$_0$ class of the distributions of positive and negative wells as observed in 6-thioguanine containing plates receiving 10^5 cells per well. This incidence, divided by 10^5, corrected by the relevant CE, yields an estimate of the TG^r T-lymphocyte M$_f$.

The results of a recent determination using peripheral blood T-lymphocytes from a normal adult are shown in Figures 2 and 3. Figure 2 shows the distribution of counts in the 96 wells of a microtiter plate that had received, on average, one cell per well. In order to include wells containing slowly growing cells, wells were scored as positive if they showed 2000 counts per minute (cpm) or more. in addition to the 40 wells with cpm $\geq$ 2000, five wells had been "picked" to obtain cells for study. Therefore, a total of 45 wells were positive in this microtiter plate. The CE (x) was therefore:

$$P_0 = e^{-x}$$

$$\frac{96-45}{96} = e^{-x}$$

$$x = 0.633$$

Similarly, five of the 96 wells containing 6-thioguanine showed 2000 or more cpm (Figure 3). In addition, four wells had been "picked" from this plate, resulting in a total of nine positive wells. The incidence of TG^r T-lymphocytes per well (x) was therefore:

$$P_0 = e^{-x}$$

$$\frac{96-9}{96} = e^{-x}$$

$$x = 0.098$$

The TG^r T-lymphocyte M_f for this determination is given as:

$$M_f = \frac{0.098}{0.633 \times 10^5} = 1.5 \times 10^{-6}$$

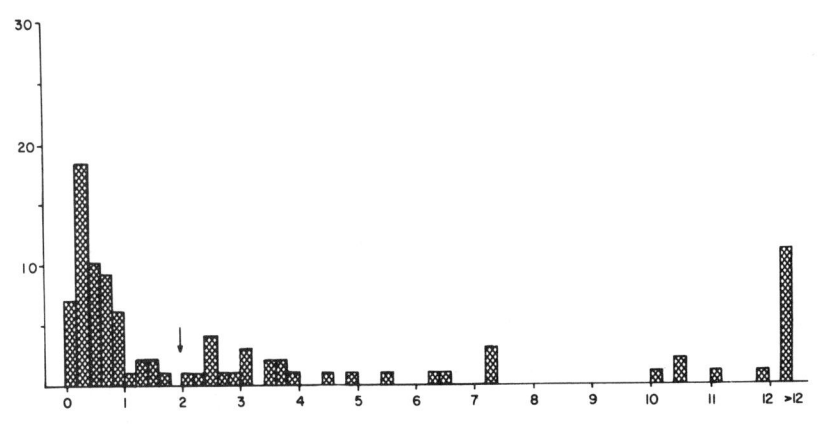

FIGURE 2: The distribution of counts per minute (cpm's) tritiated thymidine incorporation into cells of a 96 well microtiter plate which had received an average of one cell per well. The number of wells is shown on the ordinate and the cpm's x 10^3 on the abcissa. Cpm $\geq$ 2000 constitute positive wells. Forty wells are positive.

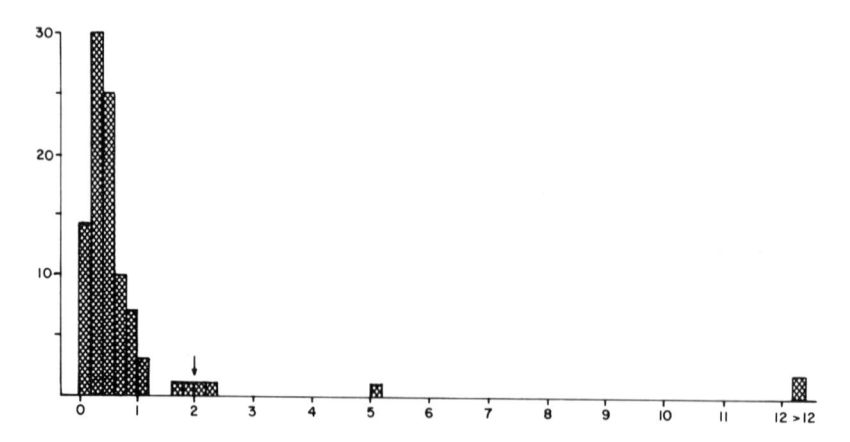

[histogram figure]

FIGURE 3 : The distribution of counts per minute (cpm's) tritiated thymidine incorporation into wells of a 96 well microtiter plate which had received an average of 10^5 cells (in 6-thioguanine) per well. The number of wells is shown on the ordinate and the cpm's x 10^3 on the abcissa. Cpm $\geq$ 2000 constitute positive wells. Five wells are positive.

Results to Date

Of most importance, characterization of TG^r T-lymphocytes that have been recovered from studies such as shown, has allowed us to conclude that these cells are somatic cell mutants as traditionally defined (Albertini and Borcherding, 1982; Albertini et al., 1982). Thus, the cells studied: (i) were deficient in HPRT activity, (ii) demonstrated heritability of the TG^r phenotype *in vitro* in the absence of selection and (iii) showed T-lymphocyte surface markers indicating both that they were T-cells and that they had been clonally derived.

Only a limited number of normal individuals have been studied quantitatively to date, as we are continuing to establish conditions for the quantitative assay. Specifically, it is recognized that CE's determined by inoculating single cells into wells are dependent on cell growth under conditions that may be quite different than those obtaining in selection wells. Although high CE's often are achieved (Figure 2), occasionally calculated CE's are low. The results of experiments in which CE's were deliberately varied showed that cell growth in selection wells did not similarly vary. Thus, if there is failure of single cell growth, an assay may show a spuriously elevated M_f due to an artificially low CE in the denominator of the calculation. Alternative methods for determining CE's are being investigated.

Nonetheless, with the assay as presented, M_f's are found to be in 10^{-6} and 10^{-5} range. When CE's are acceptable (i.e. ≥ 0.20), M_f values determined by cloning are comparable to V_f values determined simultaneously by autoradiography on the same cells, with the former being somewhat the higher. Given the heterogeneity of T-lymphocyte sub-populations and the quite different culture conditions of the two assays, there is no necessary reason why these two values should be identical.

CLONED T-LYMPHOCYTES FOR HUMAN DIRECT MUTAGENICITY STUDIES

The ability to clone and propagate human T-lymphocytes *in vitro* greatly enlarges the possibilities for using these cells for direct mutagenicity testing. Virtually any marker that currently can be used for selection in diploid mammalian cells can be adapted for use with T-lympohcytes. Also because variant cells can be recovered for further study using traditional methods of somatic cell genetics, it usually will be possible to determine if the variants truly are somatic cell mutants.

Table 1 lists tests that might be used for human mutagenicity monitoring. Some currently are available or are in an active developmental stage; others would seem to be feasible on theoretical grounds. T-lymphocytes can be exploited for testing in several ways.

Elsewhere we report that diptheria toxin resistant (dt^R) human T-lymphocytes arising *in vivo* may be detected and recovered *in vitro* using the cloning method (Albertini, 1982). Three dt^R clones have been studied and all three have maintained their variant phenotypes *in vitro*. However, the frequency of dt^R variants thus far has been disturbingly high - e.g. ten-fold or greater than simultaneously determined TG^r M_f's. Also, some apparently dt^R clones have not persisted for long intervals *in vitro*. This marker system clearly needs more work before it can be proposed as a direct mutagenicity test system. Nonetheless, the system is amenable to study. The necessary development work is really no different from that which is required for the development of any mutagenicity test system.

Other markers could be investigated for use in developing direct mutagenicity test systems using human T-lymphocytes. Ouabain resistance should be a useful marker. Furthermore, the entire area of immuno-selection is open for exploitation. Others have shown that HLA antigen loss variants arise *in vitro* in cultured human B-lymphoblasts (Pious *et al.*, 1982; Kavanthas *et al.*, 1980; Orr *et al.*, 1982). Such mutants have, in fact, been important for analyzing the structure of the HLA locus. Immunoselection methods similar to those used for B-lymphoblasts *in vitro* should be applicable to T-lymphocytes, allowing a variation of the cloning assay to be used for detecting and quantifying HLA loss mutants arising *in vivo*. Similarly, other antigens, including differentiation antigens, are present on the surface of T-lymphocytes. These too may be amenable to immunoselection. It may even be possible to detect other sorts of genetic events, such as chromosome loss, if appropriate antigens can be found for immunoselection.

As also seen in Table 1, many test systems that are available (or possible) for humans also are available (or possible) for animals. The autoradiographic detection of TG^r T-lymphocytes already has been accomplished in mice (Gocke, 1983) and in Chinese Hamster T-lymphocytes (Recio *et al., 1983*). Animal systems that are analogous to human systems will be invaluable for "bridge-building" sorts of studies. For example, only in animals can studies be designed to detect the dose-response sensitivities of the various tests to various mutagens, or to determine test parameters such as optimal expression time intervals.

TABLE 1. SOMATIC CELL BIOMONITORING SYSTEMS

Type of Endpoints	Human — Existing (or in Development)	Human — Potential	Animal — Existing (or in Development)	Animal — Potential
Chromosomal	Chromosomal aberrations SCE's	Surface antigen loss = chromosome loss; e.g. "Y" antigen Micronucleus	Chromosomal aberrations SCE's Micronucleus	Surface antigen loss = chromosome loss e.g. "Y" antigen
Specific Locus	TG^r lymphocytes Mutant hemoglobin containing RBC's	Drug resistant lymphocytes: Diptheria toxin Ouabain Surface antigen loss mutant lymphocytes: HLA Allotypes Differentiation antigen loss Glycopherin A surface mutants: MN blood group RBC's	Mouse spot test Granuloma pouch assay TG^r lymphocytes	Drug resistant lymphocytes Surface antigen loss Mutant lymphocytes e.g. H-2 Mutant hemoglobin containing RBC's Lymphocyte surface allotype mutants

Finally, human (or animal) T-lymphocytes can be propagated indefinitely *in vitro* with T-cell growth factors. *In vitro* mutagenicity test systems can thus be developed. Such developments will allow combined *in vivo-in vitro* mutagenicity testing using the same cells from the same individual. Such combined testing will allow analysis of the heterogeneity of susceptibility to genotoxins among humans - obviously an issue of much importance in relating human direct mutagenicity testing to human health risk assessments.

It also is obvious that growing mutant cells that are descendants of mutants arising *in vivo* provide a rich source of material for investigating the basis of somatic cell mutation occurring *in vivo* in humans. The "new" DNA technology should allow a molecular analysis of this sort of genetic variation occurring at the somatic level *in vivo*. It even may be possible to determine if environmentally induced somatic cell mutation results in molecular lesions which are similar to or different from those seen in spontaneously occuring somatic cell mutation. The range of possibilities for genetic analysis is quite broad indeed.

OUTSTANDING PROBLEMS

Despite the progress that had been made by using human T-lymphocytes for direct mutagenicity testing, at least three non-trivial problems remain. Two have to do with quantitation and apply primarily to "specific locus" tests. The third applies to all direct mutagenicity tests, and has to do with the relevance of test results for making estimates of human health risks.

One problem in interpreting human direct mutagenicity test results quantitatively is that test sensitivities in terms of dose-reponse characteristics currently are not known. We have shown that cancer patients receiving mutagenic therapies have elevated TG^r T-lymphocyte V_f values as compared to normals (Albertini, 1982). However, the mutagen exposures of these treated individuals is quite high. Studies of low dose mutagen exposures in humans will be necessary to directly determine test sensitivities in this regard. However, such studies will be difficult, especially in view of the wide range of potentially mutagenic agents encountered by humans in the course of daily living. Furthermore, it is likely that all elevations *in vivo* of mutant frequencies will be small in mutagen exposed versus non-mutagen exposed individuals because the mutagen concentrations to which cells are exposed *in vivo* will almost certainly be small. *In vitro* specific locus mutagenicity tests using cultured mammalian cells usually employ mutagen exposure levels that kill a large fraction of cells. Large fractions of cells usually will not be killed *in vivo* in humans during industrial exposures or, if they are, the public health concern will be one of acute illness or death rather than genotoxicity.

At present, it appears as though dose-response test sensitivities will have to be determined indirectly in animals. As noted above, T-lymphocyte direct mutagenicity test systems have already been developed for animals. Test results from animal studies will have to be correlated with test results from human studies, with the animals being used to determine minimal doses that elicit detectable responses.

One aspect of direct mutagenicity test results that often is not obvious on first consideration is the nature of the information provided. Even though it has been demonstrated that the abnormal cells scored in the TG^r T-lymphocyte assay are in fact *mutants*, such cells do not equate to *mutations*. Thus, although it is the latter - i.e. *mutations* - that are the usual events of interest in human genetic biomonitoring, it is the former - i.e. *mutants* - that actually are scored. Only where information regarding cell pool sizes and distributions *in vivo*, representativeness of test samples, *in vivo* cell kinetics, *in vivo* positive or negative selection of mutants, etc. is available can the number of *mutations* be inferred from the number of *mutants*. At present, none of these characteristics are precisely known for the human T-lymphocyte system.

Currently we are conducting studies to determine if TG^r T-lymphocytes as scored in the cloning assay, occur in the two major classes of T-lymphocytes - i.e. T4 or helper/inducer cells and T8 or suppressor/cytotoxic cells - according to expectations. This is a first step in determining if there is homogeneity of susceptibility to somatic cell mutation *in vivo* among the T-lymphocyte subsets. If there is not, yet another complication will be present in relating *mutant* to *mutation* frequencies.

At present there does not appear to be any simple way to relate mutant frequencies as determined in direct mutagenicity tests to mutation frequencies. Therefore, specific locus direct mutagenicity tests will have to be interpreted with the knowledge that changes in the number of mutants may or may not represent similar changes in the number of mutations.

Finally, the relevance of human direct mutagenicity test results to health outcomes of the individuals tested is currently unknown. Human genetic biomonitoring is performed for at least two reasons. First, the explicit justification for monitoring human populations is to determine potential exposures to deleterious genotoxic agents. If human biomonitoring data could be interpreted strictly as indicating exposure, the use of direct mutagenicity tests in human populations probably would not be controversial.

However, there is another, often implicit, interpretation put on the results of human biomonitoring. This interpretation, often made by the individuals tested, or by their representatives, relates the results of individual tests with individual future health outcomes. The specific question that has resulted in so much controversy and has effectively blocked the widespread use of human genetic biomonitoring tests is whether or not abnormal test results (e.g. chromosomal aberrations, SCE, TG^r T-lymphocytes) mean increased individual risks (e.g. for birth defects or cancer). At present the answer to this question is simply not known.

Elsewhere we have suggested a means to "validate" human direct mutagenicity tests in terms of their ability to predict subsequent human disease outcomes (Albertini, 1982; Albertini and Allen, 1981). Because these tests provide data on individuals that can be correlated with subsequent illness of these same individuals, the "receiver-operator" characteristics of the tests in terms of their ability to predict outcomes can be determined. In particular, the sensitivities and specificities of the tests in terms of indicating future disease potentials can be defined in ways that such test characteristics are usually defined for other clinical laboratory tests.

Without repeating here the details of our proposal, made elsewhere, we have suggested that cancer patients receiving mutagenic therapies currently constitute the best human populations to study in order to make this sort of validation for human direct mutagenicity tests. Many cancer patients are now cured of their cancer, or undergo long-term remissions. Many patients, formerly treated for a malignancy, have children. Happily, most cured cancer patients remain healthy but a minority experience a second malignancy, usually acute non-lymphocytic leukemia (Bender and Young, 1978; Casciano and Scott, 1979). It is thought that the second malignancies arise as a consequence of therapies given for the first.

A long-term study of cancer patients before, during and after their treatments, coupled with long-term follow-ups and computer storage of mutagenicity and clinical data, should allow the determination of test sensitivities and specificities in terms of indicating future disease. Only after this has been accomplished can results of batteries of tests performed in human populations either be used to predict likelihoods of later disease in individuals, or be dismissed as having no relevance in this regard.

No matter what is found in such a long-term study, the usefulness of direct mutagenicity tests will be enhanced. If test results are predictive of the later occurrence of disease, persons at risk may be identified before the fact and appropriate preventative measures instituted. If test results do not allow predictions in individuals regarding the later occurrence of disease, direct mutagenicity tests may be used for human biomonitoring to determine potential genotoxin exposures in populations without the attendant concern of provoking undue anxiety among the individuals tested. In either event, testing will have a greater impact on human public health.

ACKNOWLEDGEMENTS

This work was supported by NIH grant RO1 CA30688.

REFERENCES

Albertini, R. J.: Direct mutagenicity testing with peripheral blood lymphocytes. *Banbury Rep.* 2:359, 1979.

Albertini, R. J.: Drug resistant lymphocytes in man as indicators of somatic cell mutation. *Teratog. Carcinog. Mutagen.* 1:25, 1980.

Albertini, R. J.: Studies with T-lymphocytes: An approach to human mutagenicity monitoring. *Banbury Rep.* 13:393, 1982.

Albertini, R. J. and E. F. Allen: Direct mutagenicity testing in man. In *Health risk analysis: proceedings of the third life sciences symposium* (ed C. Richmond et al.), p. 131. The Franklin Institute Press, Philadelphia, PA, 1981.

Albertini, R. J., E. F. Allen, A. S. Quinn and M. R. Albertini: Human somatic cell mutation: *In vivo* variant lymphocyte frequencies as determined by 6-thioguanine resistance. In *Population and biological aspects of human mutation: Birth defects institute symposium XI.* (ed. E. B. Hook and I. H. Porter) p. 235. Academic Press, New York, 1981.

Albertini, R. J. and W. R. Borcherding: Cloning *in vitro* of human 6-thioguanine resistant peripheral blood lymphocytes arising *in vivo*. *Environ. Mutagen.* 4:371, 1982.

Albertini, R. J., K. Castle, and W. R. Borcherding: T-cell cloning to detect the mutant 6-thioguanine resistant lymphocytes present in human peripheral blood. *Proc. Natl. Acad. Sci. U.S.A.* 79:6617, 1982.

Albertini, R. J. and R. DeMars: Detection and quanitification of X-ray induced mutation in cultured diploid human fibroblasts. *Mutat. Res.* 18:199, 1973.

Albertini, R. J. and DeMars, R.: Mosaicism of peripheral blood lymphocyte populations in females heterozygous for the Lesch-Nyhan mutation. *Biochem. Genet.* 11:397, 1974.

Albertini, R. J., D. L. Sylwester, and E. F. Allen: The 6-thioguanine-resistant peripheral blood lymphocyte assay for direct mutagenicity testing in humans. *Cell Biology: Mutagenicity: New Horizons in Genetic Toxicology.* (ed. J. A. Heddle), p. 305: Academic Press, New York, 1982.

Allison, A. D., T. Hovi, R. W. E. Watts, and A. B. D. Webster: The role of *de novo* purine synthesis in lymphocyte transformation In *Purine and pyrimidine metabolism* (eds. K. Elliot and D. W. Fitzsimmons), p. 207, Elsevier/North Holland/Excerpta Medica, Amsterdam, 1977.

Balis, M. E.: Enzymology and biochemistry. B. Aspects of purine metabolism. *Fed. Proc.* 27:1067, 1968.

Bender, R. A. and R. C. Young: Effects of cancer treatment on individual and generational genetics. Semin. Oncol. 5:46, 1978.

Bigbee, W. L., E. W. Branscomb and R. H. Hensen: Counting of RBC Variants Using Rapid Flow Techniques, In: Utilization of Mammalian Specific Locus Tests in Hazard Evaluation and Estimation of Genetic Risks (ed. F. J. deSerres and W. Sheridan) p. 39, Plenom Press, N.Y. and London, 1983.

Boyum, A.: Separation of leukocytes from blood and bone marrow. Scand. J. Clin. Lab. *Invest. Suppl.* 21:51, 1968.

Brogger, A.: Chromosome damage in human mitotic cells after *in vivo* and *in vitro* exposure to mutagens. *In Genetic damage in man caused by environmental agents.* (ed. K. Berg). p. 87. Academic Press, New York, 1979.

Casciano, D. A. and J. L. Scott: Acute leukemia following prolonged cytotoxic agent therapy. *Medicine.* 58:32, 1979.

Caskey, C. T. and G. D. Kruh: The HPRT locus. *Cell 16:*1, 1979.

DeMars, R.: Genetic studies of HGPRT deficiency and the Lesch-Nyhan syndrome with cultured human cells. *Fed. Proc. 30:*944, 1971.

DeMars, R.: Resistance of cultured human fibroblasts and other cells to purine and pyrimidine analogues in relation to mutagenesis detection. *Mutation Res.* 24:335, 1974.

DeMars, R.: Suggestions for increasing the scope of direct testing for mutagens and carcinogens in intact humans and animals.
Banbury Rep. 2. 329, 1979.

DeMars, R. and K. Held: The spontaneous azaguanine-resistant mutants of diploid human fibroblasts. *Humangenetik* 16:87, 1972.

Elion, G. B.: Biochemistry and pharmacology of purine analogs.
Fed. Proc. 26:898, 1967.

Elion, G. B. and G. H. Hitchings: Metabolic basis for the actions of analogs of purines and pyrimidines. *Adv. Chemother.* 2:91, 1965.

Evans, H. J. and M. L. O'Riordan: Human peripheral blood lymphocytes for the analysis of chromosome aberrations in mutagen tests.
In *Handbook of Mutagenicity Test Procedures* (eds. B. Kilbey *et al.*), p. 261. Elsevier/North Holland, Amsterdam and New York, 1977.

Gocke, E., K. Eckhardt, M. T. King and D. Wild: Autoradiographic detection of 6-thioguanine-resistant lymphocytes of mice, *Mutat. Res.* 113:445, 1983.

Hovi, T., A. C. Allison, K. O. Raivio, and A. Vaheri: Purine metabolism and control of cell proliferation. *In Purine and pyrimidine metabolism* (eds. K. Eliot and D. W. Fitzsimmons), p. 225. Elsevier/North Hollan/Excerpta Medica, Amsterdam, 1977.

Jacobs, L., and R. DeMars: Chemical mutagenesis with diploid human fibroblasts, in: *Handbook of Mutagenicity Test Procedures,* (eds. B. Kilbey et al.), Elsevier/North Holland, Amsterdam, 1977.

Kapp, R. W., Jr., D. J. Picciano, and C. B. Jacobson: Y-chromosomal nondisjunction in dibromochloropropane-exposed workmen. *Mutat. Res.* 64:47, 1979.

Kavanthas, P., F. H. Bach and R. DeMars: Gamma ray-induced loss of expression of HLA and glyoxalase I alleles in lympho-blastoid cells. *Proc Natl. Acad. Sci. U.S.A.* 77:4251, 1980.

Kelley, W. N.: Enzymology and biochemistry. A HGPRT deficiency in the Lesch-Nyhan syndrome and gout. *Fed. Proc.* 27:1047, 1968.

Latt, S. J., J. W. Allen, W. E. Rogers, and L. A. Juerglus: *In vitro* and *in vitro* analysis of sister chromatid exchange information. In *Handbook of mutagenicity test procedures* (eds. B. Kilbey et al.), p. 275. Elsevier/North Holland, Amsterdam, 1977.

Lesch, M. and W. L. Nyhan: A familial disorder of uric acid metabolism and central nervous system function. *Am. J. Med.* 36:561, 1964.

Maizel, A. L., S. R. Mehta, S. Hauft, D. Franzini, L. B. Lachman, and R. J. Ford: Human T-lymphocyte/monocyte interaction in response to lectin: Kinetics of entry into S-phase. *J. Immunol.* 127:1058, 1981.

Orr, H. T., F. H. Bach, H. L. Ploesch, J. L. Strominger, P. Kavathas and R. DeMars: Use of HLA loss mutants to analyze the structure of the human major histocompatibility complex. *Nature.* 296:454, 1982.

Papayannopoulou, T. H., T. C. McGuire, G. Lim, E. Garzel, P. E. Nute, and G. Stamatoyannopoulos: Identification of hemoglobin S in red cells and normoblasts using fluorescent anti-Hb antibodies. *Br. J. Haematol.* 34:25, 1976.

Paul, W. E. B. Sredni, and R. H. Schwartz: Long-term growth and cloning of non-transformed lymphocytes. *Nature.* 294:697, 1981.

Perry, P. and H. J. Evans: Cytological detection of mutagen-carcinogen exposure by sister chromatid exchange. *Nature* 258:121, 1975.

Pious, D., M. S. Kransel, L. L. Dixon, P. Parham and J. L. Strominger: HLA antigen structural gene mutants selected with allospecific monoclonal antibody. *Proc. Natl. Acad. Sci. U.S.A.* 79:7832, 1982.

Recio, L., B. Chastenay, R. J. Albertini and A. W. Hsie: Detection of 6-thioguanine resistant splenocytes from Chinese Hamsters. *Environ. Mutagenesis.* 5:401, 1983.

Seegmiller, J. E., F. M. Rosenbloom and W. N. Kelley: Enzyme defect associated with a sex-linked human neurological disorder and excessive purine synthesis. *Science. 155:*1682, 1967.

Stamatoyannopoulos, G. and P. E. Nute: Detection of somatic mutants of hemoglobin in *Utilization of Mammalian Specific Locus Studies in Hazard Evaluation and Estimation of Genetic Risk.* Ed: F. J. de Serres and W. Sheridan, p. 29. Plenum Press, New York, 1983.

Steka, D. G. and S. Wolff: Sister chromatid exchange as an assay for genetic damage induced by mutagen-carcinogens. I. *In vivo* test for compounds requiring metabolic activation. *Mutat. Res. 41:*333, 1976.

Strauss, G. H., Allen, E. F. and Albertini, R. J.: An enumerative assay of purine analogue resistant lymphocytes in women heterozygous for the Lesch-Nyhan mutation. *Biochem. Genet. 18:*529, 1980.

Strauss, G. H. and Albertini, R. J.: Enumeration of 6-thioguanine resistant peripheral blood lymphocytes in man as a potential test for somatic cell mutation arising *in vivo. Mutat. Res. 61:*353, 1979.

Thilly, W. G., J. D. DeLuca, H. Hoppe IV and B. W. Penman: Mutation of human lymphoblasts by methylnitrosourea, *Chem.-Biol. Interact. 15:*33, 1976.

Thilly, W. G., J. D. DeLuca, H. Hoppe IV and B. W. Penman: Phenotypic lag and mutation to 6-thioguanine resistance in diploid human lymphoblasts, *Mutation Res. 50:*137, 1978.

Wolff, S.: Sister chromatid exchanges. *Ann Rev. Genet. 11:*183, 1977.

Wyrobek, A. J. and W. R. Bruce: The induction of sperm shape abnormalities in mice and humans. *Chem. Mutagens. 5:*257, 1978.

New Approaches in Toxicity Testing and Their Application in Human Risk Assessment, edited by A. P. Li. Raven Press, New York © 1985.

Identification of Environmental Carcinogens by Detecting the Induction of a Retrogenetic Expression

R. H. Stevens, P. A. Lindholm, D. A. Cole, P. T. Liu, and H. F. Cheng

Radiation Research Laboratory, Department of Radiology, University of Iowa, Iowa City, Iowa 52242

In 1965, the American Chemical Society initiated a Chemical Abstract Service (CAS) to assist in the indexing of chemical substances being reported in the scientific literature, and just twelve years later the CAS computer registry documented over four million distinct entities (Maugh II, 1978). While many of the chemicals are certainly esoteric materials, CAS in 1977 submitted to the Environmental Protection Agency (EPA) a list of some 33,000 substances thought to be in common use, and a corresponding conservative estimate also prepared that same year by EPA consisted of nearly 50,000 chemicals thought to be in everyday use (Maugh II, 1978). Certainly with the continued increase that has been occurring with the yearly introduction of new substances coupled along with the numbers already known to exist in our environment, it has to be considered an impossible and imaginary task for ever gathering sufficient experimental evidence regarding individual substances to assist in any sort of an assessment regarding their risk to humans. However, since substances can be generally categorized according to their potential risk based upon known chemical parameters, these smaller numbers can then be subjected to closer scrutiny for their possible mutagenicity and carcinogencity.

Once there has been categorization of a substance into a potential cancer risk group, then the choice of the proper test for evaluating its possible risk in inducing tumors is not unequivocal. The general concensus today appears to be that a battery of *in vitro* and *in vivo* systems represents the best possible strategy for the screening of possible genotoxic materials (Legator and Rinkus, 1981). Since mammalian cytogenetics represents a gross measure of the effects being exerted upon the genome, then it seems only logical that some form of an assay evaluating such effects should be incorporated into any sort of a screening program for potential genotoxic agents (Legator and Rinkus, 1981). In addition, there is also the practical experience which has been learned over the past few years in which several carcinogens that have been reported to be negative in the *in vitro* assays later were identified as carcinogens in the whole animal bioassays, for example, asbestos (Sincock, 1977), benzene (Hite *et al*, 1980), diethylstilbestrol (Sawada and Ishidate, 1978), and urethane (Wild, 1978). Another quite major consideration has to be the utilization of some measure of cytogenetics permits monitoring the actual exposure of the suspected toxic agents actually occuring in humans. For such reasons as these, it is thought by many investigators that the developed tests for mutagenicity and carcinogenicity be based upon a delineation of some sort of a genetic expression.

Retrogenetic Expression

The tendency for cancer cells to give up an originally final differentiated morphology that is associated with their adult tissues of origin, in other words, to redifferentiate was first recognized over a 150 years ago (Triolo, 1965). Speculations were later published regarding this possible event as early as 1929 that human neoplasms contained products which were similar or identical to those being initially synthesized during the eary embryonic stages of existence (Hirszfeld *et al.*, 1929). During the 1940's this idea was continually being pursued by a number of investigators resulting subsequently in conclusions such as the one stated by Greenstein, ". . . tumors tend to converge to common enzymatic patterns that in certain cases resemble those of fetal tissues" (Greenstein, 1945). Ensuing investigations support such a concept, and a landmark report was presented by Abelev and his colleagues in 1963 in which the existence of a fetal-like component, α-fetoprotein (AFP) in murine transplantable cancers was isolated (Abelev *et al.*, 1963). Two years later, the classic study of such fetal-like substances in human cancer cells was published by Gold and Freedman (1965), in which such a protein was identified in human colon cancer, and one which they termed carcinoembryonic antigen (CEA). Innumerable observations have been published following these two reports which have led to the general acceptance of the belief that most tumor cells will possess some sort of characteristic products that are similar or identical to those synthesized during fetal cell development (Alexander, 1974; Coggin and Anderson, 1974; Uriel 1976). These oncofetal substances, however, cannot be construed solely as only properties being expressed by the cancer cell as many such constituents also have been observed during periods in which normal adult tissues are undergoing nonneoplastic induction of growth. Such resumed syntheses of fetal-type components have now been considered as a reversibility occurring in the normal sequence of cell differentiation, with one concept now being put forward is that differentiation can be deemed as a particular time and space sequence for metabolic and biosynthetic patterns being expressed by the genome during developmental growth (Uriel, 1976). Thus, retrodifferentiation simply represents the reverse pathway of these nucleocytoplasmic events that normally occur during growth, and the subsequent outcome of such a reversal is the appearance of fetal-like components. The conceptual basis being a cellular reversibility of normal and cancer cells towards the less differentiated fetal state.

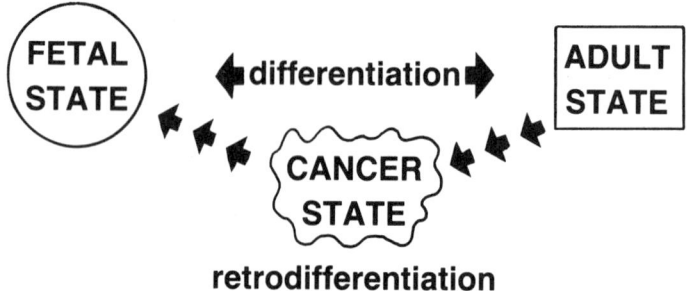

Following the recognition of this particular characteristic of tumor cells, there have been innumerable attempts to utilize the presence of fetal substances in order to diagnose the existence of cancer. The general conclusion which must be derived at present from the results of the very many animal and human cancer investigations is that at this time there exists no test for fetal products which can be used to unequivocally identify the existence of cancer. However, such tests have been employed in a very important adjunct role through monitoring the levels of fetal substances during therapy since it has been well-documented in a large number of cancer patients that successful treatment resulting in a dimishing of the concentrations of such products, then if a subsequent reappearance of the tumor occurs there will be a corresponding reoccurrence in the elevated levels of fetal materials (Oncology Review, 1981).

Observations such as these have led us to consider the possibility that such genetic re-expression with the concomitant elevation of fetal-like products might be employed as a foundation for developing short-term, inexpensive bioassays for identifying environmental carcinogens. The concept can be visualized as simply administering the test agents to the designated animal model, allowing time for the required metabolism and activation to occur, and then at a later time obtain a serum sample and analyze it for the presence of fetal products.

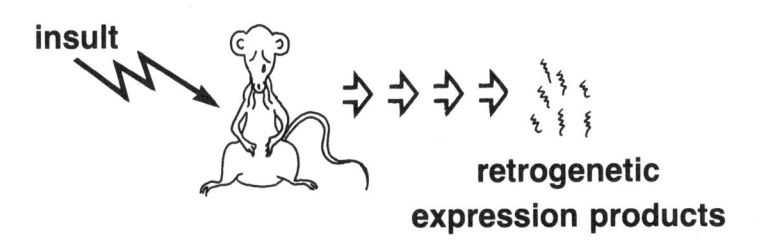

Two major assumptions underlie this concept; (1) the induced cancer cells will release sufficient concentrations of the selected fetal products to be measured into the circulatory system, and (2) the concentration of the fetal products somehow will directly complement the actual tumor burden. This latter relationship will allow a numerical value to be assigned to the test agent, and designated as its cancer inducing potential. Providing these two assumptions can be maintained, then it should be possible to develop inexpensive and rapidly performable whole-animal bioassays that are based upon retrogenetic expressions, and to then obtain numerical values which can then be indexed such that a relative risk table can be devised in which both the type of risk, that is, the particular tissue being vulnerable to the agent and the potential of risk can be reported.

Retrogenetic Expression by Animals with Cancer

The extensive efforts which have been devoted to the identification of retrogenetic expressions in animal tumor models initiated almost immediately following the report by Abelev and coworkers in which they demonstrated the existence of AFP in murine tumors (Abelev *et al.,* 1963). This particular substance has since been found to occur in every mammalian species tested including subhuman primates, carnivores, rodents, lagamorphs, ruminants, edentates, and marsupials (Tatarinow *et al.,* 1964; Gitlin and Boesman, 1967). Investigations have documented the presence of other common murine tumor associated fetal antigens (TAFA) existing in 9 to 19 day old embryos, in neoplastic lesions induced by a variety of different agents including chemicals and X-rays, as well as in spontaneously occuring mouse tumors (Stonehill and Bendick, 1970; Evans et al., 1979).

A major area of focus for many of these investigations being carried out in the early 1970's involved evaluating animal models of human colon cancer for the possible presence of such fetal antigens since CEA had previously been isolated in human tumors. Studies of cultured rat intestinal carcinomas induced *in vivo* by exposure to 1, 2-dimethylhydrazne (DMH) and N-methyl-N'-nitro-N-nitrosoguanidine (MNNG) were found to possess a common fetal-like antigen located in the membrane of the cells (Martin et al., 1975). The results indicated there was a tissue specificity since the antigen failed to be detected in non-intestinal cancer cells or other tumors such as hepatoma, glioma, and neurinoma. The possiblity for these substances being released in the animal's circulatory system was later shown to occur (Garmaise et al., 1975). It was noted that this particular fetal protein also existed in normal tissues as well, but at more than 250 times in reduced concentration (Abeyounis and Milgron, 1976).

Our studies which were intiated in 1975 revealed that like the chemically induced colon cancer model, rats which were exposed to localized X-irradiation of only their hypoxic ileum and jejunum and subsequently at a later time developed small bowel adenocarcinomas possessed fetal proteins (Stevens et al., 1975). Ensuing investigations indicated this tumor-associated fetal protein was enzymatically degraded by both endo- and exopeptidases, was soluble in detergents, and consists of at least six different glycoproteins having molecular weights ranging around a size of about 2000,000 daltons (Stevens et al., 1976). Table I summarizes our prevalent understanding about this particular fetal protein(s). Comprehensive investigations have been completed in an attempt to identify the existence of this fetal protein in normal tissues; however, in these studies which employed a xenogenic rabbit antiserum we have been unable to detect its presence in any apparently normal tissues of these X-ray induced tumor bearing animals (Table II). Later research revealed that the tumor-bearing rats generated an IgG immunoglobulin that was capable of specifically binding the fetal glyco-protein, thereby implying that it may act as an oncofetal antigen (Stevens et al., 1978). While we have yet to pursue whether this glycoprotein also acts as antigen in other types of entodermal lesions as well, we have identified its existence in rat adenocarcinomas induced by DMH in the colon and 7,12-dimethyl-benz(a)anthracene (DMBA) in the pancreas. These animals with the chemically induced tumors, unlike the rats bearing the X-ray-induced cancers, had other tissues than the primary target which also possessed the fetal protein in detectable concentrations (Table II). All three of the models consisted of animals that released the protein in detectable amounts into their circulatory system, thus fulfilling the first requirement of the proposed concept (Stevens et al., 1981). The possibility that commercially available tests could be employed for analyzing the presence of the fetal proteins was explored utilizing commerically available radioimmunoassay kits for human CEA (Lawson et al., 1979). We observed a cross-reactivity of both the tissues and serum of the tumor-bearing rats with the antiserum prepared for the human fetal protein (Table III).

TABLE I

ONOFETAL PROTEIN CHARACTERISTICS

Characteristic	Reference
Tumor-associated fetal protein (17-19 day rat old fetuses)	Stevens et al., 1975
Membrane constituent	Stevens et al., 1975
Circulating glycoprotein	Stevens et al., 1976, 1981
Heat insensitive	Stevens et al., 1976
Acid sensitive/base insensitive	Stevens et al., 1976
Enzymatically degraded with endo- and exopeptidases; resistant to nucleotidases and neuramindase	Stevens et al., 1976
Heterogenous proteins $\sim 2 \times 10^5$ daltons	Stevens et al., 1976
Accompanies partially purified blocking factors of CMI	Stevens et al., 1978, 1979
Acts as an antigen in rats bearing X-ray induced small bowel adenocarinomas	Stevens et al., 1978
Non-strain specific exists in Holtzman (outbred), Lewis Brown Norwy (F_1), and the Buffalo, and Fischer F344 inbred rats	Stevens et al., 1976, 1981
Non-tissue specific for entodermal type cancers	Stevens et al., 1981

TABLE II

EXISTENCE OF THE ONCOFETAL PROTEIN IN DETECTABLE CONCENTRATIONS

Organ   **Tumor Model**[a]

Organ	Small Bowel (X-rays)	Colon (DMH)	Pancreas (DMBA)	Mesoderm (asbestos)	Breast (spontaneous)
Small Bowel	+	+	+	−	−
Colon	−	+	−	−	−
Pancreas	−	−	+	−	−
Mesoderm	−	−	−	−	−
Breast	−	?	?	−	−
Stomach	−	−	−	−	−
Liver	−	+	+	−	−
Lung	−	+	+	−	−
Spleen	−	−	+	−	−
Kidney	−	−	−	?	?
Serum	+	+	+	?	?
Bile	−	−	+	?	?

[a] Small bowel, colon and pancreas studies reported by Stevens, Cole, and Cheng, 1981; mesoderm and breast findings represent unpublished information.

TABLE III
SERUM LEVELS OF CEA-rs IN THE RAT[a]

Animal Model	Serum level (ng/ml)
Control	0.61 ± 0.19
Small Bowel Adenocarcinoma (X-ray)	4.46 ± 0.75 (p < 0.001)
Colon Adenocarcinoma (DMH)	4.6
Pancreas Adenocarcinoma (DMBA)	3.9
X-Irradiated (Small Bowel) Non-Tumor Bearing Animals	0.60 ± 0.16

[a] Values extracted from article by Lawson et al., 1979.

In an attempt to understand what role such proteins might play in the host's immunological responses to the radiation and chemically induced tumors, investigations were focused upon the possible education of tumor-bearing animals' lymphocytes to specifically recognize various tumor target cells. Steele and colleagues in the mid-1970's reported that rats with colon tumors induced by DMH and MMNG possessed educated lymphocytes that were capable of expressing specific cytotoxicity to both colon tumor cells and to fetal colon cells (Steele and Sjögren, 1974; Steele et al., 1975). Baldwin and Vose carrying out analogous studies of animals having methylcholanthrene induced sarcomas found that fetal antigens appear to be phase specific during embryogenosis and were later expressed as common antigens in tumor cells (Baldwin and Vose, 1974). Our findings also advanced the idea that such lymphoid-cell education occurs as those rats having X-ray induced small bowel adenocarcinomas possessed lymphoid cells capable of specifically recognizing and being cytolytic to the tumor cells (Stevens et al., 1977). Blocking of such cytotoxic responses could be accomplished by adding preparations of tumor membrane extracts which contained detectable quantities of the oncofetal protein (Stevens et al., 1978), and also circulating factors which contained this fetal material (Stevens et al., 1979) that were obtained from the tumor-bearing animals (Table IV).

We have recently begun exploring the possibility that such lymphocyte education might in itself be applied for developing assays that could be used for evaluating the carcinogenic potential of various environmental carcinogens (Stevens et al., 1980a,b,; 1980 a,b; 1982a,b,; Cole et al., 1982). Our findings at the present time indicate that for those lesions which have a common germ cell origin, there is apparently a common lymphocyte education as well as the fetal protein which may be useful for developing such analyses (Table V). The role(s) which such lymphocyte education and fetal proteins may play in the animal cancer is far from being understood; although the results from a number of studies have implied that they may participate in iliciting antitumor immune responses. For examples, the immunization with fetal cells has been reported to render syngeneic animals immune to a later challenge with chemically induced transplantable tumors (LeMevel and Wells, 1973; Bansal et al., 1978). However, there have been contrasting findings negating such immunoresponsiveness also published in which no such antitumor immunity could be brought about by immunization with such products as 15-day rat embryos (Embleton and Baldwin, 1980).

TABLE IV

INHIBITION OF CELL-MEDIATED IMMUNITY BY FACTORS CONTAINING THE FETAL PROTEIN

Factor	Cell	Percent CMI Inhibition
Membrane Extracts (3M KCl)[a]	Effector	70.5 ± 17 (4)
	Target	62.5 ± 14 (4)
Ammonium Sulfate Soluble Fractions (Membrane Extracts)[a]	Effector	96.8 ± 7 (4)
	Target	10.5 ± 8 (4)
Ammonium Sulfate Insoluble Fractions (Membrane Extracts)[a]	Effector	12.5 ± 11 (4)
	Target	70.5 ± 35 (4)
Tumor Sera[b]	Effector	90 ± 12 (4)
	Target	77 ± 20 (4)
Irradiated Non-Tumor Bearing Rats' Sera[b]	Effector	69.5 ± 23 (4)
	Target	48.0 ± 15 (4)

[a] Information obtained from article by Steven et al., 1978, suggesting the blocking factors containing the fetal protein(s) act upon the lymphocyte in inhibiting CMI; whereas those factors also containing the anti IgG to the fetal protein(s) block CMI by acting in concert with the target cell.

[b] Results reported by Stevens et al., 1979.

TABLE V

CELL-MEDIATED IMMUNITY EXPRESSED TOWARDS X-RAY INDUCED SMALL BOWEL ADENOCARCINOMA

Tumor Model for Source of Effector Cells[a]	Percent CMI
Small Bowel (X-rays)	20.5 ± 8.3 (7)
Colon (DMH)	8.8 ± 4 (7)
Pancreas (DMBA)	7.4 ± 2.8 (7)
Mesothelioma (Asbestos)	0.0 (7)
Breast (Spontaneous)	0.0 (7)
Prostate (Spontaneous)	0.0 (7)
Normal Fetal Cells	15.1 ± 3.1 (3)

[a] Steven et al., 1982

The conclusion from these along with many other comparable studies is that fetal components indeed exist in animal cancer models; however, their purpose and whether there is a direct link between their concentration and tumor burden remains to be established.

Retrogenetic Expression by Humans with Cancer

Since the pioneering reports in the 1960's documenting the presence of the fetal proteins AFP and CEA, extensive amounts of evidence have accumulated, and it is now widely accepted that most human cancer cells like their animal counterparts will possess fetal substances in detectable quantities (Ibsen and Fishman, 1979; Oncology Review, 1981). The identification of such fetal-like constituents has now reached the stage of having considerable clinical usefulness. Although, assays, while not being sufficiently specific to justify indiscriminant use as cancer screening tools, have rather been found to serve as a prognosticator for evaluating the success of therapeutic intervention in the disease (Oncology Review, 1981). For example, a number of studies have shown patients with colon cancer in which the elevated CEA level was normalized following surgery, a recurrence of the disease could be successfully predicted by measuring the rising concentration of this fetal protein in their plasma (Oncology Review, 1981). Results of another type of study involving over 272 members of six different pedigrees implied that when the values of CEA were expressed as a square root value in order to correct for skewness and kurtosis, there exists a linear increase in mean $\sqrt{CEA}$ concentration which correlates directly with the known genetic cancer risk (Guirgis, 1978). The results implicated an apparent connubial effect on the meausured CEA levels that was attributed by Guirgis to a common environmental agent acting in concert with the genetic disposition to the cancer. Such representative findings as these continue to imply that the measurements of fetal substances might be useful in devising assays for quantitating genetic risks to environmental agents.

CONCLUSION

It is a currently accepted concept that many if not all tumor cells will possess fetal properties, and that with the appropriate techniques they can be detected. How these substances become increased in syntheses during carcinogenesis, and for what purpose they exist in the cancer cell still remains unclear. One question that needs to be resolved in order to utilize the measurements as a bioassay is whether those cancer cells that do express the fetal materials arise from a differentiation of a tissue reserve of stem cells or else through a process of retrodifferentiation (Uriel, 1976). The concept of a stem cell reservoir at this time seems less likely because as of yet such a repository remains to be identified, while in contrast, retrodifferentiation has been observed in a number of non-neoplastic proliferative states including those such as regenerating toxin poisoned liver, liver cells in culture, and carcinogen induced hyperplastic liver (Ibsen and Fishman, 1979). While the need for such products by the cancer cell remains a mystery, one idea that has been favorably accepted is that the fetal antigens develop during pregnancy in order to modulate the maternal immune system so that the fetus which represents a natural allograft is not rejected (Alexander, 1974; Coggin and Anderson, 1974). Cancer cells similarly re-express these products associated with early development in order to avoid an equivalent type of immunological destruction.

In summary, it is now widely believed that associated with the development of most cancers will be a concommitment increase in fetal products in concentrations that can be detected. There is evidence that similar or even possibly the same products may be induced through exposure to different types of carcinogens, acting upon tissues having a common germ cell origin, and that such products may be associated with immunological responses of the host to the presence of the cancer cells. The question that remains to be answered is whether the various analyses for such fetal products presently available can be directly applied for identifying environmental cancer causing agents, thus allowing establishment of a risk assessment index based upon induction of retrogenetic expression.

ACKNOWLEDGEMENTS

Authors are indebted to Susan Barnett for her excellent secretarial assistance. Financial support was received by grants PHS CA30967 awarded by NCI, NIOSH grants RO3-OHO-1705 and RO3-OHO-1672. Drs. P. A. Lindholm and P. T. Liu received support from training grant T32-CA-09125.

REFERENCES

Abelev, G. I.; Perova, S. D.; Khamkova, N. I.; Postnikova, Z. A.; and Irlin, I. S.: Production of embryonal α-globulin by transplantable mouse hepatomas. *Transplant., 1*:179-180, 1963.

Abeyounis, C. G. and Milgrom, E. G.: A thermostable antigen characteristic for carcinoma induced rat intestinal tumors. *J. Immunol., 116*:30-34, 1976.

Alexander, P.: Escape from immune destruction by the host through shedding of surface antigens: Is this a chracteristic shared by malignant and embryonic cells? *Cancer Res., 34*:2077-2082, 1974.

Baldwin, R. W. and Vose, B. M.: The expresion of a phase-specific foetal antigen on rat embryo cells. *Transplant., 18*:525-530, 1974.

Bansal, S. C.; Mark, R., : Bansal,B.; and Rhoade, J. E.: Immunologic surveillance against chemically induced primary colon carcinoma in rats. *J. Natl. Cancer Inst., 60*:667-675, 1978.

Coggin, Jr., J. H.; Anderson, N. G.: Cancer, differentiation and embryonic antigens: Some central problems. *Adv. Cancer Res., 19*:105-159, 1974.

Cole, D. A.; Stevens, R. H.; and Will, L. A.: Identification of carcinogens by measurement of cell-mediated immunity. III. Immunity to asbestos-induced rat peritoneal mesothelioma. Environ. Res., 28:77-83, 1982.

Embleton, M. J. and Baldwin, R. W.: Antigenic changes in chemical carcinogenesis. Brit. Med. Bull., 36:83-88, 1980.

Evans; Parker, D. V.; and Frank, M. K.: Biochemical and physical characterization of tumor associated fetal antigens. *Cancer Res., 39*:2006-2015, 1979.

Carmaise, A. B.; Rogers, A. E.; Saravis, C. A.; Zamchek, N.; Newberne, P.M.: Immunologic aspects of 1,2-dimethylhydrazine-incuded colon tumors in rats.
J. Natl. Cancer Inst., 54:1231-1235, 1975.

Gitlin, D. M. and Boesman, M.: Sites of serum α-fetoprotein synthesis in the human and in the rat. *J. Clin. Invest., 46*:1010-1016, 1967.

Gold, P. and Freedman, S.O.: Demonstration of tumor specific antigens in human colonic carcinoma by immunological tolerance and absorption techniques.

J. Exptl. Med., 121:432-462, 1965.

Greenstein, J. P.: Enzymes in normal and neoplastic tissues. In: *AAAS Research Conference* Washington, D.C., American Assoc. Adv. of Science, p. 191, 1945.

Guirgis, H. A.; Lynch, H. T.; Harris, R. E.; and Vandervoorde, J. P.: Genetic and communicable effects on carcinoembryonic antigen expressivity in the cancer family syndrome. *Cancer Res., 38*:2523-2528, 1978.

Hirzfeld, L.; Halber, N.; and Rosenblat, S.: Zeitscrift fur immunstat-s forschung und experimentelle therapie. 75:209, 1929.

Hite, M.; Pecharo, M.; Smith, I.; Thronton, S.: The effect of benzene in the micronucleus test. *Mutat. Res.,* 77:149-155, 1980.

Ibsen, K. H. and Fishman, W. H.: Developmental gene expression in cancer. *Biochem. et Biophys. Acta, 560*:243-280, 1979.

Lawson, A. J.; Cheng, H. F.; Osborne, J. W.; and Stevens, R. H.: Serum levels of a carcinoembryonic antigen-reactive substance (CEA-rs) in rats bearing X-irradiation induced small bowel adenocarcinoma. In: *Carcino-Embryonic Proteins, Vol. II,*. ed. F. G. Lehmann, Elsevier North-Holland Biomedical Press, pp. 47-56, 1979.

Legator, M. S. and Rinkus, S. J.: Mutagenicity testing: Problems in application. In: *Short-Term Tests or Chemical Carcinogens,* eds. H. F. Stich and R. H. C. San, Springer-Verlag. New York, Heidelberg, Berlin, Chapter 43, pp. 483-501, 1981.

LeMevel, B. P. and Wells, Jr., S. A.: Foetal antigens cross-reactive with tumor-specific transplantations antigens. *Nature New Biol., 244*:183-184, 1973.

Martin, F.; Knobel, S.; Martin, M.; and Bordes, M.: A carcinofetal antigen located on the membrane of cells from rat intestinal carcinoma in culture. *Cancer Res., 35*:333-336, 1976.

Maugh II, T. H.: Chemicals: How many are there? *Science, 199:162, 1978.*

Oncology Review: Carcinoembryonic Antigen (CEA) in the clinical diagnosis and treatment of colorectal cancer. U.S. Dept. of health and Human Services, 1981.

Sawada, M.; Ishidata Jr., M.: Colchicine-like effect on diethylstilbestrol (DES) on mammalian cells *in vitro. Mutat. Res., 57:175-182, 1978.*

Sincock, A.M.: Preliminary studies of the *in vitro* cellular effects of asbestos and fine glass dusts. In: *Origins of Human Cancer.* Book A. Eds. H. H. Hiatt, J. D. Watson and J. A. Nimsten, New York, Cold Springs Habor Laboratory. pp. 941-954, 1977.

Steele Jr., G. and Sjogren, H. O.; Rosengren, J. E.; Lindstrom, C.; Larsson, A.; and Leandodoer, L.: Sequential studies of serum blocking activity in rats bearing chemically induced primary bowel tumors. J. Natl. Cancer Inst., 54:959, 1975.

Stevens, R. H.; Englund, C. W.; Osborne, J. W.; Cheng, H. F.; and Richerson, H. B.: Oncofetal protein accompaying irradiation-induced small bowel adenocarcinoma in the rat. *J. Natl. Cancer Inst., 55*:1011-1013, 1975.

Stevens, R. H.; Englund, C. W.; Osborne, J. W.; Cheng, H. F.; and Hoffman, K. L.: Identification and characterization of a circulating tumor-associated oncofetal protein from a radiation induced adenocarcinoma of the rat small bowel. *Cancer Res., 36*:3260-3264, 1976.

Stevens, R. H.; Brooks, G. P.; Osborne, J. W.; Englund, C. W.; and White, D. W.: Lymphocyte cytotoxicity in X-irradiation-induced adenocarcinoma of the rat small bowel. I.

Measurement of target cell destruction by release of radioiodinated membrane proteins. *J. Natl. Cancer Inst., 59*:1315-1319, 1977.

Stevens, R. H.; Brooks, G. P.; Osborne, J. W.; Hoffman, K. L.; and Lawson, A. J.: Lymphocyte cytotoxicity in X-irradiation-induced rat small bowell adenocarcinoma. III. Blocking by 3M KC1 extract. *J. Imminol., 120*:335-339, 1978.

Stevens, R. H.; Brooks, G. P.; and Osborne, J. W.: Circulating blocking factors of lymphoid-cell cytotoxicity in X-ray-induced rat small bowell adenocarcinoma. *Radiat. Res., 80*:161-169, 1979.

Stevens, R. H.; Cole, D. A.; and Rana, R. S.: Radiation equivalency of 1, 2-dimethylhydrazine in rats. *Archives Environ. Health, 35*:69-74, 1980a.

Stevens, R. H.; Cole, D. A.; Rana, R.S.; and Graves, J. M.: Identification of carcinogens by measurement of cell-mediated immunity. I. Immunity induced by rat pancreas and colon carcinogens. *Environ. Res., 21*:143-149, 1980b.

Stevens, R. H.; Cole, D. A.; and Cheng, H. F.: Identification of a common oncofetal protein in X-ray and chemically-induced rat gastrointestinal tumors. *Br. J. Cancer, 43*:817-825, 1981.

Stevens, R. H. and Cole, D. A.: Identification of carcinogens by measurement of cell-mediated immunity. II. Assay specificity. *Environ. Res., 28*:67-76, 1982a.

Stevens, R. H. and Cole, D. A.: Detection of carcinogenic exposures by urinalysis. Induction of cell-mediated immunity. *Toxicol. Lett., 11*:299-303, 1982b.

Stonehill, E. H. and Bendich, A.: Retrogenetic expression: The reappearance of embryonal antigens in cancer cells. *Nature, 229:370, 1970.*

Tatarinov, Y. S.: Detection of embryo specific α-globulin in blood sera of patient with primary liver tumor. *Vop. med. Khim, 10*:90-91, 1964.

Triolo, V. A.: Nineteenth centurey foundations of cancer research advances in tumor pathology, nomenclature, and theories of oncogensis. *Cancer Res., 25*:75-106, 1965.

Uriel, J.: Cancer, retrodifferentation, and the myth of Faust. *Cancer Res., 36*:4269-427, 1976.

Wild, D.: Cytogenetic effects in mouse of 17 chemical mutagens and carcinogens evaluated by the micronucleus test. *Mutation Res., 56*:319-327, 1978.

New Approaches in Toxicity Testing and Their Application in Human Risk Assessment, edited by A. P. Li. Raven Press, New York © 1985.

Effects of Structurally Diverse Chemicals on Metabolic Cooperation *In Vitro*

*A. Russell Malcolm and †Lesley J. Mills

*United States Environmental Protection Agency, Narragansett, Rhode Island 02882; †Department of Microbiology, University of Rhode Island, Kingston, Rhode Island 02881

Permeable intercellular (gap) junctions allowing the direct exchange of small ions and molecules between cells in coupled populations are a common feature of most animal tissues (Cox, 1974; DeMello, 1977; Loewenstein, 1981; Pitts, 1980). Research suggests that such gap-junctional communication, defined as metabolic cooperation (Hooper, 1982; Subak-Sharpe, 1966; Subak-Sharpe et al., 1969), is necessary in plants and animals for coordination and control of cell proliferation, differentiation, and other activities which collectively result in the integration of individual cells into organized tissues (Pitts. 1980). Specifically, metabolic cooperation is implicated in developmental signalling, embryonic induction, growth control, cell nutrition, the control of hormonal responses, and general tissue homeostasis (Griepp and Revel, 1977; Loewenstein, 1981; Pitts and Finbow, 1977; Sheridan, 1977; Wolper, 1979), thus suggesting the fundamental importance of this biological process to developing and adult multicellular organisms.

The recent discovery (Murray and Fitzgerald, 1979; Yotti et al., 1979) that phorbol ester tumor promoters inhibit metabolic cooperation between several types of cultured cells suggests that inhibited metabolic cooperation is a mechanism for tumor promotion. Because metabolic cooperation appears to be important for normal embryonic development, the concept has been extended to include some reproductive system effects (Trosko et al., 1983), including teratogenesis (Trosko et al., 1982). These ideas form a general hypothesis which predicts that inhibition of metabolic cooperation in adults may result in tumor promotion, whereas its inhibition in developing embryos may induce teratogenesis.

The hypothesis that tumors may be promoted through inhibition of metabolic cooperation assumes that the carcinogenic process is mutli-step and that the growth of premalignant (initiated) cells may be regulated via signals from communicating normal cells. Multiple stage carcinogenesis is now well documented for many organs in several animal models, and is extensively reviewed (Boutwell, 1974; Slaga et. al., 1981). Regulation of initiated cell growth through metabolic cooperation with normal cells awaits demonstration, but evidence suggesting a role for metabolic cooperation in the regulation of cell growth is abundant. For example, cell strains defective for both growth control (density-dependent inhibition of replication) and metabolic cooperation have been isolated and characterized (Loewenstein, 1979; 1980). The segregation patterns of these and several other biochemical traits resulting from hybridization experiments with normal and defective cells suggest that metabolic cooperation and loss of growth control are genetically linked (Azarnia and Loewenstein 1973, 1977; Borek et al., 1969). Cells defective for both traits are also tumorigenic in appropriate animal hosts (Borek et al., 1969; Epstein et al., 1975).

Potter views carcinogenesis as a fundamental problem of local intercellular communication (Potter, 1983; 1983a) and uses the concept to propose that certain tissue-specific inhibitors of cell proliferation (chalones or chalone-like substances) might control cell growth through regulation of metabolic cooperation. Closely associated with this concept is the likely role of cyclic AMP (cAMP) and the phosphorylation of certain proteins by the kinases it activates (Prescott, 1976). Indeed, Weiner and Loewenstein recently report (Weiner and Loewenstein, 1983) that mutant Chinese hamster ovarian cells deficient for a protein kinase (cAMP receptor) are also deficient for gap-junctional communication, and that the latter deficiency is restored when the missing protein kinase is supplied exogenously.

Additional evidence suggests a connection between metabolic cooperation and cell growth regulation. Recently demonstrated (Lloyd et al., 1983) is the transfer of antiproliferative activity from interferron-induced cells to recipient cells co-cultivated *in vitro*. Transfer occurred only when donor and recipient cells were in physical contact, further implicating metabolic cooperation in the regulation of cell growth. In addition, Friedman and Steinberg report (Friedman, 1982) that early and late-stage, premalignant human colon cells communicate effectively through metabolic cooperation whereas cells from an established human colon carcinoma do not. Moreover, the tumor promoter, phorbol-12-myristate-13-acetate (PMA), inhibits metabolic cooperation between the late-stage but not early-stage cells, suggesting that promoters may facilitate the transition of some premalignant cells to malignancy by blocking metabolic cooperation. These results support recent observations that many tumor promoters and several carcinogens inhibit metabolic cooperation *in vitro* (Hartman and Rosen, 1983; Malcolm et al., 1983; Trosko et al., 1982; Williams, 1983).

We are testing the general hypothesis through correlation studies with selected tumor promoters, carcinogens, and other chemicals, some of which are also teratogenic. In this paper, we summarize results for eighteen chemicals tested in our laboratory and discuss the results in relation to general hypothesis predictions.

METABOLIC COOPERATION ASSAY

Gap junctions form between many types of cultured animal cells and metabolic cooperation between them may be measured by several techniques. We use the selection phase of the V79/HGPRT mututation assay modified to facilitate detection of chemicals which inhibit metabolic cooperation. This approach, described by Yotti, et al. (1979), and Trosko, et al. (1981), involves the co-cultivation of mutant (HGPRT$^-$) and wild-type (HGPRT$^+$) V79 Chinese hamster lung fibroblasts. The HGPRT$^-$cells are deficient for the enzyme hypoxanthine-guanine phosphoribosyl transferase (HGPRTase) and are assumed to possess mutations in the structural gene coding for the enzyme. HGPRTase is a purine salvage enzyme which catalyses the conversion of performed purine bases (hypoxanthine and guanine) into their respective nucleotides which are then incorporated into nucelic acid. In addition to these normal purine bases, HGPRTase also catalyses the conversion of certain abnormal bases, such as 8-azaguanine and

6-thioguanine, into their respective nucleotides. Because the cytoplasmic membrane is not permeable to nucleotides, such metabolites tend to be incorporated into nucleic acid in those cells within which they arise. Upon incorporation, the abnormal nucleotides are highly toxic. Consequently, 6TG is toxic to HGPRT$^+$ but not HGPRT$^-$ cells. This is the principle underlying HGPRT$^-$ cell selection by 6TG from mixed populations in mutation experiments. In such experiments, 6TG is added to the growth medium to eliminated HGPRT$^+$ cells. HGPRT$^-$ cells survive and grow into macroscopic colonies, providing they do not establish physical contact with HGPRT$^+$ cells during the selective process. If contact occurs, gap junctions will form and the toxicmetabolite of 6TG is transferred from HGPRT$^+$ to HGPRT$^-$ cells, resulting in mutant cell loss. In mutation experiments, the probability of HGPRT$^-$ cell loss is minimized by screening mixed populations at low densities where the probability of cell contact is similarly low. The loss of HGPRT$^-$ cells through metabolic cooperation with HGPRT$^+$ cells, while undesirable in mutation experiments, provides a convenient way to identify chemicals which inhibit metabolic cooperation. The assay for metabolic cooperation becomes a reconstructed selection experiment in which known numbers of HGPRT$^-$ cells are co-cultivated with enough HGPRT$^+$ cells to ensure HGPRT$^-$ cell loss unless 'rescued' by test chemicals (added simultaneously with 6TG) are measured as a function of HGPRT$^-$ cell recovery relative to the usual low recovery of these cells in solvent controls. Currently, no exogenous metabolizing system is used. Thus, because V79 cells have a limited capacity to metabolize chemicals (Bradley et al., 1981), observed responses are assumed to result from the effects of unmetabolized test substances. For results described below, the effects of chemicals on metabolic cooperation were assessed at doses permitting at least 70 percent survival in low-density, toxicity tests performed with HGPRT$^-$ cells only.

RESULTS AND DISCUSSION

Test results are summarized in Table I. Chemicals had either no effect on metabolic cooperation, inhibited metabolic cooperation, or enhanced it. Chemicals were judged to have no effect on metabolic cooperation if mutant recovery at all doses assessed was not different from that in the solvent control. Inhibition of metabolic cooperation resulted in an increase in mutant cell recovery over background, whereas enhancement was characterized by a decrease in mutant recovery relative to background.

Tumor Promoters

Five tumor promoters of varying tissue specificity and efficacy were tested. PMA, a potent promoter of mouse skin tumors, increased mutant recovery at 0.1 ng/ml and induced complete mutant recovery at 1ng/ml (Malcolm et al., 1983).
Phorbol-12,13-dibutyrate (PDBu), a much weaker promoter of similar tumors, increased mutant recovery to 60 percent at 10 ng/ml. In these experiments, background recovery averaged about 10 percent at 10 ng/ml. PMA and PDBu thus inhibited metabolic cooperation in proportion to their promoting activity *in vivo*. Inhibition of metabolic cooperation at the ng/ml level suggests that PMA and PDBu induced effects through interaction with structurally specific receptors (Korolkovas, 1970). Binding studies with specific phorbol esters provide convincing evidence for such receptors (Blumberg et al., 1982; Weiner and Loewenstein, 1983).

Butylated hydroxytoluene (BHT), a promoter of liver tumors in rats pretreated with 2-acetylaminofluorene (Peraino et al., 1977), and lung tumors in mice pretreated with urethane (Witschi, 1983), inhibited metabolic cooperation at nontoxic concentrations (25 cg/ml or less) in two experiments, but had no effect on metabolic cooperations at

TABLE I. Effects of Structurally Diverse Chemicals on Metabolic Cooperation Between Cultured V79 Chinese Hamster Lung Fibroblasts

No Effect	Inhibition	Enhancement
3,4-benzopyrene	phorbol-12-myristate-13-acetate	
	phorbol-12,13-dibutyrate	
	butylated hydroxytoluene	
	sodium cyclamate	
phenol	catechol	2-methoxyphenol
phenylglucuronide	quinol	
	hydroxyquinol	
	1,4-benzoquinone	
	phenylsulfate	
	di-(2-ethylhexyl) phthalate	
	trisodium nitrilotriacetate	
	4-chlorobiphenyl	
	ethanol	
	dimethylsulfoxide	

these same concentrations in two other experiments. Because BHT showed a dose response in those experiments where it inhibited metabolic cooperation, and because BHT is reported (Trosko et al., 1982) by others to inhibit metabolic cooperation in this assay, we classified BHT as an inhibitor of metabolic cooperation. It is possible that factors influencing the effect of BHT on metabolic cooperation were not controlled in our experiments. BHT is considered to be an atypical promoter in that it appears to promote tumorigenesis *in vivo* only if carcinogenic doses of initiator are given (Witschi, 1983). BHT promotes the *in vitro* transformation of C3H/10T1/2 cells pretreated with subtransforming doses of 20-methylcholanthrene (Djurhuus and Lillehaug, 1982). The teratogenicity of BHT is controversial (Babich, 1982).

At high doses, sodium cyclamate (SCM) promotes bladder tumors in rats pretreated with nitrosomethylurea (Hicks, 1982). SCM inhibited metabolic cooperation in a dose-dependent manner, also at high (1-4 mg/ml) concentrations. Saccharin, a similarly weak promoter (Hicks, 1982), requires similar concentrations to inhibit metabolic cooperation in V79 cells to the same extent (Trosko *et al.,* 1980). SCM reversibly inhibits electrical coupling (produced by the transfer of ions through metabolic cooperation) between human epithelial cells in culture (Enomoto *et al.,* 1981). There is no conclusive evidence that SCM is teratogenic in animals, although there is circumstantial evidence for this in humans (IARC monographs, 1982).

Phenol, a weak promoter of mouse skin tumors (Van Duuren, 1976), had no effect on metabolic cooperation at all concentrations (400 μg/ml or less) tested. Concentrations greater than 300 μg/ml were toxic. This result suggested that phenol did not fit the hypothesis that tumor promoters inhibit metabolic cooperation. Because the skin is important as a drug-metabolizing organ, seven metabolites of phenol were tested on the hypothesis that promotion by some chemicals might be mediated through metabolic products. Four minor metabolites (1,4-benzoquinone, catechol, hydroxyquinol, and quinol) weakly inhibited metabolic cooperation in a dose-related fashion at moderate (1-3 µg/ml) concentrations (Malcolm et al., 1983). Phenylsulfate, a major conjugation product, also weakly inhibited metabolic cooperation, but at high (1-4 mg/ml) concentrations and without dose response. Phenylglucuronide, another major conjugation product, had no effect on metabolic cooperation and was nontoxic at all concentrations (7.5 mg/ml or less) tested. A methylated derivative of catechol, 2-methyoxyphenol, enhanced metabolic cooperation in a dose-dependent manner between 20 and 70 µg/ml. Inhibition of metabolic cooperation by five metabolites of phenol indicates that phenol is not an exception to the hypothesis. Moreover, this result indicates the need to consider metabolites when testing the hypothesis. Recognizition of the need to consider metabolites is especially important in view of the fact that some workers have reported (Chamberlain 1982; Dorman and Boneiko, 1983; Kinsella, 1982) that inhibition of metabolic cooperation is not a property common to all tumor promoters. Some of these promoters inhibit metabolic cooperation when tested under conditions more suitable for detection of weaker substances (Trosko et al., 1981). In other cases (Dorman and Boreiko, 1983; Kinsella, 1982), effects may be mediated through metabolites.

The weakness of phenol's metabolites in inhibiting metabolic cooperation correlates with the weakness of phenol as a promoter *in vivo* (Boutwell and Bosch, 1959). The pharmacological significance of enhanced metabolic cooperation requires investigation, particularly with respect to antipromotion effects. For example, retinoic acid, an antipromoter under some conditions (Van Duuren, 1976), increases the numbers of gap junctions on the membranes of some cells (Friedman and Steinberg, 1982), thereby increasing the opportunity for metabolic cooperation. Chemicals causing cells to decrease in size may inhibit metabolic cooperation through physical disruption of gap juctions (Dorman and Boreiko, 1983). Chemicals may also effect mtabolic cooperation through effects on the size and composition of intracellular pools of transferable substances (Bianchi, 1982). Alternative explanations (e.g., cytotoxicity) for the promoting activity of phenol cannot be ruled out, particularly as catechol and quinol are reported (Boutwell and Bousch, 1959) to be inactive as mouse skin tumor promoters. These substances may, however, be promoters for other organs. Additional *in vivo* studies with catechol and quinol may be required. Phenol is not teratogenic in rats according to one study (Minor and Becker, 1971), but induces developmental defects in submammalian species, (Birge et al., 1980). Interestingly, phenol shows activity without exogenous metabolism in a recently-developed, *in vitro* test for teratogens (Braun et al., 1982).

Selected Carcinogens

3,4-Benzopyrene (BP), a complete carcinogen which may promote as well as inititate, had no effect on metabolic cooperation at nontoxic (3 µg/ml or less) concentrations (Malcolm et al., 1983). As BP is extensively metabolized and requires metabolism to a carcinogenic form, it is possible that promoting effects are mediated through metabolites. Specific metabolites should there be evaluated for their effects on metabolic cooperation. BP, however, fails to inhibit metabolic cooperation between co-cultivated HGPRTase-deficient ARL14 cells and freshly-isolated rat hepatocytes (Telang et al., 1982) which should be capable of metabolizing BP. Perhaps, in the cell culture system, not enough metabolite is produced to inhibit metabolic cooperation. BP is also teratogenic (Shum et al., 1979).

Two carcinogenic but apparently nonmutagenic chemicals were tested. The trisodium salt of nitrilotriacetic acid (NTA), a carcinogen at high doses in rats (Goyer et al., 1983), inhibited metabolic cooperation in a dose-related manner at high (1-3 mg/ml) concentrations (Malcolm et al., 1983). NTA may inhibit metabolic cooperation by chelating calcium, an important element in the regulation of metabolic cooperation (Anderson et. al., 1982). Evidence from animals studies (Anderson et al., 1982) indicates that the toxic effects of NTA correlate with the extraction of calcium via chelation from tissue intercellular spaces. With the exception of clastogenic effects at high doses in somatic cells (Bora, 1975), NTA is not genotoxic in a variety of assays (Dunkel and Simmon, 1980; Epstein et al., 1975; Kramers, 1976). NTA does not appear to be teratogenic in mammals (Wilson, 1977), but developmental defects are reported (Birge et. al., 1980) for nonmammalian species.

Di(2-ethylhexyl) phthalate (DEHP) presents a similar situation. DEHP is carcinogenic at high doses in F344 rats and B6C3F1 mice, but, with the possible exception of chromosomal effects, is not genotoxic (IARC monographs, 1982). DEHP inhibited metabolic cooperation in a dose-dependent fashion at moderate (1-30 µg;ml) concentrations (Malcolm et. al. 1983). DEHP promotes JB-6 epidermal cells to anchorage indendence and tumorigenicity (Diwan et al., 1983), and is a potent promoter of hepatic tumors in B6C3F1 mice (Ward et al., 1983). DEHP is also teratogenic at high doses in rats and mice (Shiota and Nishimura, 1982).

As a class, polychlorinated biphenyls (PCBs) induced a broad range of biological effects, including carcinogenesis (IARC monographs, 1978), teratogenesis (Watanabe and Sugahara, 1981), and tumor promotion (Ito et al., 1973; Preston et al,, 1981), but not genotoxicity (Shorny, 1982). In addition, some are strong inhibitors of metabolic cooperation (Tsushimoto et al., 1983). The monochlorinated biphenyl, 4-chlorobiphenyl (4-CBP), was tested for comparative purposes. 4-CBP inhibited metabolic cooperation in a dose-dependent manner at moderate (3-20 µg/ml) concentrations (Malcolm et al., 1983). Concentrations greater than 20 µg/ml were toxic. Inhibition of metabolic cooperation by 4-CBP indicates that monochlorinated biphenyls may have tumor-promoting or teratogenic potential.

Solvents

Ethanol (ETOH) and dimethylsulfoxide (DMSO) were evaluated for their effects on metabolic cooperation as they are frequently used to prepare chemicals for testing. ETOH had no effect on metabolic cooperation at concentrations of 5 mg/ml or less (Malcolm et al., 1983), but inhibited metabolic cooperation in a dose-dependent fashion at high (10-20) mg/ml) concentrations. Concentrations greater than 20 mg/ml) were toxic. ETOH is considered to be cocarcinogenic in humans (Wolper, 1979), is perhaps teratogenic in humans (Smith, 1980), and is teratogenic in rats and mice (Chernoff, 1977; Mankes et al., 1982). In addition, ETOH is a surface-active agent and is predicted to have tumor promoting properties for this reason (Boyland, 1983).

DMSO had no effect on metabolic cooperation at concentrations of 2.5 mg/ml or less (Malcolm et al., 1983), but inhibited metabolic cooperation in a dose-related manner between 5 and 25 mg/ml. DMSO is teratogenic in mice and hamsters, but apparently not rats (Juma and Staples, 1967), suggesting species differences. DMSO is not carcinogenic for mouse skin according to one study (Stenback and Garcia, 1975), and, in fact, strongly inhibit the promoting activity of PMA on mouse skin (Slaga et al., 1981). In view of the rapid and complete absorption of DMSO through the intact dermis and other membranes, inhibition of PMA-induced promotion by DMSO may reflect the rapid absorption of dissolved PMA beyond the zone of initiated cells. Moreover, the fact that DMSO inhibits promotion by PMA infers little about the promoting potential of DMSO, as other promoters (e.g., BHT and acetic acid also inhibit promotion by PMA (Slaga *et al.,* 1975; 1981). Were are unaware of any studies in which the promoting potential of DMSO has been evaluated.

SUMMARY

The effects on metabolic cooperation of eighteen chemicals, summarized and discussed in this paper, largely support the general hypothesis that tumor promoters and some teratogens inhibit metabolic cooperation. Consequently, *in vitro* assays designed to assess the effects of chemicals on metabolic cooperation may be predictive of these events. If so, such assays may be useful as screening tests to identify chemicals requiring risk evaluation.

The inhibiting effects on metabolic cooperation by metabolites of phenol, but not phenol, indicates the importance of considering metabolites when testing the hypothesis. The discovery that chemicals enhance was well as inhibit metabolic cooperation requires pharmacological evaluation and suggest the need to understand how chemicals influencing metabolic cooperation differently might interact to produce an effect. Also needed are more specific predictions of those reproductive system effects likely to arise through disturbances of metabolic cooperation so that this aspect of the general hypothesis can be adequately tested. Additional studies are required to better establish the role of metabolic cooperation in biological systems and the biological consequences of effects on this process. In our judgment, results from correlation studies presently support the general hypothesis sufficiently well to justify further investigation into the role of metabolic cooperation as a possible mechanism underlying some apparently different but perhaps related toxicological events.

REFERENCES

Anderson, R. L.; Alden, C. L.; and Merski, J. A.: The effects of nitrilotriacetate on cation disposition and urinary tract toxicity.
Food. Chem. Toxicol., 20:105-122, 1982.

Azarnia, R.; Larsen, W.; and Lowewnstein, W. R.: The membrane junctions in communicating and non-communicating cells, their hybrids and segregants.
Proc. Natl. Acad. Sci. USA, 71:880-884, 1974.

Azarnia, R.; and Loewenstein, W. R.: Parallel correction of cancerous growth and of a generic defect of cell-to-cell communication.
Nature, 241:455-457, 1973.

Azarnia, R.; and Loewenstein, W. R.: Intercellular communication and tissue growth. VIII. A genetic analysis of junctional communication and cancerous growth. *J. Membrane Biol., 34*:1-37, 1977.

Babich, H.: Butylated hydroxytoluene (BHT): A review.
Environm. Res., 29:1-29, 1982.

Bianchi, V.: Nucleotide pool unbalance induced in cultured cells by treatments with different chemicals. *Toxicol., 25*:13-18, 1982.

Birge, W. J.; Black, J. A.; and Bruser, D. M.: Toxicity of organic chemicals to embryo-larval stages of fish. EPA-560/11-79-007, U.S. EPA, Washington, D.C., 1979.

Birge, W. J.; Black, J. A.; and Kuehne, R. A.: Effects of organic compounds on amphibian reproduction. Res. Report 121, Univ. of Kentucky Water Resources Res. Inst., Lexington, 1980.

Blumberg, P. M.; Delclos, K. B.; Dunphy, W. G.; and Jaken, S.: Specific binding of phorbol ester tumor promoters to mouse tissues and cultured cells. In Hecker, E.; et al. (eds.): Carcinogenesis - A Comprehensive Survey, Vol. 7. New York, Raven, 519-535, 1982.

Bora, K. C.: Effects of nitrilotriacetic acid (NTA) on chromosome replication and structure in human cells. Mut. Res., 31:325, 1975.

Borek, C.; Higashino, S.; and Loewenstein, W. R.: Intercellular communication and tissue growth. IV. Conductance of membrane junctions of normal and cancerous cells in culture. J. Membrane Biol., 1:274-293, 1969.

Boutwell, R. K.: The function and mechanism of promoters of carcinogenesis. CRC Crit. Revs. Toxicol., 2:419-443, 1974.

Boutwell, R. K.; and Bosch, D. K.: The tumor-promoting action of phenol and related compounds for mouse skin. Cancer Res., 19:413-424, 1959.

Boyland, E.: Surface active agents as tumor promoters. Environm. Health. Perspect., 50:347-350, 1983.

Bradley, M. O.; Bhuyan, B.; Francis, M. C.; Langenbach, R; Peterson, A.; and Huberman, E.: Mutagenesis by chemical agents in V79 Chinese hamster cells: A review and analysis of the literature. Mut. Res., 87:81-142, 1981.

Braun, A. G.; Buckner, C. A.; Emerson, D. J.; and Nichinson, B. B.: Quantitative correspondence between the in vivo and in vitro activity of teratogenic agents. Proc. Natl. Acad. Sci. USA, 79:2056-2060, 1982.

Chamberlain, M.: The influence of mineral dusts on metabolic cooperation between mammalian cells in tissue culture. Carcinogenesis, 3:337-338, 1982.

Chernoff, G.: The fetal alcohol syndrome in mice: An animal model. Teratology, 15:223-230, 1977.

Cox, R.P. (ed.): Cell Communication. New York, J. Wiley & Sons, Inc., 1974.

DeMello, W. C. (ed.): Intercellular Communication. New York, Plenum, 1977.

Diwan, B.; Ward, J. M.; Colburn, N.; Spanger, F.; Creasia, D.; Lynch, P.; and Rice, J. M.: Promoting effects of di(2-ethylhexyl) phthalate in mouse liver, skin and JB-6 epithelial cells. Proc. Am. Assoc. Cancer Res., 24:105, 1983.

Djurhuus, R.; and Lillehaug, J. R.: Butylated hydroxytoluene: Tumor-promoting activity in an *in vitro* two-stage carcinogenesis assay. Bull. Environm. Contam. Toxicol., 29:115-120, 1982.

Dorman, B. H.; and Boreiko, C. J.: Limiting factors of the V79 cell metabolic cooperation assay for tumor promoters. Carcinogenesis, 4:873-877, 1983.

Dunkel, V. C.; and Simon, V. F.: Mutagenic activity of chemicals previously tested for carcinogenicity in the National Cancer Institute Bioassay Program.

In Monsanto, R; Bartsch, H.; and Tomatis, L. (eds.): *Molecular and Cellular Aspects of Carcinogen Screening Tests.* IARC Scientific Pub. 27. Lyon, WHO, 283-302, 1980.

Enomoto, T.; Saski, Y.; Shiba, Y.; Kanno, Y.; and Yamasaki, H.: Tumor promoters cause a rapid and reversible inhibition of the formation and maintenance of electrical coupling in culture. *Proc. Natl. Acad. Sci. USA,* 78:5628-5632, 1981.

Epstein, S. S.; Arnold E.,; Andrea, J.; Bass, W; and Bishop, Y.: Detection of chemical mutagens by the dominant lethal assay in the mouse. *Toxicol. Appl. Pharmacol.,* 23:288-325, 1975.

Feldman, J.; Gilula, N. B.; and Pitts, J. D. (eds.): Intercellular Junctions and Synapses. London, Chapman and Hall, 1979.

Ferm V. H.: Congenital malformations induced by dimethylsulfoxide in the golden hamster. *J. Embryol. Exp. Morphol.,* 16:49-54, 1966.

Friedman, E. A.; and Steinberg, M.: Disrupted communication between late-stage premalignant human colon epithelial cells by 12-0-tetradecanoylphorbol-13-acetate. *Cancer Res.,* 42:5096-5105, 1982.

Gelboin, H.V.: Benzo(a)pyrene metabolism, activation and carcinogenesis: Role and regulation of mixed-function oxidases and related enzymes. Physiol. Revs., 60:*1107-1166, 1980.*

Goyer, R. A.; Falk, H. L.; Hogan, M.; Feldman, D. D.; and Richter, W.: Renal tumors in rats given trisodium nitrilotriacetate acid in drinking water for 2 years. *J. Natl. Cancer Inst.,* 66:869-880, 1981.

Griepp, E. B.; and Revel, J.-P.: Gap junctions in development. In DeMello, W. C. (ed.): *Intercellular Communication.* New York, Plenum, 1-32, 1977.

Hartman, T. G.; and Rosen, J. D.: Inhibition of metabolic cooperation by cigarette smoke condensate and its fractions in V79 Chinese hamster lung fibroblasts. *Proc. Natl. Acad. Sci. USA, 80:*5305-5309, 1983.

Hicks, R. M.: Promotion in bladder cancer. In Hecker, E.; et al. (eds.): Carcinogenesis - A Comprehensive Survey, Vol. 7. New York, Raven, 139-153, 1982.

Hooper, M. L.: Metabolic cooperation between mammalian cells in culture. *Biochemica et Biophysica Acta,* 651:85-103, 1982.

IARC monographs on the evaluation of the carcinogenic risk of chemicals to humans. Vol. 18. Polychlorinated and polybrominated biphenyls. Lyon, WHO, 43-103, 1978.

IARC monographs on the evaluation of the carcinogenic risk of chemicals to humans. Vol. 22: Some non-nutritive sweetening agents. Lyon, WHO, 90, 1980.

IARC monographs on the evaluation of the carcinogenic risks of chemicals to humans. Vol. 29. Some industrial chemicals and dyestuffs. Lyon, WHO, 269-294, 1982.

Ito, N.; Nagasaki, H.; Arai, M.; Makiura, S.; Sugihara, S.; and Hirao, K.: Histopathologic studies on liver tumorigenesis induced in mice by technical polychlorinated biphenyls and its promoting effect on liver tumors induced by benzene hexachloride. *J. Natl. Cancer Inst.,* 51:1637-1646, 1973.

Juma, M. B.; and Staples, R. E.: Effect of maternal administration of dimethyl sulfoxide on the development of rat fetuses.
Proc. Soc. Exp. Biol. Med., 125:567-569, 1967.

Kinsella, A. R.: Elimination of metabolic cooperation and the induction of sister chromatid exchanges are not properties common to all promoting or cocarcinogenic agents. *Carcinogenesis,* 3:499-503, 1982.

Korolkovas, A.: *Essentials of Molecular Pharmacology.* New York, John Wiley & Sons, Inc., 1-11, 1970.

Kramers, P. G. N.: Mutagenicity studies with nitrolotriacetic acid (NTA) and citrex S-5 in Drosophila. *Mut. Res.,* 40:277-280, 1976.

Lloyd, R. E.; Blalock, J. E.; and Stanton, G. J.: Cell-to-cell transfer of interferon-induced antiproliferative activity. *Science,* 221:953-955, 1983.

Loewenstein, W. R.: Junctional intercellular communication and the control of growth. *Biochem. Biophys Acta,* 560:1-65, 1979.

Loewenstein, W. R.: Junctional cell-to-cell communication and growth control. *Annals New York Acad. Sci.,* 339:39-45, 1980.

Loewenstein, W. R.: Junctional intercellular communciation: The cell-to-cell membrane channel. *Physiol. Revs.,* 61:829-913, 1981.

Malcolm, A. R.; Mills, L. J.; and McKenna, E. J.: Inhibition of metabolic cooperation between Chinese hamster V79 cells by tumor promoters and other chemicals. In Williams, G. M.; Dunkel, V. C.; and Ray, V. A. (eds.): *Cellular Systems for Toxicity Testing. Annals New York Acad. Sci.,* 407 :448-450, 1983.

Mankes, R. F.; Rosenblum, I.; Benitz, K. F.; LeFevre, R.; and Abraham, R.: Teratogenic and reproductive effects of ethanol in Long-Evans rats.
J. Toxicol. Environm. Health, 10:267-276, 1982.

Minor, J. L.; and Becker, B. A.: A comparison of the teratogenic properties of sodium salicylate, sodium benzoate, and phenol.
Toxicol. Appl. Pharmacol., 19:373, 1971.

Murray, A. W.; and Fitzgerald, O. J.: Tumor promoters inhibit metabolic cooperation in cocultures of epidermal and 3T3 cells.
Biochem. Biophys. Res. Commun., 91:395-401, 1979.

Peraino, C.; Fry, R. J. M.; Stadtfeldt, E.; and Christopher, J. P.: Enhancing effects of phenobarbital and butylated hydroxytoluene on 2-acetylaminofluorene-induced hepatic tumorigenesis in the rat.
Food Cosmet. Toxicol., 15:93-96, 1977.

Pitts, J. D.; and Finbow, M. E.: Junctional permeability and its consequences. In DeMello, W. C. (ed.): *Intercellular Communication.* New York, Plenum, 61-86, 1977.

Pitts, J. D.: Role of junctional communication in animal tissues. *In Vitro,* 1049-1056, 1980.

Potter, V. R.: Alternative hypothesis for the role of promotion in chemical carcinogenssis. *Environm. Health Perspect., 50*:139-148, 1983.

Potter, V. R.: Cancer as a problem in intercellular communication: Regulation by growth-inhibiting factors (chalones). Prog. Nucelic Acid Res. Molec. Biol., 29:161-173, 1983.

Prescott, D. M.: Reproduction of Eukaryotic Cells. New York, Academic Press, 107-118, 1976.

Preston, B. D.; Van Miller, J. P.; Moore, R. W.; and Allen, J. R.: Promoting effects of polychlorinated biphenyls (arochlor 1254) and polychlorinated dibenzofuran-free arochlor 1254 on dimethylnitrosamine-induced tumorigenesis in the rat. *J. Natl. Cancer Inst., 66*:509-515, 1981.

Schoeny, R.: Mutagenicity testing of chlorinated biphenyls and chlorinated dibenzofurans. *Mut. Res., 101*:45-56, 1982.

Sheridan, J. D.: Cell coupling and cell communication during embryogenesis. In Poste, G.; and Nicholson, G. L. (eds.): *The Cell Surface in Animal Embryogenesis and Development.* New York, Elsevier-North Holland, 409-447, 1977.

Shiota, K.; and Nishimura, H.: Teratogenicity of di-(2-ethylhexyl) phthalate (DEHP) and di-n-butyl phthalate (DBP) in mice. *Environm. Health Perspect., 45*:65-70, 1982.

Shum, S.; Jensen, N. M.; and Nebert, D. W.: the murine Ah locus: *in utero* toxicity and teratogenesis associated with genetic differences in benzo(a)pyrene metabolism. *Teratology, 20*:365-376, 1979.

Slaga, T. J.; Bowden, G. T.; and Boutwell, R. K.: Acetic acid, a potent stimulator of mouse skin epidermal macromolecular synthesis and hyperplasia but with weak tumor-promoting ability. *J. Natl. Cancer Inst., 55*:983-987, 1975.

Slaga, T. J.; Fischer, S. M.; Weeks, C. E.; and Klein-Szanto, A. J. P.: Cellular and biochemical mechanisms of mouse skin tumor promoters. *Rev. Biochem. Toxicol., 3*:231-281, 1981.

Smith, D.: Alcohol effects on the fetus. In Schwartz, R.,; and Yaffe, S. (eds.): *Drug and Chemical Risks to the Fetus and Newborn.* New York, A. R. Liss, 73-82, 1980.

Staples, R. E.; and Pecharo, M. M.: Species specificity in DMSO teratology. *Teratology, 8*:238, 1966.

Stenback, F.; and Garcia, H.: Studies on the modifying effect of dimethylsulfoxide and other chemicals on experimental skin tumor induction. *Annals New York Acad. Sci., 243*:209-227, 1975.

Subak-Sharpe, H.; Burk, R. R.; and Pitts, J. D.: Metabolic cooperation by cell-to-cell transfer between genetically different mammalian cells in tissue culture. *Heredity, 21*:342-343, 1966.

Subak-Sharpe, H.; Burk, R. R.; and Pitts, J. D.: Metabolic cooperation between biochemically marked mammalian cells in tissue culture. *J. Cell Sci., 4*:353-367, 1969.

Telang, S.; Tong, C.; and Williams, G. M.: Epigenetic membrane effects of a possible tumor promoting type on cultured liver cells by the non-genotoxic organochlorine pesticides chlordane and heptachlor. *Carcinogenesis,* *3*:1175-1178, 1982.

Trosko, J. E.; Chang, C. C.; and Metzloff, M.: The role of inhibited cell-cell communication in teratogenesis. *Teratogenesis, Carcinogenesis, and Mutagenesis,* 2:31-45, 1982.

Trosko, J. E.; Dawson, B.; Yotti, L. P.; and Chang, C. C.: Saccharrin may act as a tumor promoter by inhibiting metabolic cooperation between cells. *Nature,* *285*:109-110, 1980.

Trosko, J. E.; Jone, C.; and Chang, C. C.: The role of tumor promoters on phenotypic alternations affecting intercellular communication and tumorigenesis. In Williams, G. M.; Dunkel, V. C.; and Ray, V. A. (eds.): *Cellular Systems for Toxicity Testing. Annals New York Acad. Sci.,* *407*:316-327, 1983.

Trosko, J. E.; Yotti, L. P.; Dawson, B.; and Chang, C. C.: In vitro assay for tumor promoters. In Stich, H. F.; and San, R. H. C. (eds.): *Short-Term Tests for Chemical Carcinogens.* New York, Springer-Verlag, 420-427, 1981.

Trosko, J. E.; Yotti, L. P.; Warren, S. T.; Tsushimoto, G.; and Chang, C. C.: Inhibition of cell-cell communication by tumor promoters. In Hecker, E.; et al. (eds.): *Carcinogenesis - A Comprehensive Survey,* Vol. 7. New York, Raven, 565-585, 1982.

Tsushimoto, G.; Asano, S.; Trosko, J. E.; and Chang, C. C.: Inhibition of intercellular communication by various congeners of polybrominated biphenyl and polychlorinated biphenyl. In D'Imitri, F.; and Kamrin, M. (eds.): *PCB's: Human and Environmental Hazards.* Ann Arbor, Ann Arbor Sci. Publs., 241-252, 1983.

Van Duuren, B. L.: Tumor-promoting and cocarcinogenic agents in chemical carcinogenesis. In Searle, C. E.; (ed.): Chemical Carcinogens. Washington, D. C., ACS Monograph, 173, 24-51, 1976.

Van Duuren, B. L.; Orris, L.; and Arroyo, E.: Tumor-Enhancing activity of the active principles of *Croton tiglium L. Nature,* *200*:1115-1116, 1963.

Van Duuren, B. L.; Sivak, A.; Katz, C.; and Melchionne, S.: Cigarette smoke carcinogenesis: Importance of tumor promoters. *J. Natl. Cancer. Inst.,* *47*:235-240, 1971.

Verma, A. K.; Slaga, T. J.; Wertz, P. W.; Mueller, G. C.; and Boutwell, R. K.: Inhibition of skin tumor promotion by retinoic acid and its metabolite 5,6-epoxyretinoic acid. *Cancer Res,,* *40*:2367-2371, 1980.

Ward, J. M.; Rice, J. M.; Creasia, D.; Lynch, P.; and Riggs, C.: Dissimilar patterns of promotion by di(2-ethylhyxyl) phthalate and phenobarbital of hepatocellular neoplasia initiated by diethylnitrosamine in B6C3F1 mice. *Carcinogensis,* *4*:1021-1029, 1983.

Watanabe, M.; and Sugahara, T.: Experimental formation of cleff palate in mice with polychlorinated biphenyls. *Toxicol.,* *19*:49-53, 1981.

Weiner, E. C.; and Loewenstein, W. R.: correction of cell-cell communication defect by introduction of a protein kinase into mutant cells. *Nature,* *305*:433-435, 1983.

Williams, G. M.: Epigenetic effects of liver tumor promoters and implications for health effects. Environm. *Health Perspect., 50*:177-183, 1983.

Wilson, J. G.: Environmental chemicals. In Wilson, J. G.; and Fraser, F. C. (eds.): *Handbook of Teratology.* Vol. 1. New York, Plenum, 357-385, 1977.

Witschi, H. P.: Promotion of lung tumors in mice. *Environm. Health Perspect., 50*:267-273, 1983.

Wolper, L.: Gap junctions; channels of communication in development. In Feldman, J.; Gilula, N. B.; and Pitts, J. D. (eds.): *Intercellular Junctions and Synapses.* London, Chapman and Hall, 81-96, 1979.

Yotti, L. P.; Chang, C. C. and Trosko, J. E.: Elimination of metabolic cooperation in Chinese hamster cells by a tumor promoter. *Science, 206*:1089-1091, 1979.

Use of Formalin-Treated Cells in the DNA-Cell Binding Assay for Genotoxic and Carcinogenetic Chemicals

H. Kubinski, Z. O. Kubinski, and J. Shahidi

University of Wisconsin School of Medicine, Madison, Wisconsin 53706

Our earlier observations indicate that the DNA-cell binding (DCB) assay predicts the chemical's potential to induce neoplasia in humans and in experimental animals (Kubinski et al. 1981). This assay is based on the observation that isolated radioactive DNA binds *in vivo* to proteins in the presence of activated carcinogens. Such proteins include those present on the surface of mammalian cells or gram-negative bacteria. The percentage of correct identifications (carcinogens vs. non-carcinogens) was found to be somewhere between 86 and 96%, dependent on the quality of available data on carcinogenic potential of the chemical studied. Although this system seems to be superior in many respects to other methods of quick detection of carcinogens, several aspects of the assay could be further improved. For example, the cells used in the original protocol had to be grown every day and used fresh. However, preparation of large batches of cells well in advance would be clearly advantageous, especially if such cells were stable for a considerable period of time. For this reason, we investigated the possibility that bacteria stabilized with formaldehyde may be useful for this test. The results of our preliminary experiments indicated that *Escherichia coli* cells treated with formaldehyde are at least as good as the non-treated cells. In many cases, the amounts of radioactively labeled DNA associated with cell sediment in the presence of carcinogens are higher than in untreated controls, thus increasing the changes of detection of only marginally active genotoxic chemicals.

MATERIALS AND METHODS

Cells

Escherichia coli cells were grown overnight in nutrient broth and then collected by centrifugation. The sediment was washed twice with TSM buffer (10 mM Tris-HCl, pH 7.2; 0.14M NaCl; 2 mM $MgSO_4$) and resuspended in the same buffer.

Radioactive DNA

Our previous experiments indicated than DNA from either bacterial or eucariotic sources can be used for the purpose of testing. In present experiments, Escherichia coli cells were labeled with radioactive phosphorus (^{32}P) for at least 10 generations. DNA was then extracted by the modified technique of Marmur (Kubinski et al., 1966).

DCB Assay

The technique has been described earlier (Kubinski et al., 1981). The cells were mixed with the radioactive nucleic acid and with the tested chemical and incubated at 37°C. At 0 and 60 minutes samples were withdrawn, washed several times with TSM, and the amount of radioactivity associated with the bacterial sediment was determined and compared with the total amount of radioactivity known to be present in the sample. Some carcinogenic chemicals are known to increase the DNA binding only in the presence of lysozyme. Thus, this protein was routinely added to a set of tubes during the assay (120 µg/ml). Another set of tubes contained liver extract prepared as described by Ames and his collaborators (Ames et al., 1973) for the activation of non-ultimate carcinogenic chemicals (approximately 100 µg of membrane protein/ml).

RESULTS

Our experiments indicate that in the case of a simple alkylating agent, betapropiolactone, the 1% formalin-treated cells were superior to their untreated counterparts (Table 1): more radioactivity was found associated with cellular sediment in the presence of the tested carcinogen and less in control samples and samples containing liver extract. The 1% concentration of 39-40% formalin solution was subsequently used for our assays. We do not know whether this particular concentration of formaldehyde is indeed the optimal one for all kinds of chemicals which we tested.

TABLE 1

EFFECTS OF FORMALIN ON ESCHERICHIA COLI CELLS AS INDICATORS IN DCB TEST; IN THE PRESENCE AND IN THE ABSENCE OF 10 uM BETAPROPIOLACTONE (BPL).

Formalin Concentration, %*	BPL	+ Lysozyme	+ Liver Extract**	% Radioactivity Retained
0	—	—	—	0.48
0	—	+	—	1.39
0	—	—	+	13.40
0	+	—	—	6.89
0.1	—	—	—	0.06
0.1	—	+	—	0.77
0.1	—	—	+	2.99
0.1	+	—	—	38.60
1	—	—	—	0.04
1	—	+	—	0.48
1	—	—	+	0.86
1	+	—	—	80.51
2	—	—	—	0.11
2	—	+	—	0.65

TABLE 1 (continued)

Formalin Concentration, %*	BPL	+ Lysozyme	+ Liver Extract**	% Radioactivity Retained
2	—	—	—	1.01
2	+	—	—	67.08
5	—	—	—	17.53
5	—	+	—	6.40
5	—	—	+	5.42
5	—	—	—	40.07

*Overnight culture, washed twice in TSM, concentrated 10x and resuspended in TSM. Incubated with the indicated concentration of formalin (39-40% formaldehyde; analytical grade) for 15 minutes at 37°C.

**Freshly prepared.

In most experiments summarized in Table 2, the formalin-treated cells appeared to be either superior or at least as good as the cells which were not treated with this chemical. A few exceptions to this rule demonstrate that at some rather extreme concentrations of tested chemicals the dose-response of the assay system becomes non-linear. A single experiment seems to indicate that the formalin-treated cells can better distinguish between carcinogenic chemicals and compounds which are mutagenic but not carcinogenic (or weakly carcinogenic), such as provflavine. Further studies are required to confirm this preliminary observation.

TABLE 2

EFFECT OF VARIOUS CHEMICAL ON DNA BINDING TO ESCHERICHIA COLI CELLS TREATED AND NOT TREATED WITH 1% FORMALIN (15 MINUTES, 37°C)

Chemical	Concentration	Formalin		+ Lysozyme	+ LE*
1,3 propane-sultone	10 uM	—	8.9	ND**	ND
"	"	+	21.9	ND	ND
Formaldehyde	0.02%	—	3.0	39.7	69.2
"	"	+	53.0	61.8	47.4
1-methyl-3-nitro-1-nitrosoguanidine (MNNG)	50 uM	—	1.5	1.9	0.0
"	"	+	1.9	11.3	10.9
"	250 uM	—	1.0	3.3	0.0
"	"	+	6.0	14.5	16.7
2-aminonaphthalene	50 uM	—	0.0	ND	6.7
"	"	+	0.0	ND	7.4
2-acetylaminofluorene	30 uM	—	0.7	ND	3.5
"	"	+	0.0	ND	10.5
"	150 uM	—	2.1	ND	7.5
"	"	+	1.1	ND	22.2
Adriamycin	50 uM	—	6.7	42.3	18.7
"	"	+	22.3	49.3	20.1
"	250 uM	—	21.0	44.1	22.2
"	"	+	29.7	102.1	29.9
5-fluorouracil	50 uM	—	0.0	0.1	0.0
"	"	+	0.8	0.0	0.3
"	250 uM	—	0.2	0.1	0.7
"	"	+	0.1	0.4	0.0
Proflavine	50 uM	—	2.0	4.2	2.3
"	"	+	0.5	0.5	0.2

TABLE 2 (continued)

Chemical	Concentration	Formalin	+ Lysozyme		+ LE*
"	250 uM	—	7.3	13.9	10.0
"	"	+	2.8	1.0	1.1
8-hydroxyquinoline	50 uM	—	0.0	1.8	1.0
"	"	+	0.1	1.2	7.5
"	500 uM	—	1.0	2.1	3.5
"	"	+	1.1	4.7	11.7
Acridine orange	30uM	—	6.6	6.0	2.9
"	"	+	4.9	2.2	2.6
"	300 uM	—	33.0	35.9	28.7
"	"	+	43.0	57.0	24.3
BeSO4	1 mM	—	83.6	96.9	74.5
"	"	+	3.9	2.8	59.6
"	5 mM	—	101.0	99.8	87.3
"	"	+	100.1	10.2	80.4
CrCl2	0.1 mM	—	83.8	63.0	49.9
"	"	+	73.2	103.8	32.0
"	0.5 mM	—	76.2	29.8	66.2
"	"	+	99.1	77.5	40.3

*LE: liver extract
**ND: not determined

From the separate experiments (not shown) we have learned that such properties of the formalin-treated cells as the ability to bind larger amounts of radioactive DNA in the presence of carcinogenic and genotoxic chemicals and the ability to bind less DNA in their absence remains unchanged even after 20 days of storage in TSM buffer at +4°C.

DISCUSSION

We believe that the DNA-cell binding (DCB) assay system which we described earlier may be useful for the detection of carcinogenic and genotoxic chemicals for several reasons. Firstly, this assay quantitizes chemical reactions between biologically important cellular macromolecules. A large body of experimental evidence indicates that formation of macromolecular complexes is the first step in the development of tumors in humans and in experimental animals (Morin *et al.*, 1977). Secondly, the available information indicates that the assay has a good record of predicting the carcinogenic potential of chemicals, including mixtures of chemicals (see, for example, Morin and Kubinski, 1978; Athas *et al.*, 1979; Kubinski *et al.*, 1982). Thirdly, it is rapid, inexpensive and not falsifiable by common laboratory errors. Finally, there are several ways to improve our present assay protocol and increase the sensitivity and accuracy. Treatment of the indicator cells with formaldehyde seems to be one of the ways to accomplish this task. We recommend that formalin-treated bacterial cells should be used in DCB assay either in parallel to or instead of the untreated bacteria.

REFERENCES

Ames, B. N.; Durston, W. E.; Yamasaki, E., and Lee, F. D.: Carcinogens are mutagens: a simple test system combing liver homogenates for activation and bacteria for detection. *Proc. Natl. Acad. Sci.*, 70:2231-2235, 1973.

Athas, W. F.; Gutzke, G. E.; Kubinski, Z. O., and Kubinski, H.: In vitro studies on the carcinogenic potential of orthodontic bonding materials. *Ecotoxicol. Environ. Saf., 3*:401-410, 1979.

Kubinski, H.; Gutzke, G. E., and Kubinski, Z. O.: DNA-cell binding (DCB) assay for suspected carcinogens and mutagens. *Mutation Res., 89*:95-136, 1981.

Kubinski, H.; Kubinski, Z. O., and Javid, M.: Suspected cancer-causing agents in the hospital environment. *Ecotoxicol. Environ. Saf., 6*:9-18, 1982.

Kubinski, H.; Kubinski, Z. O., and Szybalski, W.: Patterns of Interaction between polyribonucleotides and individual DNA strands derived from several vetebrates, bacteria and bacteriophages. *J. Mol. Biol., 20*:313-319, 1966.

Morin, N. C., and Kubinski, H.: Potential toxicity of materials used for home insulation. *Ecotoxicol. Environ. Saf., 2*:133-141, 1978.

Morin, N. C.; Zeldin, P. E.; Kubinski, Z. O.; Bhattacharya, P. K, and Kubinski, H.: Macromolecular complexes produced by chemical carinogens and ultraviolet radiation. *Cancer Res., 37*, 3802-3814, 1977.

Discussion

Al Li: Dr. McCormick, with regard to the human cell system, you mentioned that the cells do not have the ability to metabolize xenobiotics. How would you foresee incorporating an exogenous metabolic activation system with your human cells to constitute a relevant system?

Justin McCormick: Well, we have incorporated metabolic activation using human tumor cells. We have various human tumor cell lines which have various types of metabolic activation abilities. We have some lines that will do very well with hydrocarbons and some lines that will do well with aromatic amines and some will do well with alkylating agents. Such assays work but they're clumsy assays in our terms in the sense that one must use fairly long periods of time to co-incubate the cells by comparison of what you do when you use a direct-acting agent with a time of incubation on the order of an hour or two. If you have to, when you're using metabolic activation systems of this sort you have to incubate the cells together for 48 to 72 hours. If you're using repair positive cells then you have a dynamic process in which the adducts are being put under the DNA and taken off the DNA and it's hard to know where to start an experiment. How to do the actual measurements and do very refine kind of measurements of adducts present and the relationship of adducts to particular types of things. So, it depends precisely on what your interests are and it certainly can be done. Our interests have been more in modeling systems where one could use a very short pulse chemical that one added like one does radiation studies, and then begin to study at that point and determine precisely what happens to the cells. So we've tended not to use activations if we could get around it by using chemically synthesized direct-acting chemicals. But for other people's studies, for different endpoints that's a very relevant point and one can certainly couple them. There's no more problem in doing that with human cells than there is with any rodent cell or other cell system. You can also use S9 fractions.

Bob Naismith: I think one of the take home messages at least that I see based on some of the data you've presented at this point is that maybe we're doing well with mutation as an endpoint. Using transformation as an endpoint in short term testing may be premature and maybe not necessary.

Justin McCormick: Let me repeat your question since those in the other room may not have heard it. Comment was whether we may not be doing just as well looking at mutations rather than moving on to transformation assay. Since the data I presented, showed a parallel between thioguanine resistance and mutation and anchorage independence in all cases we've looked at so far. What I didn't say when I presented the data this morning is if I had showed you ouabain resistance data or diptheria toxin resistance data the induction of that in human cells, it would not have paralleled anchorage independence data. Thioguanine resistance is a mutational marker, its a forward mutational marker that measures all types of mutation simultaneously and anchorage independence closely parallels that in our hands so far, in everything that we've done. But, if you chose other markers it would not be so and that's because the other types of markers only pick up particular types of mutant classes as has been discussed by a number of workers in the literature. Now what we don't know is we don't know what the other steps to carcinogenesis are and what types of mutational markers will reflect those adequately but since thioguanine seems to reflect the broadest category of mutational markers, presumably that's in general an adequate category but one would have to be a little hesitant to comment upon that because the rest of the process is relatively unknown as you well know. And second of all, we don't really know the transformation as measured in some assays is really equivalent to mutations. There are certainly mutational-transformational assays in those same cells and that suggests that there are steps in transformation that are not adequately modeled by mutational type assays, at least in those cells of interest. It's hard to know what to make of those at the moment I think because we don't understand in general the basis of many transformation assays. We're hardput to know how to evaluate them I think.

Dennis Flaherty: I have a question for Dr. Albertini. The fact that your lymphocyte assay is really picking up helper T lymphocytes and you're picking up more of those mutational events in that subpopulation. Do you have any evidence to indicate that those particular helper cells which you do pick up are fully functional or whether they are functionally impaired as a consequence of mutation event?

Albertini: Again, to repeat, the question was that in the looking at the surface or the functional chracteristics of the mutants there appear to be more in the T4 class or helpers than were in the non-sensitized clones. That really is what we initially thought, but what I just showed is that the T4's clone better than the T8's but if you look at the non-selective clones, that is those that are without 6-thioguanine resistance, the 4:8 ratio is about the same as is in the 4:8 ratio of those that we pick up. Now we've only looked at 20 or 30 clones so far so statistically I think that's going to be the case. On the other hand, we do pick up more of the undifferentiated, that's the 4H's which either may be the poisson doublet or they may be true 4A's which do exist and that we have to look at. We know nothing about the functional characteristics at the present time. I do think though that looking at the 0^6-methyl transferase is going to be possible now in cloned cells. It is my understanding that some of the lymphocyte work initially is that there is really a difference in B and T cells now I think we can look at clonal heterogeneity of the cell. Basically, I don't have functional answers and we really don't have the answer yet whether there is heterogeneity or homogeneity amongst the cell types for mutability.

Wil Ridley: I have a question for Dr. Butterworth. In attempting to distinguish between agents that act by a direct genetic mechanism as opposed to those that act by some non-genetic mechanism. One marker you might use would be replication and I was wondering if in your hepatocyte system you looked at agents like for, example TCDD dioxin, which apparently don't interact directly with DNA and wouldn't increase UDS but might affect replication. Could this approach be used to distinguish between agents that act by genetic and non-genetic mechanisms.

Butterworth: Well, we think that this is a valuable way to go about it. The compounds that we have looked at so far that appear to induce replication but not repair are carbon tetrachloride and chloroform. We've looked at other agents like DEHP which looks like it induces a very slight amount of replication and we see no DNA repair whatsoever. We're currently in the process of doing TCDD but I think that this is a very nice way of distinguishing between those two types of carcinogens.

Salvatore Biscardi: I'm with the Environmental Protection Agency in the Office of Pesticides Programs. Quite recently we did a number of oncogenicity studies where we had negative results. The negative results of oncogenicity because the tumors we get in the treated groups do not exceed significantly with the instances of the control animals. However, strangely enough with all the kind of tumors that we have, we found the same tumors you see in the control groups. What we say is the chemical in that particular situation statistically is not significant and I was wondering whether the tumors observed were compound related or not compound related. I would like to present this question to Dr. Preston.

Preston: I don't think that I can provide a very satisfactory answer to the question. I think that the short term, all the short term human subjects or cell culture subjects at this point in time are giving you just a plus and minus answer, the mutagenicity test, the chromosome aberrations and the mutations. So if you want to use that information subsequently when you have observed tumors in a situation, I think that there is a time gap in here which makes it very difficult to relate observations that are essentially immediatey induced events which all the short term tests are with some type of subsequent events. So I don't know of much help except telling you that this agent under these sets of circumstances has the potential to produce a specific end point which in short term cultures could go as far as cell transformation. I'm a little dubious about cell transformation assays, by the way. Taking the like some of the radiation studies where you get the same frequency of transformants irrespective of the dilutions that you do on the cultures which is a rather misleading observation and until that is sorted out I think the transformation assay is not a predictive assay and not very easy to do. So I don't think we can help out. That's always a problem in germ cell studies where you're not looking at an induced event. When you're looking at treatment of a germ cell stage you're always analyzing it somewhere further down th road. Either in spomatocytes or in F1 generation. It's always very difficult where you're trying to predict subsequent events or you're measuring subsequent events trying to predict what frequencies of the particular endpoint you are interested in. We can tell you what the induced frequencies are but we can't predict for you what recovered frequencies are likely to be.

Metabolic and Pharmacokinetic Approaches

Section Editor: A. G. E. Wilson

ns in Toxicity Testing and Their
Application in Human Risk Assessment, edited by
A. P. Li. Raven Press, New York © 1985.

Significance of Metabolism Studies in Toxicity Testing and Risk Assessment

Rick G. Schnellmann and I. Glenn Sipes

Department of Pharmacology and Toxicology, College of Pharmacy, University of Arizona, Tucson, Arizona 85721

During the past thirty years significant progress has been made in understanding the importance of metabolism in the toxicity produced by chemicals foreign to the body. Until recently metabolism was viewed mainly as a detoxification process, since metabolism of most foreign chemicals resulted in the formation of more water soluble metabolites; forms of the chemical that were more readily excreted. Thus, the process of biotransformation is a key event in determining the rate of elimination of lipophilic foreign chemicals. Those lipophilic chemicals that are resistant to metabolism will tend to accumulate in the body with continued exposure. Ultimately, this accumulation may lead to the expression of toxicity.

Because of the pioneering work of the Millers' and Brodie and his colleagues, it is now widely recognized that biotransformation is also involved in the toxification of foreign chemicals. Biotransformation may result in the production of a toxicologically or pharmacologically active metabolite. It may also result in the formation of reactive intermediates of selected chemicals. The interaction of these reactive intermediates with critical cellular macromolecules is thought to initiate the events that ultimately lead to tissue injury and cell death or to permanent genomic alternations that can ultimately be expressed as cancer. Thus, it is important to understand the process of biotransformation of chemicals and how it relates to their toxic potential. This process may involve the lack of biotransformation of particular lipophilic chemicals, which would allow one to predict bioaccumulation of these chemicals, if other means of elimination are lacking. For those chemicals that are metabolized, it is important to know the pathways, mechanisms, rates of metabolism, and the subsequent disposition of the metabolites. Knowledge of these parameters may permit one to predict if particular pathways may become saturated, if reactive intermediates are produced, and the nature of the toxicity that may result.

Obtaining such knowledge on the biotransformation of chemicals is relatively straightforward. A voluminous amount of information is available concerning the various enzymes systems involved in biotransformation and the nature of many of the metabolites that are produced. However, problems arise when one wants to extrapolate data generated in animal systems to the human situation. Because of the key role of metabolism in toxicity, there is a need to develop systems that will permit us to determine how humans biotransform chemicals.

A number of systems to study biotransformation are available. These include whole animal studies, isolated perfused organs, isolated cells and cells in culture, tissue slices, tissue homogenates, subcellular fractions and isolated enzymes. *In vivo* experiments and isolated perfused organs are not usually viable options for human studies. Isolated cells and tissue slices have potential, but they also have limitations, including availablity on a routine basis, viablity and maintenance of cellular integrity and biotransformation enzymes. However, during the past three years, considerable progress has been made in maintaining the concentration and activity of cytochrome P-450, and the concentration of glutathione in these preparations. Therefore, preparations are available that maintain the normal intracellular distribution of the various enzyme systems involved in biotransformation. Since the integration of these systems is important in the overall biotransformation of a chemical, use of isolated cells and tissue slices will undoubtedly become important tools for assessing biotransformation of chemicals in humans.

During the past two years we have studied the metabolism of environmental contaminants using subcellular fractions obtained from human livers. These systems are useful because they can identify the sites(s) of metabolism, the nature of the metabolites, and the rates of metabolism. Also, the preparations are stable for prolonged periods when maintained at -70° or less. Data obtained using this human system can then be compared to identical preparations from various animal species. Once the relationship between these *in vitro* animal preparations and *in vivo* animal data is determined, it is our belief that using the *in vitro* human data and the relationship between the *in vitro* and *in vivo* animal data, the most appropriate animal model to predict the disposition and the potential toxicity in humans can be determined.

To test the concept of *in vitro/in vivo* extrapolation, we have studied the metabolism of polychlorinated biphenyls (PCBs) by human liver microsomes and compared these results to those obtained in other species. In addition, we have extrapolated our results to those obtained in epidemiological studies of individuals exposed to PCBs.

PCBs were chosen because 1) of their environmental and toxicological relevance, 2) of their epidemiological data in humans, 3) of the pharmacokinetic data base in rodents, 4) of the species variation in the rates and routes of biotransformation, 5) their structure allows for many similar cogeners which may help to unravel the reasons for the species differences, and 6) essentially only metabolites are excreted (1-6).

The degree of biotransformation of PCBs depends on three factors. The first factor is the number of chlorines on the phenyl rings. For example, Matthews and Anderson (7) found that the excretion half-life in rats of four PCBs with 1, 2, 5, and 6 chlorines increased as the number of chlorines increased (Figure 1). This decreased rate of excretion with increasing chlorination was directly related to the decreased metabolism of the more highly chlorinated congeners. The second factor is the position of the chlorines on the phenyl rings. For example, Sipes *et al.,* (8) found that the dog eliminated four hexachlorobiphenyls (HCB) at different rates depending on the positions of the chlorines (Table 1). In this case, as the number of unsubstituted meta-position increased or the number of adjacent unsubstituted carbon atoms increased, the percent of the dose eliminated within three days increased. Again, the rate of elimination was directly related to the degree of metabolism. Finally, the degree of biotransformation depends on the animal species (Table 2). For example, the dog and rat eliminated 50% of a dose of 2,2',3,3',6,6'-hexachlorobiphenyl (236-HCB) in one day, while the monkey eliminated the same amount in six days. In contrast, the dog eliminated 50% of a dose of

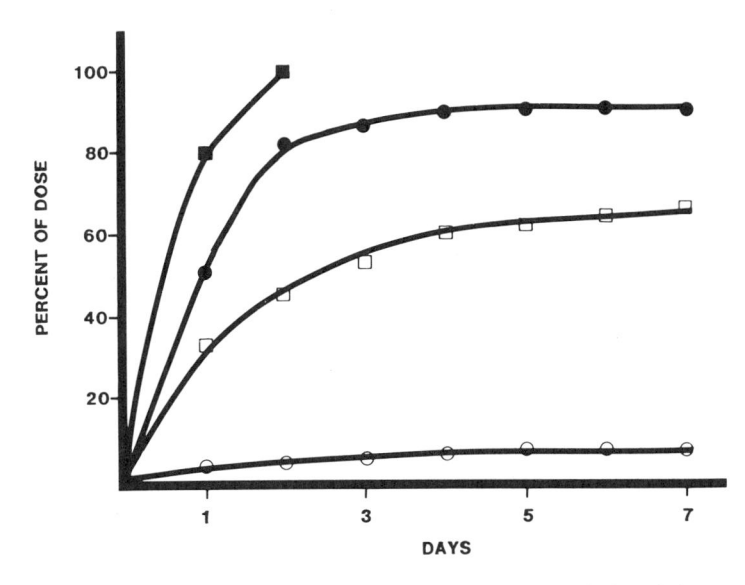

FIGURE 1: Cumulative percentage recovery of four polychlorinated biphenyls from urine and feces of rats for seven days following intravenous administration. (■), 4-chlorobiphneyl; (●), 4,4'-dichlorobiphenyl; (□), 2,2',4,5,5'-pentachlorobiphenyl, and (○), 2,2',4,4',5,5'-hexachlorobiphenyl. Graph drawn from data published by Matthews and Anderson (7).

2,2',4,4',5,5'-hexachlorobiphenyl (245-HCB) in eight days, while the monkey and rat were incapable of eliminating 50% of the administered dose during their remaining lifespan (5,6,9). This species variation in the degree of biotransformation was also seen with 4,4'-dichlorobiphenyl (4-DCB). The dog and rat eliminated 50% of a dose in one day, while the monkey required 20 days to eliminate the same amount (2,4). Since a large variation in the metabolism of these compounds exists among these animal species, it is difficult to choose the appropriate species for extrapolation to humans. This paper will report the results of our *in vitro* experiments using human, dog, and monkey liver microsomes to examine PCB metabolism. Such *in vitro data* can then be used to strengthen the interspecies extrapolation of the disposition of these chemicals by humans.

Table 1. The effect of chlorine position on the excretion of hexachlorobiphenyls by the dog after intravenous administration.

Hexachlorobiphenyl	Percent of Dose Eliminated in 3 Days
2,2',3,3',5,5'-HCB	4
2,2',4,4',5,5'-HCB	28
2,2',4,4',6,6'-HCB	50
2,2',3,3',6,6'-HCB	70

Data taken from Sipes *et al.,* (8).

Table 2. Species differences in the elimination of PCBs.

Species	PCB	Time to 50% Excretion (Days)
Rat	236-HCB	1
	245-HCB	—*
	4-DCB	1
Dog	236-HDB	1
	245-HCB	8
	4-DCB	1
Monkey	236-HCB	6
	245-HCB	—*
	4-DCB	20

* The rat only excreted 5.5% of the dose in 7 days and the monkey only excreted 18% of the dose in 90 days. 2,2′,3,3′,6,6′-hexachlorobiphenyl, 236-HCB; 2,2′,4,4′,5,5′-hexachlorobiphenyl, 245-HCB; 4,4′-dichlorobiphenyl, 4-DCB. Data taken from Sipes *et al.,* (5); Sipes *et al.,* (6); and Kato *et al.,* (9).

METHODS

Hepatic tissue was obtained from cancer patients undergoing partial liver resection at the University of Arizona and the Veterans Administration in Tucson, Arizona. In all cases, the patients had a grossly visible tumor of metastatic origin. Tissue was selected from areas of the liver which were visually free of tumor, and was obtained within minutes after loss of total blood flow to that lobe. Hepatic tissue was also obtained from adult male cynomolgous monkeys (3-5 kg) and adult male beagle dogs (8-12 kg). Both the monkeys and the dogs were anesthetized with ketamine and then were terminated by intravenous potassium chloride. The livers were immediately removed and placed in ice-cold 50 mM Tris buffer containing 150 mM potassium chloride (pH 7.4). Microsomes from all species were prepared by differential centrifugation and stored at -70° as previously described (10,11). Cytochrome P-450 concentrations were determined by the method of Omura and Sato (12). In addition, cytochrome c reductase activity, and several enzymatic activities were determined and were found to be similar to those reported by other researchers (10).

Microsomal metabolism of PCBs was determined under conditions of linearity as previously described (10,11). Briefly, various concentrations of the ^{14}C-labeled PCB were incubated with 1 or 2 mg of microsomal protein, a NADPH generating system, 0.25 mM EDTA and 50 mM Tris buffer containing 150 mM potassium chloride in a final volume of 2 ml. After a 2 minute pre-incubation, the reactions were initiated by the addition of the PCB. Incubations were performed at 37° under air in a shaking metabolic incubator. The reactions were stopped by the addition of 2.5 ml of 0.5 N sodium hydroxide, and the mixture was heated at 70° for ten minutes. To determine the amount of metabolism that occurred, the parent PCB was removed by extracting repeatedly with 5 ml aliquots of hexane-ethanol (19:1) until no radioactivity appeared in the organic layer. The ^{14}C remaining in the aqueous phase was determined by liquid scintillation spectrometry and was used to quantify the amount of metabolism. Activity was determined by subtracting the amount of product formed in the control incubations (without NADPH generating system) from the corresponding incubation with the NADPH generating system. The results of this work were analyzed by the method of Hofstee and by nonlinear regression analysis (13,14). The procedures for isolation of individual metabolites, metabolite identification, and covalent binding were as previously described (10,11).

RESULTS

We examined three PCB congeners as models for the metabolism of PCBs. The first congener, 4,4'-dichlorobiphenyl (4-DCB) has a low molecular weight with chlorines substituted in the para-positions (Figure 2). This compound was chosen because the preferred site of metabolism on the phenyl rings is blocked. The second congener 236-HCB, is highly chlorinated but contains two adjacent unsubstituted carbon atoms on each ring. This congener was chosen because two adjacent unsubstituted carbon atoms have been shown to facilitate the metabolism of these compounds in most species (5,6,9). The third PCB, 245-HCB, is also highly chlorinated but does not contain any adjacent unsubstituted carbon atoms. This pattern of chlorine substitution severely hinders metabolism (5,9).

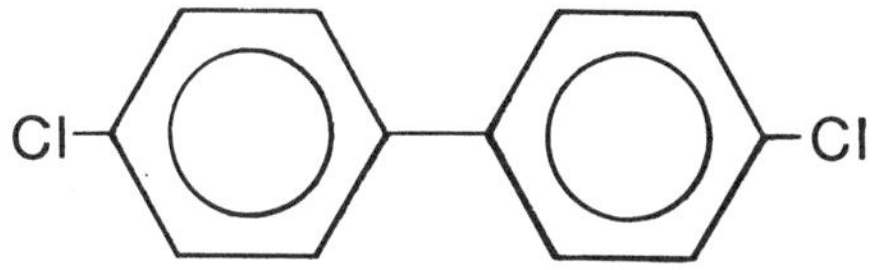

4,4'-DICHLOROBIPHENYL

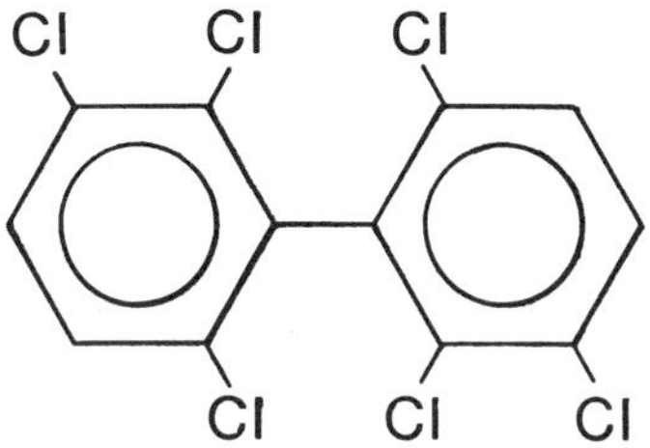

2,2',3,3',6,6'-HEXACHLOROBIPHENYL

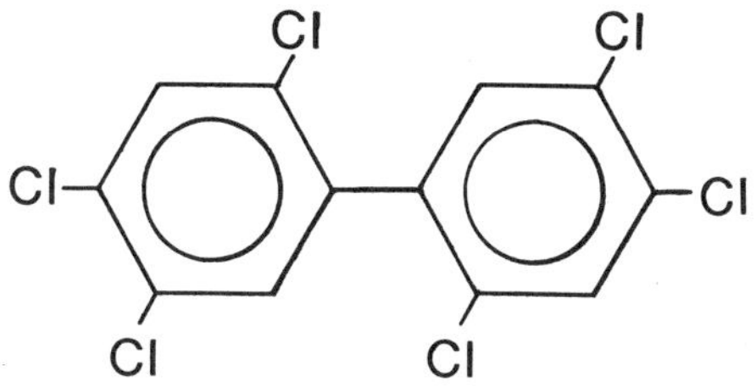

2,2',4,4',5,5'-HEXACHLOROBIPHENYL

FIGURE 2: Structures and names of three model polychlorinated biphenyl congeners.

Under our incubation conditions, 245-HCB was not metabolized by human or monkey liver microsomes (limit of detection 0.2 pmoles/mg microsomal protein/min). However, dog liver microsomes metabolized 245-HCB with an apparent Km of 9.5 µM and a Vmax of 5.8 pmoles/nmole P-450/min (Table 3). All three species metabolized 4-DCB and 236-HCB (Table 3). The apparent Km values ranged from 0.43 - 1.3 µM for 4-DCB and from 0.12 - 8.8 µM for 236-HCB. In all cases, the Km of the monkey was closer to that of the human than the dog. While the Km of 4-DCB in the monkey and human was lower than the Km of 236-HCB, the Km of 4-DCB in the dog was higher than that of 236-HCB. These apparent Km values suggest that these compounds have a relatively high affinity for the cytochrome P-450 enzymes. However, it is known that PCBs readily partition into the lipid matrix of the microsomal membrane (10,11,15). Thus, the concentration of PCB at the enzyme site may be much higher than that calculated for the incubation mixture. When the partitioning of these compounds into the lipid matrix is taken into consideration, the calculated Km values are in the millimolar range and may reflect a more accurate Km (10,11). The Vmax values for 236-HCB metabolism by the human and monkey microsomes are similar (19.3 vs 13.9 pmoles/nmole P-450/min) and are approximately one-half the Vmax value found in the dog (29 pmoles/nmole P-450/min). The Vmax values of 4-DCB in the human and monkey are also similar (4.4 vs 4.3 pmoles/nmole P-450/min) and are approximately one-fortieth the Vmax value found in the dog (160 pmoles/nmole P-450/min).

Table 3. PCB metabolism by human, monkey and dog hepatic microsomes.

Enzymatic Constant	Human	Monkey	Dog
Apparent Km (µM)			
236-HCB	8.8 ± 2.1	5.2 ± 4.1	0.12 ± 0.05
4-DCB	0.43 ± 0.13	0.92 ± 0.86	1.3 ± 0.2
245-HCB	—	—	9.5 0.8
Vmax (pmoles/nmole P-450/min)			
236-HCB	19.3 ± 4.0	13.9 ± 8.3	29.0 ± 6.9
4-DCB	4.4 ± 1.4	4.3 ± 2.1	160 ± 52
245-HCB	—	—	5.8 ± 2.1

Metabolism was determined as described in the text. The data were analyzed by the method of Hofstee (13) and by nonlinear regression analysis (14). Values are the mean ± S.D. 245-HCB metabolism was not detected in human and monkey liver microsomes.

To identify and confirm the nature of the PCB metabolites, extracts from human microsomal incubations were subjected to HPLC analysis. HPLC analysis revealed two major peaks of radioactivity for 236-HCB (Figure 3). Similarly HPLC analysis of monkey microsomal incubations containing 236-HCB resulted in two major peaks of radioactivity that coeluted with those of human incubations. The compounds identified in these peaks for 236-HCB have been identified for the human by gas chromatography-mass spectrometry (Table 4), (10). The two metabolites of 236-HCB are 2,2',3,3',6,6'-hexachloro-4-biphenylol (peak A) and 2,2',3,3',6,6'-hexachloro-5-biphenylol (peak B).

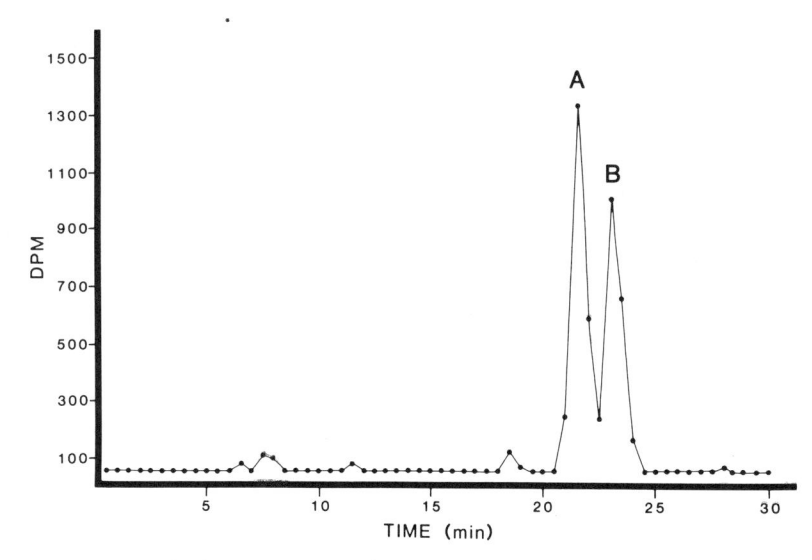

FIGURE 3: HPLC radiochromatogram of 236-HCB aqeous soluble metabolites generated by human liver microsomes. HPLC conditions were previously described (10). Peak A and B are 2,2',3,3',6,6'-hexachloro-4-biphenylol and 2,2',3,3',6,6'-hexachloro-5-biphenylol, respectively.

Table 4. Metabolites of 236-HCB and 4-DCB catalyzed by human liver microsomes.

Parent	Peak	Metabolite
236-HCB	A	2,2',3,3',6,6'-hexachloro-4-biphenylol
	B	2,2',3,3',6,6'-hexachloro-5-biphenylol
4-DCB	B	4,4'-dichloro-3,3'-biphenyldiol
	C	4'-chloro-3-biphenylol
	C	4'-chloro-4-biphenylol
	E	4,4'-dichloro-2-biphenylol
	E	4,4'-dichloro-3-biphenylol
	E	3,4'-dichloro-4-biphenylol

The metabolites of 4-DCB were more complex. HPLC analysis of human microsomal incubations containing 4-DCB metabolites revealed five peaks of radioactivity (Figure 4). Similarly, analysis of 4-DCB metabolites generated by monkey liver microsomes results in four peaks of radioactivity that coeluted with A, B, C, and E in the human. The compounds found in these peaks for 4-DCB have been identified for the human by gas chromatography-mass spectrometry, coelution with synthetic standards on HPLC and by coelution with synthetic biphenylols on HPLC following dechlorination (Table 4). Peaks A and D were not identified. Peak B coeluted with the synthetic standard 4,4'-dichloro-3,3'-biphenyldiol. Following methylation of peak B, selective ion monitoring GC-MS analysis confirmed a dimethoxy-dichlorobiphenyl. Based on the HPLC and GC-MS data and that 4,4'-dichloro-3,3'-biphenyldiol could result from the further hydroxylation of the major metabolite 4,4'-dichloro-3-biphenylol, we have tentatively assigned peak B the structure 4,4'-dichloro-3,3'-biphenyldiol. Although peaks C and E coeluted with the synthetic standards, 4'-chloro-4-biphenylol and 4,4'-dichloro-3-biphenylol respectively, a C_{18} reverse phase column cannot readily separate 3-hydroxylated-DCBs and 4-hydroxylated-DCBs (15). Therefore, to conclusively identify the metabolites in peaks C and E, each peak was reductively dechlorinated and subjected to normal phase HPLC. Peak C was found to contain two peaks of radioactivity that coeluted with the synthetic biphenyl metabolites, 4-biphenylol and 3-biphenylol. Thus peak C actually contained the metabolites 4'-chloro-3-biphenylol and 4'-chloro-4-biphenylol. When Peak E was subjected to dechlorination and normal phase HPLC, three peaks of radioactivity were obtained that coeluted with 2-biphenylol, 3-biphenylol and 4-biphenylol. Thus the actual metabolites in peak E were 4,4'-dichloro-2-biphenylol, 4,4'-dichloro-3-biphenylol (most abundant metabolite), and 3,4'-dichloro-4-biphenylol. Studies to identify the metabolites generated by dog liver microsomes are currently in progress.

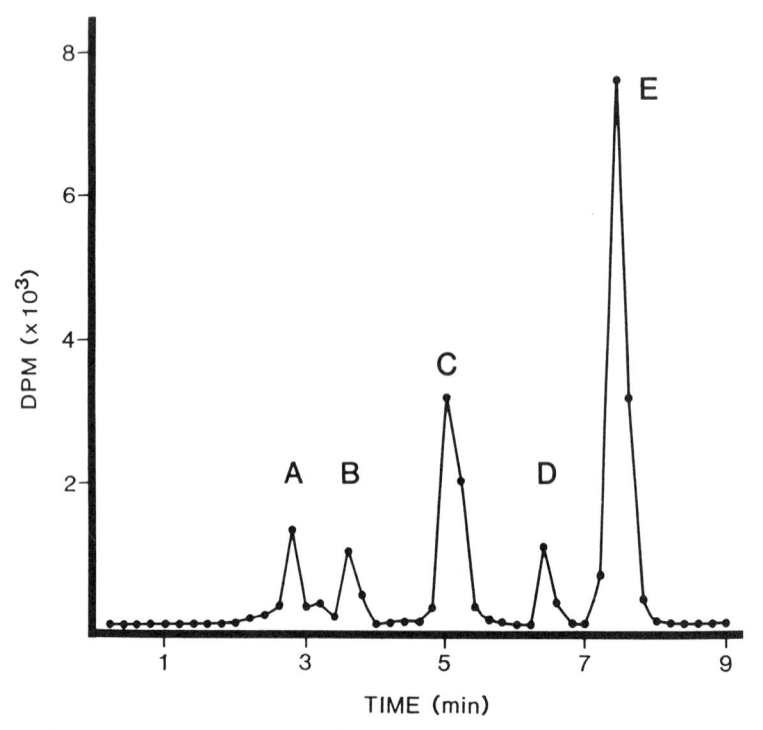

FIGURE 4: HPLC radiochromatogram of 4-DCB aqueous soluble metabolites generated by human liver microsomes. HPLC conditions were previously described (11). See text for identification of peaks.

In order to determine if the reactive intermediates formed during metabolism of these PCBs are capable of binding to macromolecules, covalent binding of PCB-equivalents to microsomal protein was determined. The extent of covalent binding of 4-DCB and 236-HCB was time, protein, and NADPH dependent. In addition, 236-HCB was found to covalently bind to a greater extent than 4-DCB (Figure 5). The addition of 1 mM reduced glutathione to the microsomal incubations resulted in a reduction of covlent binding for both compounds.

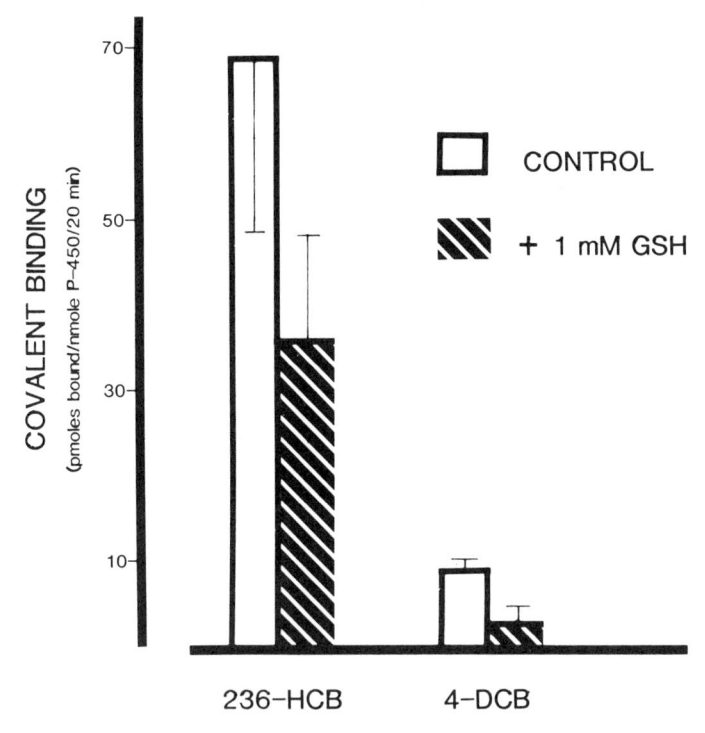

FIGURE 5: Covalent binding of 236-HCB and 4-DCB equivalents to human microsomal protein in the presence and absence of 1 mM reduced glutathione (GSH).

DISCUSSION

These results illustrate 1) the similarity in the rates of metabolism of PCBs between monkeys and humans *in vitro,* 2) the importance of unsubstituted meta- and para-positions in facilitating the rate of metabolism in the monkey and human, and 3) the major qualitative and quantitative differences in the metabolism of PCBs by the dog. The *in vitro* metabolism data from the human and monkey agree quite well. Both species did not metabolize 245-HCB, but did metabolize 236-HCB at a faster rate than 4-DCB. These data are consistent with the general rules of PCB metabolism for most species (1). That is, two adjacent unsubstituted carbon atoms are necessary for PCBs to be readily metabolized and an unsubstituted para-position facilitates the metabolism.

The *in vitro* results in the monkey are consistent with the *in vivo* results. The PCB congener 245-HCB was not metabolized *in vitro*. This is not surprising since only 18% of a dose of 245-HCB was excreted over 90 days after *in vivo* administration. The excretion half-life of 236-HCB and 4-DCB is 1 and 19 days, respectively. Since the *in vivo* half-lives of 236-HCB and 4-DCB in the monkey are qualitatively similar to the *in vitro* Vmax values and since the *in vitro* human Vmax values are similar to the *in vitro* monkey results, one would predict that the disposition results in the monkey would better extrapolate to humans than the disposition results obtained in the dog.

However, while the qualitative *in vitro* metabolism of these compounds is similar, the overall *in vivo* disposition may be different between the human and monkey. The monkeys used in this study had a 4-fold higher concentration of cytochrome P-450 per milligram microsomal protein than the concentration found in human microsomes (1.2 vs. 0.3 nmoles cytochrome P-450/mg microsomal protein). This difference, particularly if it is reflected as a difference in the cytochrome P-450 isozymes that metabolize PCBs, may influence the overall rate of excretion.

The question of whether the *in vitro* human results actually apply *in vivo* still exists. We have two lines of evidence that our *in vitro* results are in agreement with the *in vivo* situation. Firstly, after a recent accidental exposure of a group of people in Taiwan to PCBs, Chen *et al.*, (16) found that the blood levels of 245-HCB only decreased 10% over a 300-500 day period (Figure 6). These minimal changes in blood concentrations over a long period of time, suggest that this compound is not metabolized or metabolized very slowly and thus essentially cannot be eliminated from the body. Secondly, Jensen and Sundstrom (17) found that 245-HCB was the PCB found in the greatest concentration in human adipose tissue, while 236-HCB was apparently not present. Since both compounds are found in the environment and have been reported in the commercial PCB mixtures, the difference in adipose tissue concentrations most likely results from differences in the body to metabolize and excrete these compounds (17-19). Thus, the *in vitro* results obtained with human liver microsomes predicted the fate of these two PCB congeners following their absorption by humans.

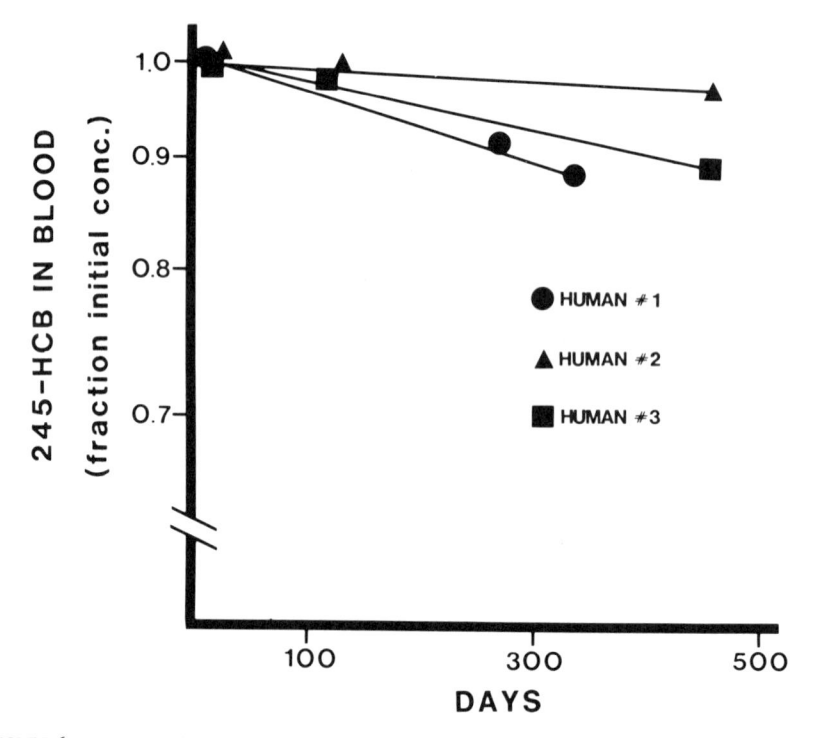

FIGURE 6: Fraction of initial concentration of 245-HCB found in human blood after an accidential exposure. Graph drawn from data published by Chen *et al.*, (16).

Our results suggest that the human and probably the monkey primarily metabolize these compounds through an arene oxide intermediate. The formation of 2,2'3,3'6,6'-hexachloro-4-biphenylol and 2,2',3,3',6,6'-hexachloro-5-biphenylol could result from the rearrangement of the 4,5-epoxide of 236-HCB. For 4-DCB, the 3,4'-dichloro-4-biphenylol metabolite most likely resulted from an arene oxide intermediate followed by intramolecular migration of the chlorine (NIH shift). In addition, the covalent binding of 236-HCB and 4-DCB equivalents to microsomal protein and the inhibition of this binding by reduced glutathione are suggestive of an arene oxide intermediate. The toxicological consequences of PCB metabolism via an arene oxide intermediate remains to be determined. However, there is evidence that the arene oxide is capable of binding to DNA, RNA and protein (20).

When compared to humans and monkeys, there are major qualitative and quantitative differences in the metabolism of PCBs by the dog. The dog was found to elminate all three PCBs at a faster rate than the monkey and was capable of reducing its body burden of 245-HCB (5,8). In addition, the excretion half-lives of 4-DCB and 236-HCB in the dog are equivalent (one day). These results suggested that the dog may be metabolizing these compounds by an alternate pathway not found, or only found to a limited extent, in other species. This hypothesis is further supported by the *in vitro* data. Unlike the monkey and human, the dog was found to metabolize 245-HCB *in vitro* and metabolized 4-DCB at a faster rate than 236-HCB. Thus, a substituted para-position does not hinder the rate of metabolism in the dog as it did in the other species. Additional evidence for an alternate pathway of metabolism in the dog can be found in a study that focused on how the position of the chlorine affected the elimination of selected symmetrical hexachlorobiphenyls (Table 1). As the number of unsubstituted meta-positions increased, the rate of elimination increased. Furthermore, when the hexachlorobiphenyl had an unsubstitued meta- and para-position the rate of elmination further increased. Again, these data support the hypothesis that the dog has an additional pathway of PCB metabolism which allows the dog to eliminate these compounds more rapidly than most other species. Elucidation of the mechanism of PCB hydroxylation by the dog will further our understanding of hydroxylation reactions. Whether or not this alternative pathway involves an arene oxide is of considerable interest, since a pathway which does not involve an arene oxide may result in less toxicity. Clearly, the combined *in vitro/in vivo* results obtained for the dog, indicate it would be an inappropriate choice for extrapolation of the disposition of PCBs in humans.

We believe that the use of these relatively straightforward *in vitro/in vivo* studies will greatly aid in the selection of the most appropriate animal model for extrapolation of chemical disposition studies to humans. Major savings in time, money and animal life would be gained if the results of initial *in vitro* studies directed the *in vivo* studies. The metabolic constants could be used in physiological pharmacokinetic modeling which would predict how these animals would handle the compound over time. The reliability of the model could then be tested *in vivo* for a few time points. If the model is predictive for animals, then the *in vitro* metabolic constants obtained for humans would be critical for using this model to extrapolate to humans.

It should be emphasized that these *in vitro* studies have certain limitations. Chemicals which are excreted unchanged or metabolized in extrahepatic tissues would not predict well in these studies. In addition, diffusional and transport effects are not taken into consideration. For example, it has been suggested that cytosolic proteins may actually promote the transport of lipophilic compounds to the endoplasmic reticulum and thus increase the rate of their metabolism (21). Since primary metabolites are not removed from the system, they may be further hydroxylated by the monooxygenase enzymes. The dihydroxy-metabolite of 4-DCB (4,4'-dichloro-3,3'-biphenyldiol) probably resulted from recycling of the monohydroxy-metabolite in our system. Finally, the absence of conjugating enzymes may influence the rate of metabolism, particularly if primary metabolites recycle and inhibit the metabolism of the parent compound. However, it is possible to add conjugating enzymes to the microsomal incubations and/or the necessary cofactors to better simulate the intact cellular system. In fact, we have shown that 4,4'-dichloro-3-biphenylol readily undergoes glucuronidation by microsomal preparations of human liver (11). Despite these difficulties, valuable information can be obtained from metabolic studies that use subcellular preparations. One must be aware of these difficulties when extrapolating to *in vivo* studies.

ACKNOWLEDGEMENTS

The authors would like to thank Dr. Charles W. Putnam of the Veterans Administration Medical Center, Tucson, Arizona for providing the human liver tissue. This work was supported by ES-82130 and ES-07091 from the National Institutes of Health.

REFERENCES

1. Kimbrough, R. D.: (ed.), *Halogenated Biphenyls, Terphenyls, Napththalenes, Dibenzodioxins and Related Products*, Elsevier/North Holland, Amsterdam, 1980.

2. Lutz, R. J., Dedrick, R. L., Matthews, H. B., Eling, T. E., and Anderson, M. W.: A preliminary pharmacokinetic model for several chlorinated biphenyls in the rat. *Drug Metab. Disp.* 5:386-396, 1977.

3. Tuey, D. B. and Matthews, H. B.: Use of a physiological pharmacokinetic model for the rat to describe the pharmacokinetics of several chlorinated biphenyls in the mouse. *Drug Metab. Disp.* 8:397-403, 1980.

4. Sipes, I. G., Slocumb, M. L., Perry, D. F., and Carter, D. E.: 4,4'-Dichlorobiphenyl: Distribution, metabolism, and excretion in the dog and the monkey. *Toxicol. Appl. Pharmacol.* 55:554-563, 1980.

5. Sipes, I. G., Slocumb, M. L., Perry, D. F., and Carter, D. E.: 2,4,5,2',4',5'-Hexachlorophenyl: Distribution, metabolism and excretion in the dog and the monkey. *Toxicol. Appl. Pharmacol.* 65:264-272, 1982.

6. Sipes, I. G., Slocumb, M. L., Chen, H-S.G., and Carter, D. E.: 2,3,6,2',3',6'-Hexachlorobiphenyl: Distribution, metabolism, and excretion in the dog and monkey. *Toxicol. Appl. Pharmacol.* 62:317-324, 1982.

7. Matthews, H. B. and Anderson, M. W.: Effect of chlorination on the distribution and excretion of polychlorinated biphenyls. *Drug Metab. Disp.* 3:371-380, 1975.

8. Sipes, I. G., McKelvie, D. H., and Collins, R.: Excretion of hexachlorobiphenyls and 2,4,5,2',4',5'-hexabromobiphenyl in the dog. *Toxicol. Appl. Pharmacol.* 48:A155, 1979.

9. Kato, S., McKinney, J. D., and Matthews, H. B.: Metabolism of symmetrical hexachlorobiphenyl isomers in the rat. *Toxicol. Appl. Pharmacol.* 53:389-398, 1980.

10. Schnellmann, R. G., Putnam, C. W., and Sipes, I. G.: Metabolism of 2,2',3,3',6,6'-hexachlorobiphenyl and 2,2',4,4',5,5'-hexachlorobiphenyl by human hepatic microsomes. *Biochem. Pharmacol.* 32:3233-3239, 1983.

11. *Schnellmann, R. G., Volp, R. F., Putnam, C. W., and Sipes, I. G.*: The hydroxylation, dechlorination, and glucuronidation of 4,4'-dichlorobiphenyl (4-DCB) by human hepatic microsomes. *Biochem. Pharmacol. 33:*3503-3510, 1984.

12. *Omura, T. and Sato, R.*: The carbon monoxide binding pigments of liver microsomes. I. Evidence for its hemoprotein nature. *J. Biol. Chem. 239*:2370-2378, 1964.

13. *Hofstee, B. H. J.*: Non-inverted versus inverted plots in enzyme kinetics. *Nature 184*:1296-1298, 1959.

14. *Metzler, C. M., Elfring, G. L., and McEwan, A. J.*: A users manual for NONLIN. The Upjohn Company, Kalamazoo, MI, 1974.

15. *Kennedy, M. W., Carpentier, N. K., Dymerski, P. P., and Kaminsky, L. S.*: Metabolism of dichlorobiphenyls by hepatic microsomal cytochrome P-450. *Biochem. Pharmacol. 30*:577-588, 1981.

16. *Chen, P. H., Luo, M. L., Wong, C. K, and Chen, C. J.*: Comparative rates of elimination of some individual polychlorinated biphenyls from the blood of PCB-poisoned patients in Taiwan. *Food Chem. Toxicol. 20*:417-425, 1982.

17. *Jensen, S. and Sundstrom, G.*: Structures and levels of most chlorobiphenyls in two technical PCB products and in human adipose tissue. *Ambio. 3*:70-76, 1974.

18. *Sissons, D. and Welti, D.*: Structural identification of polychlorinated biphenyls in commerical mixtures by gas-liquid chromatography, nuclear, magnetic resonance and mass spectrometry. *J. Chromatogr. 60*:15-32, 1971.

19. *Albro, P. W., Corbett, J. T., and Schroeder, J. L.*: Quantiative characterization of polychlorinated biphenyl mixtures (Aroclors®) 1248,1254 and 1260 by gas chromatography using capillary columns. *J. Chromatogr. 205*:103-111, 1981.

20. *Morales, N. M. and Matthews, H. B.*: *In Vivo* binding of 2,3,6,2',3',6'-hexachlorobiphenyl and 2,4,5,2',4',5'-hexachlorobiphenyl to mouse liver macromolecules. *Chem.-Biol. Interact. 27*:99-110, 1979.

21. *Dixit, R., Bickers, D. R., and Mukhtar, H.*: Binding of benzo(a)pyrene to hepatic cytosolic protein enhances its microsomal oxidation, *Biochem. Biophys. Res. Commun. 104*:1093-1101, 1982.

New Approaches in Toxicity Testing and Their Application in Human Risk Assessment, edited by A. P. Li. Raven Press, New York © 1985.

Drug Metabolizing Enzyme Systems and Their Relationship to Toxic Mechanisms

*M. R. Boyd, *V. Ravindranath, *,[1]L. T. Burka, *,[1]J. S. Dutcher, *R. B. Franklin, *,[1]C. N. Statham, †,[1]W. M. Haschek, †,[1]P. J. Hakkinen, †C. C. Morse, and †H. P. Witschi

*National Cancer Institute, Bethesda, Maryland 20205; †Biology Division, Oak Ridge National Laboratory, Oak Ridge, Tennessee 37830

Consistent with the purpose of this meeting, this paper will address the topic "Drug Metabolizing Enzyme Systems and their Relationship to Toxicity" with an emphasis toward possible implications for human risk assessment. We shall illustrate our particular approach by discussing a specific toxicological problem which has been a focus of our efforts over the past few years. We should preface this discussion too with the qualifier that, although in the example we shall discuss the studies to date appear to have certain implications for human risk, we still cannot assess whether this risk is vanishingly small, or whether it is of substantial public health significance. Nevertheless, we do believe we have established a path that may ultimately provide critical information needed to extrapolate from observations of phenomena in experimental animals to valid predictions of effects in humans.

A few months ago, shortly after receiving the invitation to participate in this symposium and while in the stage of attempting to identify an appropriate example to discuss, we received a telephone inquiry from scientists at the Monsanto Company who were concerned with the possible toxicological significance of 3-methylfuran. This material apparently had been detected under certain conditions as a by-product generated during production and/or storage of a product under development. This inquiry was a rather paradoxical coincidence, not to mention also a somewhat humbling experience to us. Here we were, being consulted as presumed "experts" (by virtue of over 10 years

---

[1]Present addresses: (L. T. B.) Toxicology and Research Testing Program, NIEHS, P. O. Box 12233, Research Triangle Park, NC 27709; (J.S.D.) Inhalation Toxicology Research Institute, Albuquerque, NM 87105; (R. B. F.) Eli Lilly and Co., 307 E. McCarty St., Bldg. 28, S-208, Indianapolis, IN 46285; (C.N.S.) Toxicology Branch, 10th Medical Laboratory, A.P. O. NY 09180; (W. M. H.) Department of Veterinary Pathobiology, University of Illinois, 2001 S. Lincoln, Urbana, IL 60801; (P. J. H.) Procter & Gamble Co., Sharon Woods Technical Center, Cincinnati, OH 45241;

research work and numerous publications on the subject) on the toxicity of furan compounds, and being asked for advice concerning a "real world" problem. Unfortunately we really were not able to provide any of the ultimate answers needed to adequately evaluate human risk in this example. Nevertheless, in the interim, we have had the opportunity to reflect upon the problem in this new light. Therefore, we could think of no better example to discuss here than that of 3-methylfuran.

METABOLIC ACTIVATION AND TOXICITY

Clearly, one of the major advances in recent years concerning toxicological mechanisms is the elucidation of the importance of metabolic activation and of the role chemically reactive metabolites play in determining target organ toxicity. There are many examples of relatively "inert" chemicals which are transformed in the body to highly electrophilic products that may react extensively with cellular macromolecules. This in turn may lead to various adverse effects including necrosis or neoplastic transformation. The primary metabolic pathway involved often is an oxidative one involving the cytochrome P-450 system. However, metabolic activation may also occur by other pathways such as reduction, conjugation and/or combinations thereof. As might be anticipated, toxicities involving reactive metabolites occur predominantly in tissues containing the enzymes capable of mediating the requisite metabolism. Thus, tissues such as the liver, the lungs and the kidneys frequently are sites of toxicity by reactive metabolites formed *in situ*. Moreover, since drug-metabolizing enzymes tend to be concentrated in specific families of cells, such individual cell populations may be particularly susceptible to damage. Because of the dependency of these kinds of toxicities upon metabolism, variations in drug-metabolizing enzymes (toxifying and/or detoxifying) among species, strain, sexes, ages, and/or due to prior exposure to inducing or inhibiting agents may markedly alter the intensity of target organ damage, or may even totally alter organ or cell specificity. Such factors complicate our chances of extrapolating experimental data from animals to predictions of susceptibility and/or target organ or cell specificity in other species, including man. However, it is only through observations made in animals that we have been able to identify critical factors that may modify target organ metabolism and therefore target organ susceptibility. These precedents also suggest, at least in those specific instances in which it is known or can be proven, that highly reactive metabolites must be generated *in situ* within the target tissues in order to case damage, that the absence of such a necessary metabolic pathway in a test tissue of interest (e.g., from a different species) would predict nonsusceptibility of that tissue to this type of toxicity. This of course presumes the test tissue was prepared in such a way that any pre-existing metabolic activity of interest was not destroyed by the prior experimental manipulations.

One final caution should be made to qualify the above lines of reasoning. Although the absence of the necessary metabolic activity would predict nonsusceptibility of a given target tissue, the *presence* of such activity, especially as might be observed in an *in vitro* test, does *not* necessarily predict susceptibility. For example, the simple observation that a chemically unreactive compound becomes bound colvanently to particular target tissues *in vitro* or *in vivo* does not necessarily mean toxicity is present or is likely to develop. Although covalent binding indicates that the parent compound has undergone transformation to a more reactive product, there are some other important criteria that need to be met before we can say first that the covalent binding does in fact reflect the formation of a reactive metabolite and secondly (and even more importantly), whether or not the reactive metabolite is toxic. We must always be cautious not to imply that "covalent binding" has any direct causative role in the toxic response in question. With our present state of insight (or lack thereof), we prefer to think "covalent binding" simply as a way to detect or measure the formation of reactive metabolites that are generally too labile to actually isolate. Although, in some instances it may be possible to examine reactive metabolites more directly (e.g., through chemical trapping), in most cases this may be technically much more difficult, if not impossible.

In studying the relationships between metabolism, covalent binding (e.g., reactive metabolite formation) and toxicity, there are a logical and interrelated series of questions that are the focus of the approach that we, and many other laboratories, typically might pursue. These are summarized in Tables I and II. Operationally, we usually define "covalent binding" in our studies as the irreversible binding of radioactivity to tissue macromolecules (usually protein and/or nucleic acids) following *in vivo* administration or *in vitro* exposure to the radiolabeled parent compound of interest. Assuming we see covalent binding of a given compound after a dose or a concentration relevant to the toxicity of interest, we are then concerned about whether the binding indeed represents the formation of a reactive metabolite; there may be other alternatives to consider, such as carbon incorporation tritium exchange or possibly nonspecific binding of radiolabeled impurities present in our original compound. As indicated in Table I we may tackle these questions from several fronts. With the tissue preparations of interest (e.g., isolated organs, slices, cells, subcellular fractions, purified enzymes) we may examine *in vitro* how the "colvalent binding" measure is affected by enzyme inactivation or modification by heat, cofactors, or chemical inhibitors or inducers. We may even wish to compare the kinetics of the binding pathway in target vs. nontarget tissue preparations. With studies *in vivo,* we are concerned about dose- and time-dependency of covalent binding, effects of inducers or inhibitors of metabolism, tissue and cell-specificity and the possible correlations with presence of enzyme activities in specific tissues and cells, comparisons of studies using various labeling positions within a given compound, and in some cases, the possible effects of inhibitors of endogenous biosynthetic pathways.

TABLE I

Approaches to Establishing that the Covalent Binding of Radioactive Material After Exposure to Radiolabled Compound is due to Formation of Highly Reactive Metabolites (s)

In vitro

1. Effects of heat-denaturation of enzyme of tissue preparations
2. Cofactor effects
3. Effects of enzyme inhibitors and inducers
4. Kinetic studies

In vivo

1. Dose- and time-dependency studies
2. Effects of enzyme inducers and inhibitors
3. Tissue and cell specificity; correlations with known presence of enzyme activities in specific tissues and/or cell types
4. Comparison of different types of radiolabel of different positions of label in a given compound
5. Effects of inhibitors of endogenous biosynthetic pathways

TABLE II

Approaches to Establishing the Role of Reactive Metabolites in Toxicity *In Vivo*

1. Correlations of dose- and time-dependencies of covalent binding and toxicity
2. Correlations of effects on covalent binding and toxicity after treatments with enzyme inducers and inhibitors
3. Correlations of organ- and cell-specificities of covalent binding and toxicity
4. Correlations of covalent binding and toxicity of structurally related compounds
5. Effects of manipulations of tissue levels of nonprotein sulfhydryl compounds

Then, assuming we are convinced that the covalent binding we observe with a given compound does in fact result from the formation of a reactive metabolite, we now must evaluate its relationship to toxicity. As shown in Table II, these critical studies may include correlations of dose- and time-dependencies of binding and toxicity, the modifying effects of inhibitors or inducers, organ and cell specificities of binding and toxicity, comparisons with structurally related compounds, and, where possible, the effects of compromised detoxification pathways. A more detailed discussion of these approaches and their applications to variety of toxicological problems may be found in another review (1). The remainder of this presentation will be devoted to the example of 3-methylfuran introduced earlier. This example illustrates several of the more important points we have raised concerning the approaches we have used to these kinds of problems.

3-METHYLFURAN: A TOXIC COMPOUND ACTIVATED BY METABOLISM

Background

Compounds containing the furan nucleus are ubiquitous in nature (2). Many hundreds of furan derivatives have been found in terrestrial and marine organisms. Many good and beverage materials contain furan compounds. For example, coffee alone contains nearly 100 different furan derivatives.

Some furans are highly toxic. Several have been shown to metabolized in the body to reactive electrophilic intermediates. These compounds typically cause necrosis within target tissues such as the liver, the lungs or the kidneys (3-5). There are varying degrees of tissue specificity, depending upon if or how a potential target tissue metabolizes a given furan compound. Thus, target organ specificity may be dependent both upon host factors (e.g., species, sex, strain, age, etc.) as well as chemical factors (structure of parent compound, nature of reactive intermediate, and substrate specificities for toxifying and detoxifying metabolic pathways) (4).

Our particular interest in 3-methylfuran (3-MF) was intially stimulated by a report by Saunders *et al.,* (6) describing the analysis of organic constituents present in the atmosphere during the late-summer smog/haze alerts typically occurring in Washington, D.C., and many other east-coast cities. Quite surpisingly, they found 3-MF to be a major (if not *the* major) component present. This seemed especially unusual, since the presence of this compound could not be acribed to any known industrial or other man-made source. The current speculation is that the 3-MF arises from atmospheric photo-decomposition of naturally-occuring terpenoids, such as those produced by large tracts of leaf-bearing trees (e.g., like those found in forests of the Appalachian mountain chain).

Because of our long-standing interest in the metabolism and toxicity of furans, we were naturally interested in the biological fate and activity of 3-methylfuran. Therefore, after the important step of synthesizing the quantities of radiolabeled and unlabled compounds needed, we carried out a series of studies which we briefly summarize as follows.

Metabolic activation in vitro

Since we already had good reason to suspect 3-MF might be similar to other toxic furans known to require activation by metabolism, we first performed an experiment to see if mouse livers and lungs possessed the microsomal enzymes necessary to catalyze the covalent binding (i.e., metabolism to a reactive intermediate) of 3-MF. Microsomes from these tissues clearly were active, and the metabolic pathways in both had characteristics typical of cytochrome P-450 monooxygenases (7). Thus, maximal activity (rates of covalent binding) required the presence of NADPH and oxygen in addition to the microsomes. Activity was markedly decreased by the known cytochrome P-450 inhibitors, carbon monoxide and piperonyl butoxide. Additionally, the nucleophilic trapping agent, reduced glutathione, prevented the covalent binding, as typically might be expected if it reacted with some electrophilic intermediate to form a conjugate and thereby prevent the covalent binding of the intermediate to the microsomes.

Because we hoped that the elucidation of the structure of a glutathione conjugate formed in such systems might help us identify the chemical structure of the reactive intermediates(s), we expended considerable effort to isolate and purify such conjugates from incubation mixtures using both 3-MF and its related isomers, 2-MF, as the parents substrates. Unfortunately, even though adducts were apparently rapidly formed with nucleophilic reagents including glutathione, N-acetyl cysteine and cysteine, in our hands they were not stable enough to allow isolation. We also looked for other non-conjugate metabolites, such as unsaturated lactones or dihydrodiols which might have implicated the initial formation of an epoxide-type intermediate followed by the further metabolism and/or nonenzymatic rearrangement or degradation (8). However, we were unable to detect any of these hypothetical products, and thus, were unable to make any substantial case for the involvement of an epoxide.

Recently, Drs. Ravindranath and Burka have reexamined this problem has have obtained some very illuminating new results (9,10). Their studies were based upon the hypothesis (11) that an unsaturated aldehyde intermediate was a likely product which, even though it could conceivably be formed via epoxide, it could also be formed directly from the parent furan. The latter hypothetical pathway could involve an initial one-electron oxidation by a cytochrome P-450 ferryl oxide intermediate to form a furan radical cation species stabilized by the furan oxygen. Subsequent reaction with the Fe^{IV}-O species might be expected to given an intermediate which could then either form the epoxide, or, perhaps via a more energetically favorable pathway, form an unsaturated aldehyde directly without going through the epoxide. In either case, the unsaturated aldehyde would likely be potentially hazardous were it to be formed in living cells, since it would be expected to have high reactivity with cellular constituents (e.g., via Michael addition to the double bond or by nucleophilic additions to the aldehyde).

To explore the unsaturated aldehyde hypothesis, a suitable trapping agent was needed. Semicarbazide proved to be the answer. The disemicarbazones of the suspected unsaturated aldehyde products from 2-MF and 3-MF (acetyl acrolein [AA] and methylbutenedial [MB], respectively) were first prepared by chemical synthesis. Rat hepatic microsomal incubations were then performed in the presence and absence of NADPH, semicarbazide and 2-MF or 3-MF. High-pressure liquid chromatographic [HPLC] analyses of extracts from these incubations showed peaks from incubations with 2-MF and 3-MF correspondings to the synthetic standards AA and MB, respectively. When NADPH was deleted, no such peaks were observed. A similar experiment performed with rat lung microsomes and 3-MF also showed a peak corresponding to MB, and again only from incubations containing NADPH. Subsequent preparative HPLC, purification by gel permeation chromatography, and mass spectral analyses confirmed the identities of the AA and MB disemicarbazones produced in the microsomal incubations.

Another experiment addressed the question of whether these unsaturated aldehydes were responsible for the "covalent binding" of 3-MF observed *in vitro*. Thus, when a comparison was made of the covalent binding and the amounts of MB disemicarbazone produced in hepatic microsomal incubations in the presence and absence of NADPH and semicarbazide, there clearly was an inverse relationship between the two measures. Semicarbazide strongly inhibited the NADPH-dependent covalent binding of 3-MF, presumably by trapping the reactive dialdehyde intermediate (MB) before it could react and bind irreversibly to the microsomal macromolecules.

Metabolic activation in vivo.

Not surprisingly, when 3-MF and 2-MF were administered *in vivo* to laboratory animals, large amounts of radioactivity were bound covalently to the livers and lungs, and much smaller or insignificant amounts were bound to tissues with little or no known cytochrome P-450 mono-oxygenase activity (7,12). Moreover, in the lungs the covalently bound 3-MF metabolite was shown by autoradiography to be most heavily bound in the bronchiolar Clara cells. It is known from other studies that a very active cytochrome P-450 enzyme system is concentrated in this specific family of lung cells (13). Not surprisingly therefore, many Clara cells were destroyed in the lungs by 3-MF. Also, as could be anticipated, the metabolism inhibitor, piperonyl butoxide, prevented the *in vivo* covalent binding and toxicity of 3-MF in the lungs of mice. Conversely, diethylmaleate treatment, which removes glutathione (presumably an alternate, "nontoxic" site for reaction of the active 3-MF metabolite), resulted in the enhancement of pulmonary covalent binding and toxicity of 3-MF in mice.

Target tissue toxicity

Drs. Haschek, Hakkinen, Morse and Witschi at the Oak Ridge National Laboratory have extensively studied the toxicity of single-dose and multi-dose regimens of 3-MF administered by inhalation. Several detailed reports of these results are in press (14-16) and others are forthcoming. A few of the major observations from this work are particularly noteworthy in the present context.

In all the species studied, including mice, rats and hamsters, the bronchiolar Clara cells were a prominent site of acute damage in the lungs after a single 1 hr exposure to 3-MF. As indicated before, this is exactly what we would anticipate based on the knowledge that 3-MF must be activated by metabolism, and that the necessary enzymatic machinery is present in these cells. The exposure concentrations studied were in the range of 300-900 ppm for mice and 3600-7900 ppm in rats and hamsters.

In mice, the Clara cell damage was followed by bronchiolar cell proliferation and airway repair which was essentially complete within 21 days. In the hamster, after nonlethal exposures, the selective necrosis of pulmonary Clara cells was repaired within about 14 days. In contrast, in the rat, the pulmonary bronchiolar damage was more extensive and was followed by scattered peribronchiolar fibrosis and epithelial mucous metaplasia suggestive of "small airway disease" of man. Also as might be expected, the higher concentrations of 3-MF caused centrilobular liver necrosis in all three species. Only in mice did 3-MF cause kidney necrosis, and this result was consistent with studies with another furan compound, 4-ipomeanol, that causes nephrotoxicity only in mice and not in rats and hamsters (17). Metabolism studies with 4-ipomeanol showed that only the kidneys of adult male mice (as used in the present studies) and not those of rats or hamsters contained a cytochrome P-450 enzyme activity which catalyzed the covalent binding of the compound to renal macromolecules.

Another striking lesion that occured in all three species was a relatively selective necrosis of the nasal olfactory epithelium. In rats, the olfactory damage was more severe and still not resolved even after a month, and a partial occlusive fibrosis of the nasal cavity was present (16). Although we have not yet studied directly the metabolilsm of any furan compound in olfactory tissue, it seems likely that this target tissue damage by 3-MF is also a result of the capacity to metabolically activate the compound *in situ.* Interestingly, there have been several recent reports of cytochrome P-450 dependent mixed function oxidase activity in the nasal epithelium of various animal species (18).

CONCLUSIONS

At this point we should like to conclude with a few comments concerning the possible relevance of such studies to the problem of human risk assessment. Obviously, we still lack much critical knowledge before we could yet make any really quantitative extrapolations for human risk with 3-methylfuran. Nevertheless, what we have learned is potentially useful at least in a *qualitative* sense. For example, some knowledge of the biochemical mechanism of toxicity and, in particular, the importance of target tissue metabolism, may alert us not only to possible target tissues for damage but also in some cases the characteristic pattern of cellular damage we might expect to see in a given tissue. Indeed, if, as if the case if 3-methylfuran, we know that target tissue susceptibility depends upon the capacity of that tissue to metabolize the compound to a reactive intermediate *in situ,* we may directly compare animal and human tissues in this respect. This requires, of course, that we have access to suitable samples of human material. For example, an inability of human kidney to metabolize 3-methylfuran to methylbutenedial might predict that humans would more likely resemble rats and hamsters, rather than mice, with respect to susceptibility to renal damage by 3-methylfuran.

However, our ability to make more quantitative projections based on these kinds of studies still is difficult or impossible due to many critical gaps in our knowledge. These gaps not only concern toxic mechanisms but also the question of actual exposure concentrations encountered and what they may really mean with a particular compound. For example, even if we had accurate quantitative data on actual human exposure to 3-methylfuran (which we do not presently have) and could therefore relate this to animal exposures, we would still need to relate this in turn to the resultant concentrations to which the target tissues are subjected. This information, while relatively straightforward to obtain in laboratory animals, is difficult, if not practically impossible, to obtain in humans. Moreover, the target tissue concentrations of the parent compound alone are not sufficient to allow any kind of extrapolation in terms of expected toxicity. We need also to know how to quantitatively relate exposure concentrations to the amounts of the ultimate toxic metabolites(s) produced at the target sites. Even then, given our present state of knowledge, we must realize that it is still impossible to place any *quantitative* significance on the actual amounts of reactive metabolite(s) produced in a potential target tissue. How much or how little of a particular metabolite in a particular tissue is required to produce toxicity in a given animal species is subject to the effects of a plethora of biological variables, only a few of which we are yet able to identify.

Thus, it clearly appears that, for any given compound whose target tissue toxicity depends upon *in situ* metabolic activation, we may have a long way to go in terms of quantitative risk extapolations from laboratory animals to man. Nevertheless, we do seem to be gaining new knowledge of metabolism and toxicity mechanisms that may lead to improvements in our ability to make such predictions in the future. At the very least, this new knowledge can presently both help us predict likely target tissues for a given compounds, as well as also help us to predict what other compounds might produce similar kinds of target organ toxicity.

ACKNOWLEDGEMENT

Research partially sponsored jointly by the Office of Health and Environmental Research, U. S. Department of Energy, under contract W-7405-eng-26 with the Union Carbide Corporation, University of Tennesee-Oak Ridge Graduate School of Biomedical Sciences under subcontract 3322 from the Biology Division or ORNL to the University of Tennessee and PHS Grant CA-33765 from NCI.

REFERENCES

1. *Boyd, M. R.*: Biochemical mechanisms of chemical-induced lung injury: Roles of metabolic activation. *CRC Crit. Rev. Toxicol.* 7:103-176, 1980.

2. *Dunlop, A. P. and Peters, F. N.*: *The Furans*, Reinhold Publishing Co., New York (1953).

3. *Boyd, M. R.*: Biochemical mechanisms in pulmonary toxicity of furan derivatives. In Bend, J. R. *et al.* (eds.): *Reviews in Biochemical Toxicology.* New York, Elsevier/North Holland, 1980, pp. 71-101.

4. *Boyd, M. R.*: Toxicity mediated by reactive metabolites of furans. In Snyder, R., *et al.*, (eds.): *Biological Reactive Intermediates*, Vol. 2. New York, Plenum Press, 1982, pp. 865-879.

5. *Boyd, M. R., Grygiel, J. G. and Michin, R. F.*: Metabolic activation as basis for organ-selective toxicity. *Clin. Exp. Pharmacol. Physiol.* 10:87-107, 1983.

6. *Saunders, R., Griffith, J. and Saalfeld, F.*: Identification of some organic smog components based on rain water analysis. *Biomed. Mass. Spectrom.* 1:192-195, 1974.

7. *Boyd, M. R., Statham, C. N., Franklin, R. B. and Mitchell, J. R.*: Pulmonary bronchiolar alkylation and necrosis by 3-methylfuran, a potential atmospheric contaminant derived from natural sources. *Nature* 272:270-271, 1978.

8. *Franklin, R. B., Dutcher, J. S. and Boyd, M. R.*: Studies on toxic alkylating metabolites of 2-methylfuran. *Toxicol. Appl. Pharmacol.* 45:279, 1978.

9. *Ravindranath, V., Burka, . T. and Boyd, M. R.*: Isolation and characterization of the reactive metabolites of 2-methylfuran (2-MF). *Pharmacologist* 25:171, 1983.

10. *Ravindranath, V., Burka, L. T. and Boyd, M. R.*: Identification of reactive metabolites from the bioactivation of toxic methylfurans. *Toxicologist.* (in press).

11. *Burka, L. T. and Boyd, M. R.*: Furans. In M. W. Anders (ed.): *Bioactivation of Foreign Compounds.* Academic Press, (in press).

12. *Statham, C. N., Franklin, R. B. and Boyd;, M. R.*: Pulmonary bronchiolar alkylation and necrosis by 3-methylfuran, a potential atmospheric contaminant derived from natural sources. *Toxicol. Appl. Pharmacol.* 45:111, 1978.

13. *Boyd, M. R.*: Evidence for the Clara cell as a site of cytochrome P-450-dependent mixed-function oxidase activity in lung. *Nature 269* :713-715, 1977.

14. *Haschek, W. M., Morse, C. C., Boyd, M. R. Hakkinen, P. J. and Witschi, H. P.*: Pathology of acute inhalation exposure to 3-methylfuran in the rat and hamster. *Exp. Mol. Pathol.*, (in press).

15. *Haschek, W. M. Boyd, M. R., Hakkinen, P. J. and Witschi, H. P.*: Acute inhlation toxicity of 3-methylfuran in the mouse: Pathology, cell kinetics and respiratory rate effects. *Toxicol. Appl. Pharmacol.*, (in press).

16. *Morse, C. C., Boyd, M. R. and Witschi, H.*: The effect of 3-methylfuran inhalation exposure on the rat nasal cavity. *Toxicology.* (in press).

17. *Boyd, M. R. and Dutcher, J. S.*: Renal toxicity due to reactive metabolites formed *in situ* in the kidney: Investigations with 4-ipomeanol in the mouse. *J. Pharmacol. Exp. Ther. 216*:640-646, 1981.

18. *Hadley, W. M. and Dahl, A. R.*: Cytochrome P-450-dependent monooxygenase activity in ansal membranes of six species. *Drug Metabolism Disp. 11*:275-280, 1983.

*New Approaches in Toxicity Testing and Their
Application in Human Risk Assessment,* edited by
A. P. Li. Raven Press, New York © 1985.

Physiological Pharmacokinetics: Relevance to Human Risk Assessment

R. J. Lutz and R. L. Dedrick

Chemical Engineering Section, Biomedical Engineering and Instrumentation Branch, Division of Research Services, National Institutes of Health, Bethesda, Maryland 20205

The growing public awareness of the widespread distribution of anthropogenic chemicals in the environment has led to an increased concern about their effects on animals and man. This concern has produced demands that the risks of such chemicals be estimated in some rational way and that exposure be limited if the risks are judged excessive. We are thus faced with the problem of assessing risk quantitatively based on observations that we can make. Surveillance of selected populations, such as occupational groups, has produced important data and will continue to be an important epidemiological tool. But surveillance is not adequate because it is inherently retrospective and because certain affects, such as cancer, may not be observed for many years. We must conduct studies in experimental systems, and the quantitative interpretation of these studies poses important and challenging scientific questions. Quantitative risk assessment involves the use of mathematical models which are designed to predict the probability of a toxic response as a function of the dose of chemical agent. These models must consider problems such as: (1) the extrapolation of high-dose toxicity studies to low-dose predictions, (2) interspecies extrapolation, e. g. predictions of effects of human exposure from studies with experimental animals, and (3) the temporal variation in exposure. Low dose experiments in animals are either statistically intractable, too time consuming, or too expensive when the probability of response is 10^{-2} or less (1).

The mathematical models referred to can be viewed as having distinct but interacting components as illustrated in Figure 1. One component, which we call a pharmacokinetic model, describes the time courses of concentration of the toxic agent at any location in a subject after exposure to a known dose of chemical. A second component is a biological model that describes the toxic agent's interaction with the susceptible tissue's biochemical elements. The third component is a risk assessment model which correlates the probability of a response, such as carcinogenesis, as a function of the local concentration of toxic agent. The supposition in many dose-response risk assessment models is that the response is directly related to the magnitude of the administered dose of parent chemical rather than to the concentration of the effective chemical species at the site of action. The former and the latter are not always linearly related for numerous reasons which we will discuss later. However, their inter-relationship can often be described by a pharmacokinetic model. A risk assessment model which incorporates more relevant correlates such as local metabolite concentration or DNA-adduct formation, rather than administered dose, can be used more effectively to predict the response due to low levels of exposure.

This paper deals primarily with the first component of Figure 1, in the overall risk assessment scheme, namely the usefulness of the pharmacokinetic model. It describes the fundamental principles in pharmacokinetic model development which include concepts such as animal scale-up, interspecies metabolism difference, *in vitro* or *in vivo* correlation, and physiologic transport mechanisms. The discussion of the pharmacokinetic model development is rather general and draws upon examples of previous work which includes pharmacokinetic studies of environmental contaminants as well as other agents such as anti-cancer drugs. However, the same principles are applicable. Some of the unique and interesting findings of the pharmacokinetic model analysis can serve as guidelines for use in further development of improved risk assessment models.

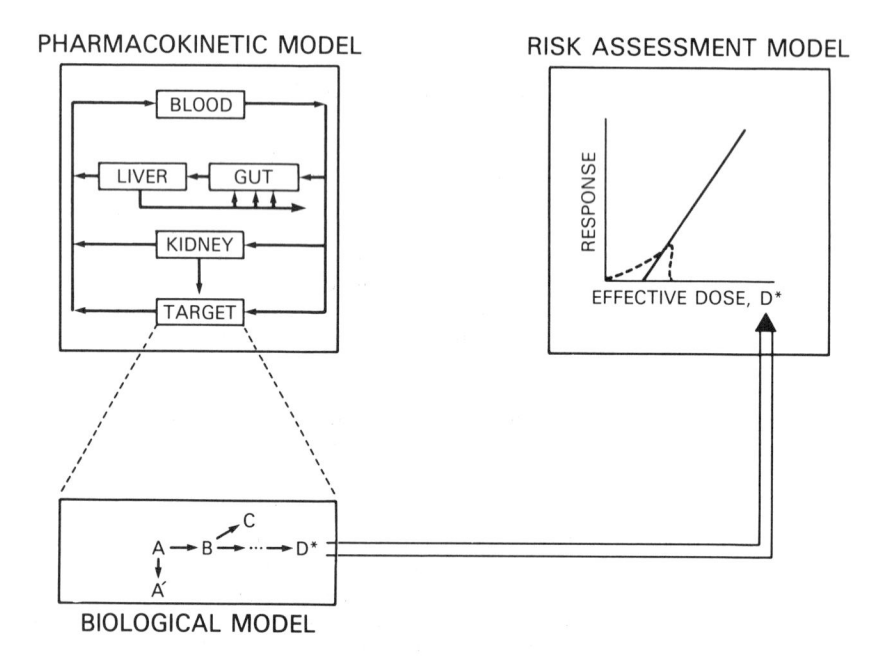

FIGURE 1: Schematic representing the interactions of pharmacokinetic models to risk assessment models via biological interpretation in target tissues.

PHARMACOKINETIC MODELS

Pharmacokinetic models are designed to describe and predict the time course of drug or other chemical concentration throughout the body. Classical pharmacokinetics yield parameters which usually have no obvious relationships to anatomical structure or physiological function. In essence, they represent curve fits of data. Physiological pharmacokinetic models apply basic physiological, anatomical, and biochemical information to determine chemical distribution and disposition. Our discussion here deals strictly with physiological pharmacokinetic models. Only a brief discussion of such models is presented here. More detailed descriptions are available (2,3).

The basic unit of construction for a physiological model is a lumped-compartment which is illustrated in Figure 2. A compartment respresents a region of the body at some uniform chemical concentration. It may be a single capillary with surrounding tissue, a discrete organ, like the kidney or liver, or a widely distributed anatomical region such as muscle or fat. Numerous compartments can be arranged according to a proper anatomical scheme in order to simulate an entire body system. The compartments that are included are major sites for disposition of the chemical or for elimination by clearance or metabolism, or are regions that are suspect for possible toxic response. Figure 3 represents a physiological pharmacokinetic model of polychlorinated biphenyl distribution that has been applied to the mouse, rat, dog, and monkey. The mathematical formulation of the model consists of mass balances on each compartment. The balance equations account for the influx and efflux of chemical by blood flow, for transport across cells membranes, for intracellular or extracellular binding to proteins or other cellular elements such as DNA, for clearance by specific organs such as the liver or kidney, and for metabolism in any tissue. The availability of such a seemingly powerful mathematical tool is not without drawbacks. To make *a priori* predictions of chemical distribution, a rather larger number of parameters is required. The parameters can be put into four general categories: (1) anatomical, such as tissue blood flow rates and tissue or organ volumes; (2) thermodynamic, such as equilibrium relationships between free and bound chemical in intracellular and extracellular compartments; (3) physiological, such as clearances and metabolism rates; and (4) transport, such as diffusion coefficients, cell membrane permeabilities, and absorption rates. A considerable body of literature is available to obtain many of these necessary parameters, while others can be determined from properly designed experiments.

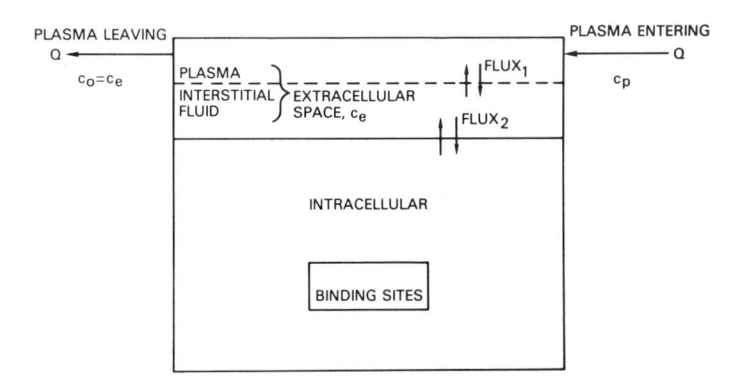

FIGURE 2: Representation of a single compartment in a pharmacokinetic model.

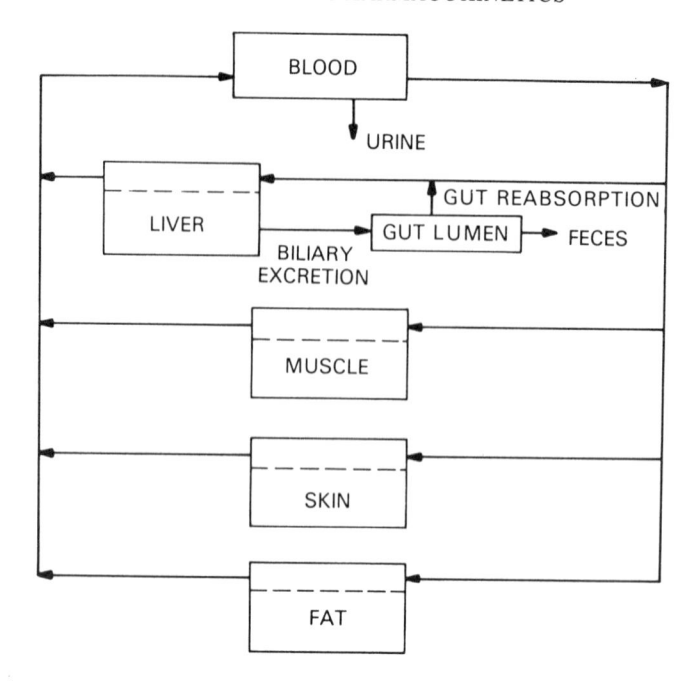

FIGURE 3: Compartmental flow diagram for polychlorinated biphenyls (11).

Since these parameters have physiological significance, interspecies correlations are possible, and herein lies the utility of physiological pharmacokinetic models. As we shall see from the upcoming discussion, the methods for scaling some parameters from one species to another are rather direct and well-documented, while other parameters require some novel approach for interspecies correlation. We can discuss the parameter scale up procedures according to the four generic categories.

Anatomical

There are many similarities in the anatomy of mammalian species including a remarkable geometric similarity. The same blood flow diagram could be used for all mammals, and most organs and tissues are similar fractions of body weight. Adolph (4) summarized the orderly variation of numerous anatomic properties of some mammalian species as a function of body weight. Bischoff *et al.,* (5) have presented a number of correlations for these parameters in mammals. For example, the blood flow rate to various organs varies as body weight to approximately the 0.8 power. Volumes of organs and tissues also correlated well with (body weight)^n, where the exponent, n, varies somewhat, for example, 0.85 for kidney, 0.87 for liver, 0.94 for small intestine, and 1.0 for muscle. Other data are often available for compartment spaces, organ sizes, and blood flow rates, in standard reference handbooks (e.g. 6). The applicability of the scale-up procedure in a physiological model is not restricted to mammalian species as long as the requisite parameters can be obtained for the system of interest. For example, Bungay *et al.,* (7) have successfully modeled phenol red distribution in the dogfish shark and Zaharko *et al.,* (8) have simulated the pharmacokinetics of methotrexate in the sting ray. Zaharko *et al.,* used a physiological pharmacokinetic model developed originally for the mouse. There are numerous reports where the scale-up procedure has been sucessfully applied from small mammals all the way to humans, e.g. (5,9,10). Anatomical similitude among various

Thermodynamic

Thermodynamic parameters relate primarily to terms which describe purely physical interactions of exogenous chemicals with biological tissues and fluids in the form of equilibrium distribution such as protein binding and tissue partitioning. In many cases, these parameters are quite similar from species to species as the following examples can attest. Lutz et al., (11) have estimated the tissue to blood distribution coefficients for four congeners of polychlorinated biphenyls (PCB's) in the rat. Adipose tissue consistently exhibited the highest distribution coefficient of all tissues; skin was second. Similar results have been observed in the mouse, dog, and monkey. In all four species, the fat had the highest distribution coefficient, and it was similar from species to species. This effect reflects the fat solubility of PCB. Fat represents a primary depot for PCB distribution and as such has a significant influence on the time course of the distribution. An example of this influence is illustated in Figure 4, which compares experimental data for 2,2',4,4',5,5' hexachlorobiphenyl in blood and fat tissue of the rat with pharmacokinetic model simulations. The dotted lines represent simulations using compartments of constant volume. However, during the 42-day time course of the experiments, the data indicated a more rapid decline in concentration than these initial simulations. It was determined that during this time interval, the young rats were growing considerably, and much of the increase in total body mass was attributed to an increase in adipose tissue size. This increase in fat content provided a gradually increasing volume of distribution for the PCB and resulted in a dilution of its concentration in the fat and a shift of the compound from blood to fat. When the time increase in fat volume was incorporated into the model, a better simulation of the long term data was achieved, as shown by the solid lines (Figure 4). The effective "volume" of the fat is much larger than its anatomical volume because of its larger partition coefficient, R.

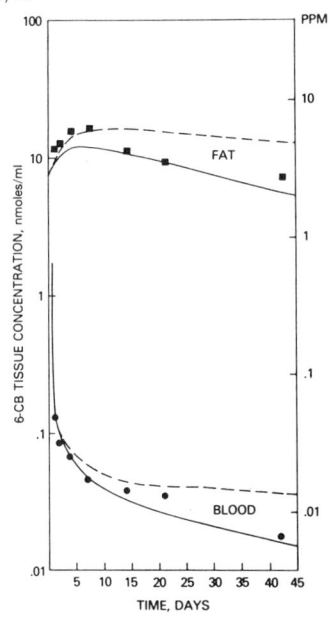

FIGURE 4: Concentration of 2,2',4,4',5,5'-hexachlorobyphenyl versus time in fat and blood of a rat after a single *iv* dose of 0.6 mg/kg (11).

Another method for estimating thermodynamic parameters for any animal species involves the use of *in vitro-in vivo* correlations. For example, Bischoff and Dedrick (9) developed a pharmacokinetic model for thiopental that used protein binding data from the cow and rabbit, and fat solubility from peanut oil-water partitioning to successfully predict the distribution of thiopental in the dog and in humans. Lindstrom *et al.,* (12) have presented a mammalian model of dieldrin pharmacokinetcs that is based on the lipid content of tissue and on the lipid fraction of blood flow to each tissue. They applied this approach to a simulation of dieldrin distribution in rats and in humans. Their model should be valid for highly lipid-soluble compounds, and its allows for data interpretation and experimental design.

A scheme for estimating *in vivo* tissue-to-blood partitioning coefficient has been proposed by Lin *et al.,* (13) using *in vitro* drug-protein binding data. Binding studies of a model drug (ethoxybenzamide) were performed with homogenates of numerous tissues in the rat. The partition coefficients calculated in this way correlated very well with the partition coefficients determined by standard *in vivo* pharmacokinetic studies.

Nonspecific binding of drugs to plasma protein or tissue is not necessarily the sole determinant of *in vivo* distribution. Binding to specific intracellular elements may affect the overall distribution of drugs or exogenous chemicals, and, indeed, this binding may be influential in eliciting a carcinogenic or toxic response. Terasaki *et al.,* (14) suggest that the characteristic tissue distribution of adriamycin can be associated with the tissue concentration of DNA to which it binds. They found a good correlation between the tissue-to-blood partition coefficient and the tissue DNA content in the rat, and a reasonably good similar correlation in the rabbit except for gut, lung, and spleen. Heart and liver showed a 10-fold difference in partition coefficient between the rats and rabbits, but the authors suggest that this species difference can be explained by the different DNA concentration in these tissues. Another species comparison of non-specific protein binding and specific saturable binding to intracellular enzymes was reported by Bischoff *et al.* (5) for methotrexate binding to dihydrofolate reductase in the mouse, rat, dog, monkey, and man. There was a fair degree of similarity in binding characteristics among tissues from all five species. Data from our laboratory showed a good correlation between the maximum binding capacity parameter in the methotrexate pharmacokinetic model and the activity of dihydrofolate reductase (DHFR) that was measured in several tissues of the rat. Also, the same dissociation constant for methotrexate-DHFR binding was applied in the methotrexate model for all five species, and this dissociation constant was determined by Weikheiser (15) from *in vitro* binding studies of liver tissue homogenates.

Bungay *et al.,* (16) summarized tissue-to-blood distribution coefficients for Kepone in the rat and human and found better than order of magnitude agreement in all tissues examined. The liver showed the greatest discrepancy, and this may reflect the liver metabolizing ability.

In summary, then, it appears plausible that distribution of many drugs and xenobiotics will follow principles of thermodynamic partitioning, and that these principles will be predictable from tissue to tissue and from species to species, so that distribution studies conducted in animals can be extrapolated to humans especially if physiological pharmacokinetic models are available. Numerous techniques have proven useful for correlating these thermodynamic parameters.

Physiological

The model parameters that fall under the physiological category show very significant tissue-to-tissue and species-to-species variation. These include clearances and metabolism rates. Since they are among the more difficult to predict or extrapolate, estimation of these model paramaters often confounds pharmacokinetic model predictability. In spite of the seeming restrictions, a number of useful correlations have been reported for kinetic parameters which can be readily incorporated into the physiologic model structure.

Adolph (4) presented correlations for clearances in mammals as a function of body weight as shown in Table 1. Dedrick et al., (17) have demonstrated this correlation in their pharmacokinetic study of the anticancer drug 1-β-D arabinofuranosylcytosine (Ara-C). Figure 5 shows clearance values for mice, monkey, dogs, and humans on a log-log plot. The slope of the line is 0.8 which agrees well with the exponent for clearance of inulin and PAH in Table 1. Dedrick et al., (18) also showed a correlation for the plasma half life of methotrexate in mouse, rat, monkey, dog and man which show a 0.2 power dependence of half life on body weight, in good agreement with their theoretical estimate of 0.25 based on residence-time considerations. We have noted in our own work that methotrexate clearance is approximately 30% greater than creatinine clearance in humans, and likewise the methotrexate clearance reported by Bischoff et al., (5) for rats is just slightly larger (20%) than the rat inulin clearance given by Bourne and Barba (19). If the predominate mechanism for clearance is the same from species to species, then extrapolation from one species to another would seem feasible by correlations such as those listed above.

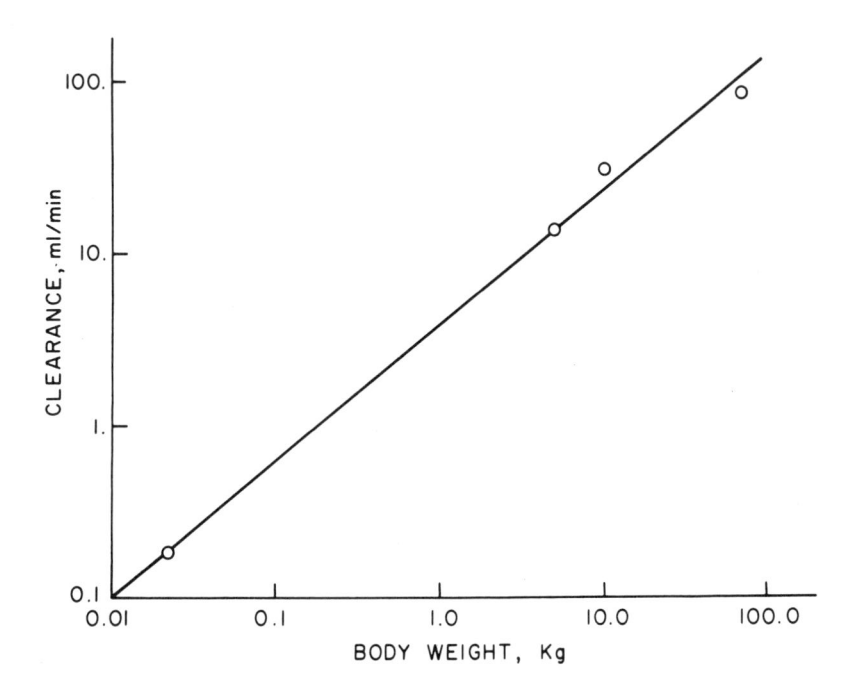

FIGURE 5: Kidney clearance of Ara-C and Ara-U versus body weight for mice, monkeys, dogs, and man. (17)

TABLE 1

Property	Exponent
Creatinine clearance	0.69
Inulin clearance	0.77
PAH clearance	0.80
Basal O_2 consumption	0.73
Endogeneous N output	0.72
O_2 consumption by liver slices	0.77
Kidney weight	0.85
Heart weight	0.98
Liver weight	0.87
Stomach and intestines weight	0.94
Blood weight	0.99

Relationship between properties and body weights among mammals, Property = (Body Weight)^{Exponent} from (4).

One of the most unpredictable physiological mechanisms is metabolism. A good example of this variability is evident from our recent work with polychlorinated biphenyls (PCB). In our studies with four PCB congeners in mice, rats, dogs, and monkeys, we utilizied a physiological pharmacokinetic model to estimate intrinsic metabolism constants and found no correlation with body weight for either slowly or rapidly metabolized PCB's. The dog had a much greater metabolism rate than the monkey although they are of comparable body size. The metabolism rate parameters for Ara-C for mouse, monkey, dog, and man reported by Dedrick et al., (17) showed no apparent correlation from species to species. Indeed, localization of metabolic activity in specific tissues was quite variable; e.g., the largest metabolic rate for man was assigned to the liver whereas mice had a low metabolic rate in the liver but a very high rate in the kidney.

Though it may not be possible to generalize about metabolism rates in various species, one method that shows considerable potential for overcoming this limitation in in vitro - in vivo correlation. The metabolism of most foreign organic compounds in the body occurs by enzymatic pathways whose activities can be determined by several systems such as tissue homogenates, cell suspensions, microsomal preparations, and even isolated, perfused whole organs. The enzymatic activities, converted to the proper basis, can be incorporated into physiological pharmacokinetic models. Examples of in vitro - in vivo correlations for metabolism have already been reported in the literature.

As discussed earlier, Dedrick et al., (17) have reported the large variability of deaminase activity in various tissues in mouse, monkey, dog, and man. However, they used this in vitro data (10) to obtain the Vmax and Michaelis constant for the deamination of Ara-C and with the aid of a physiologic pharmacokinetic model were able to simulate the tissue concentrations of Ara-C and its metabolic product Ara-U (1-β-D-arabinofuranosyluracil) in the four species. Caution must be exercised in evaluating in vitro and in vivo metabolic data. If reaction rates in specific organs, like the liver, are very high then metabolism of parent compound may be controlled by the blood flow rate to that organ rather than by local enzyme kinetics. Predictions of drug concentrations would be insensitive to the enzyme kinetic parameters, and estimate of in vivo enzyme activities may prove erroneous. This concept is known as blood flow limitation and its interpretation with regard to *in vivo* enzyme kinetics has been illustrated by Dedrick and Forrester (20). Figure 6 shows the results of a flow model for ethanol pharmacokinetics and illustrates how changes in the liver blood flow alone can effect the predicted ethanol concentration and lead to incorrect *in vivo* estimates of the Michaelis constant for the alcohol dehydrogenase-ethanol reaction in the liver. The flow rates of 6.3 ml/min and 13.2 ml/min represent a range of values reported for liver blood flow in rats.

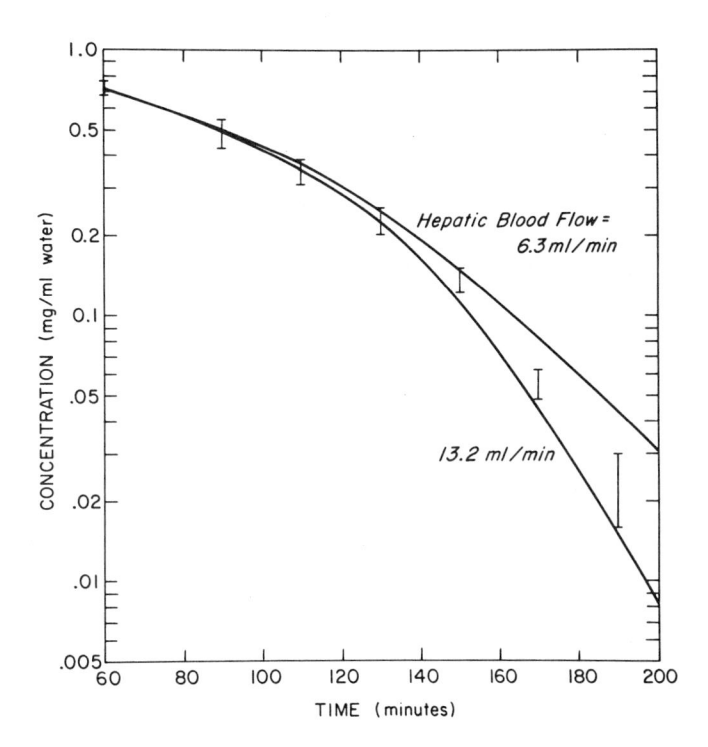

FIGURE 6: Concentration of ethanol in rat body water versus time showing the effect of hepatic blood flow on liver clearance of ethanol (20).

In vitro - in vivo correlations for other drugs have been performed for which organ blood flow limitations have not been a factor. For example, Collins *et al.,* (21) predicted the clearances and half lives of phenytoin in pregnant and non-pregnant female rats based on *in vitro* liver homogenate reaction data. Lin *et al.,* (22) used *in vitro* data from rat and rabbit liver microsomes to estimate Vmax and Michaelis constants for the deethylation of ethoxybenzamide and incorporated these parameters into a physiologic pharmacokinetic model to simulate plasma and tissue concentrations of ethoxybenzamide.

Estimates of metabolic parameters can also be derived from studies with isolated perfused organs. McManus *et al.,* (23) investigated the elimination of the radiation sensitizer misonidazole (MISO) and its metabolite, desmethylminsonidazole (DESMISO) in isolated rat liver. A pharmacokinetic model was formulated to describe the dose-dependent elimination of both MISO and DESMISO. Most of the kinetic parameters in the model were determined from least square regression analysis of the liver perfusate data, although several reaction rate parameters were previously estimated from *in vitro* microsomal assays. These parameters were incorporated into a physiological pharmacokinetic model to simulate the drug distribution.

Use of isolated, perfused organ studies allows the investigator to fractionate the pharmacokinetic problem by studying interactions of a chemical in a specific organ without the added complication of pharmacokinetic events in the remainder of the body. Conclusions made from such studies are valid to the extent that the milieu of the isolated organ mimics the *in situ* environment that the chemical would experience in that tissue whole-body studies.

It is important to note that both linear and nonlinear reaction kinetics can easily be handled in the framework of a pharmacokinetic model. As in the misonidazale example cited above, the nonlinear kinetics is usually written in the form of saturable, Michaelis-Menten equations. The notion of saturable metabolism has important implications in risk assessment analysis as Gehring *et al.,* (24) have recently pointed out, since it is often the reactive form of a metabolite rather than the parent compound that leads to a toxic reponse. The ability of pharmacokinetic models to calculate levels of metabolites can greatly improve the predictability of risk assessment models since the latter can be based on exposure levels of metabolite rather than doses of parent compound.

Transport

Another concept that should be considered in risk assessment analysis is the time-dependent concentration of the toxic agent at the site of action. The site of action is often an intracellular element such as DNA or a microsomal enzyme. The concentration of toxic agent at this site is not always proportional to the dose or even to the plasma levels of administered chemical, thus making direct correlations between reponse and dose a tenuous procedure in dose-response models. Aside from nonlinear metabolism considerations, transport processes such as blood perfusion (flow rate per unit volume of tissue) or cell membrane diffusion can also significantly influence the amount and the time course of tissue uptake of a toxic chemical agent. Some examples will be discussed to illustate this point.

A compartment, tissue, or organ is said to be flow-limited with regard to its uptake of a chemical agent when the rate of tissue uptake is controlled by the rate at which the chemical is carried to the tissue by the blood flow. In contrast, a compartment, tissue, or organ is said to be membrane-limited with regard to its uptake of a chemical agent when the rate of uptake is controlled by capillary or cell membrane permeability. It is the relative magnitude of the flow rate per unit volume of tissue (Q/V) compared to the product of the cell membrane permeability and cell membrane area per unit volume of tissue (PA/V) that determines which process dominates the uptake. Transport is said to be flow-limited, e.g., if Q/V is much less than PA/V.

Different tissues in the body do have different perfusion rates per unit volume. The perfusion rates per unit volume for the liver and kidney are quite high (Q/V of the order 1 min^{-1}) for example, compared to the skin and fat Q/V of the order 0.1 to 0.01 min^{-1}. The effect of these different perfusion rates on tissue uptake can be demonstrated by model simulations. Figure 7 shows the concentrations in three tissues, each with a different Q/V, when all are exposed to a constant plasma concentration of 1.0 µg/ml. The tissue with Q/V = 0.05 min^{-1} obviously responds more slowly to the imposed plasma concentration and takes much longer to reach its equilibrium value compared to the tissue with Q/V = 0.5 min^{-1}. Figure 8 illustrates the transient response of three tissues with different Q/V to a declining plasma concentration. This simulates the result from a single exposure to a chemical that is gradually cleared from the body. The concentration in the compartment with the largest Q/V (1.0 min⁻¹) is seen to track the plasma concentration quite readily, and it has the highest peak value. The compartment with $Q/V = 0.1$ min⁻¹ is similar to the previous curve, though its peak concentration is not as high. The compartment with the lowest perfusion rate has a "sluggish" response to the plasma concentration. Although its peak concentration is the lowest, we notice that its concentration persists for a much longer time than the other two compartments in response to the same plasma curve. In this example, if a tissue concentration of 0.05 µg/ml happened to be a toxic level of chemical, then the "sluggish" compartment would be exposed to levels greater than 0.05 µg/ml for a longer time than the compartments with higher perfusion rates. The "sluggish" compartment also may serve as a reservoir for the chemical which results in a slow release back into the body.

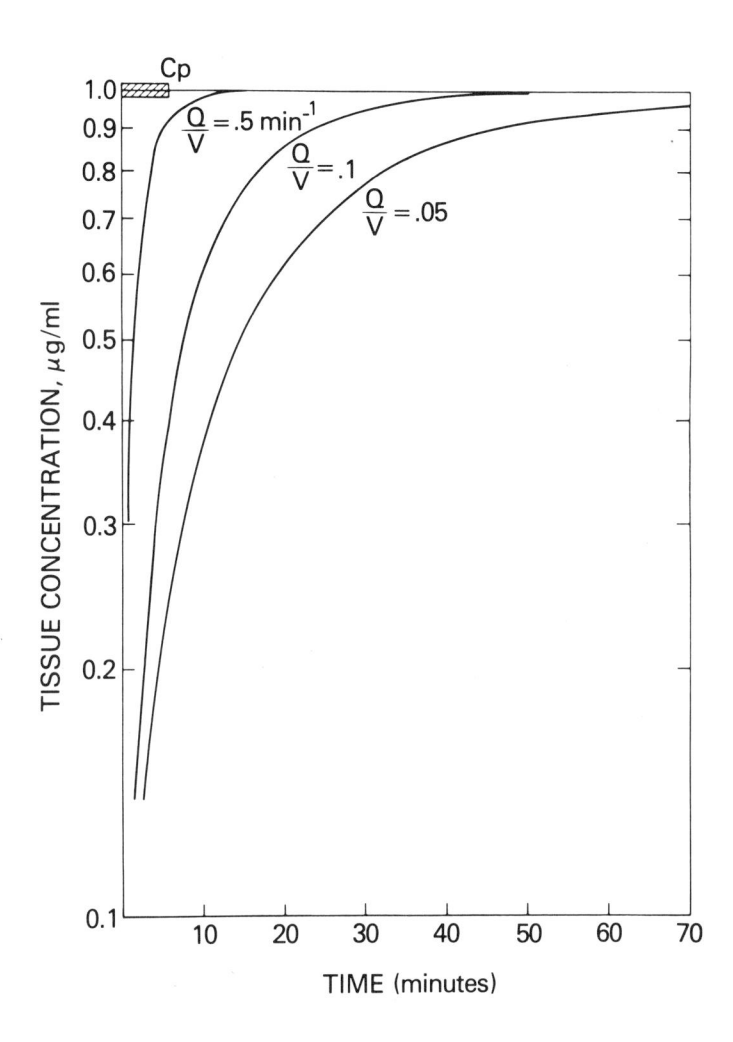

FIGURE 7: Simulation in a flow-limited compartment showing the effects of plasma perfusion rate on the time course of tissue concentration when exposed to a constant plasma concentration of 1.0 g/ml.

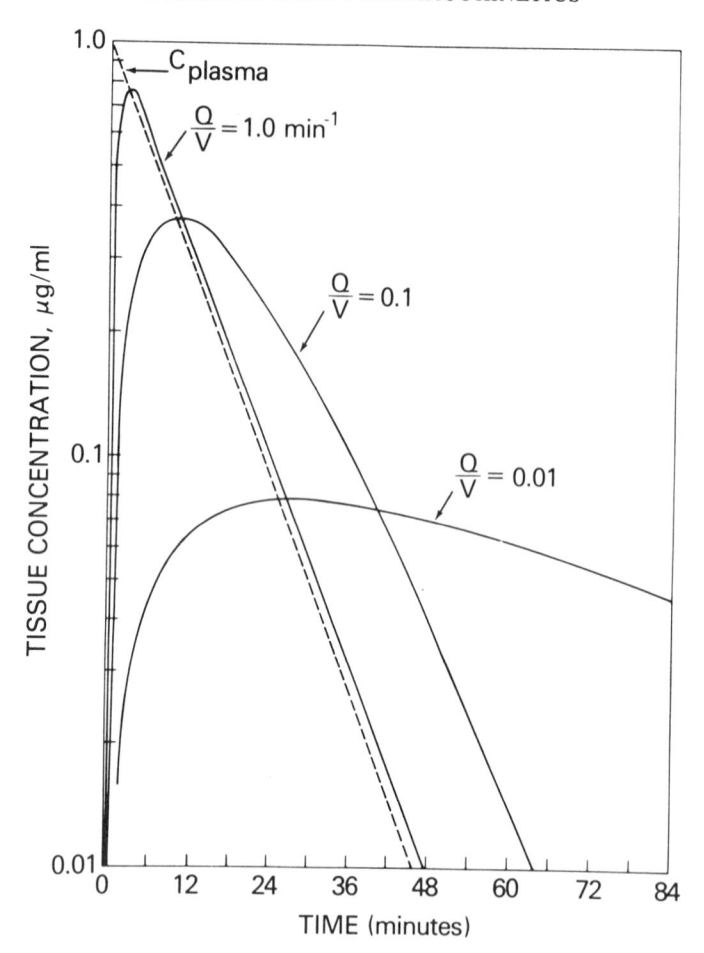

FIGURE 8: Simulation in three flow-limited compartments each with a different relative perfusion rate (1:10:100) showing the effects of perfusion rate on the time couse of tissue concentration when exposed to a single, iv bolus injection.

It should be pointed out that the area under each tissue curve is the same in all three cases if, as assumed in the simulations above, the chemical is not metabolized in the tissues. Unless one knows about the pharmacodynamics (i.e., the mechanism for toxicity), then it is difficult to assess which of the three curves represents the more serious toxic threat. For example, tissue reponse to alkylating agents is thought to correlate well with the area under the curve, whereas chemicals or drugs that are cell cycle specific are more influential when they exceed a minimum level for a particular period of time.

The effective volume or space of a compartment depends on the product of its anatomic volume V, and its tissue-to-blood partition coefficient R. If RV for one compartment is large compared to the summation of the RV's for the remaining compartments, then that compartment can actually dominate the whole body chemical disposition, and the long term transient of the plasma and other tissues would result in overall body persistence of the chemical. Such was the case with our analysis of PCB's in mouse, rat, dog, and monkey, as illustrated in Figure 9 which gives the time course of

2,2',4,4',5,5' hexachlorobiphenyl (2,4,5-HCB) in the rat after an intravenous bolus injection of 0.6 mg/kg. After four days the fat compartment still has not reached equilibrium, and the blood and other tissues have a long half-time, approximately 27 days (25), which is dictated by the fat compartment. As discussed above, much of the concentration decrease results from dilution caused by growth so that the actual elimination from the animal is much slower than implied by the 27-day half life. The arguments that we have listed regarding time-scaling of blood flow limited materials apply rigorously to non-metabolized compounds. The 2,4,5-HCB is so slowly metabolized, that it fits this analysis well.

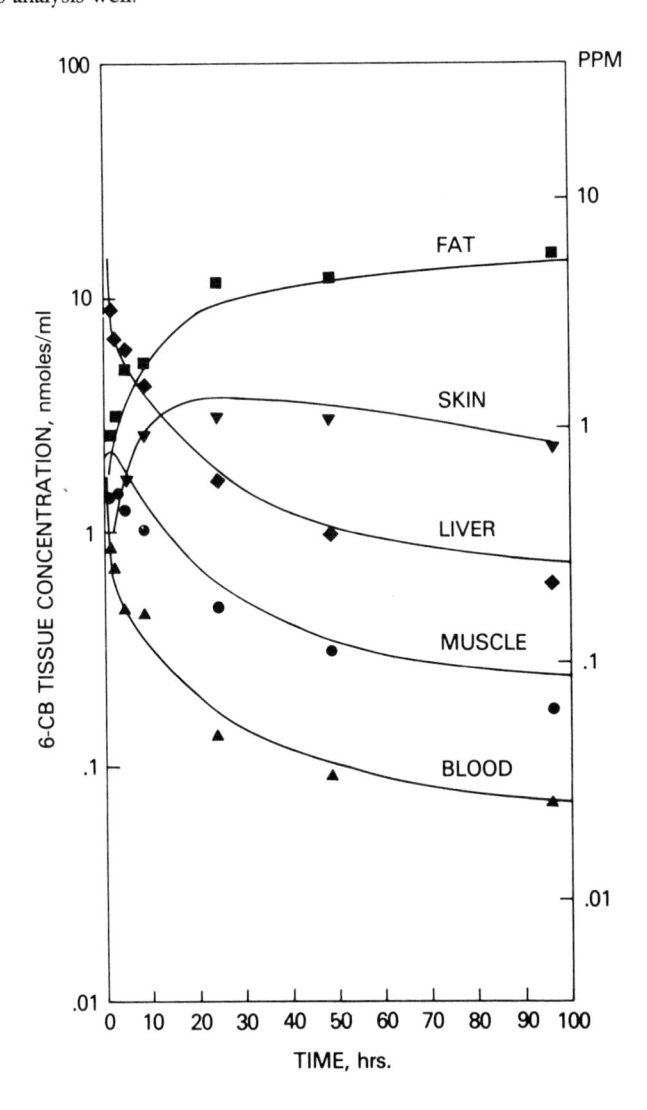

FIGURE 9: Concentration of 2,2',4,4'5,5'-hexachlorobiphenyl versus time in several tissues of the rat after a 0.6 mg/kg *iv* dose (11)

The pharmacokinetic effects in membrane-limited tissues can be similar to those of flow-limited tissues, especially when the permeability is independent of blood concentration. Nonlinear effects, often evident in membrane-limited intratissue transport, can lead to other interesting results in tissue uptake. Figures 10 and 11 illustrate the effects of saturable membrane transport. Figure 10 is a model simulation of a well-perfused compartment with linear cell membrane transport properties. The shaded bars represent three levels of constant plasma concentration of a chemical, and the curves represent the respective intracellular tissue concentrations which are seen to be directly proportional to the plasma concentration. Figure 11 represents model simulations of saturable membrane transport (Michaelis-Menten form) of a tissue exposed to the same constant plasma concentrations of chemical as in Figure 10. At the lowest dose (i.e. lowest plasma level) the linear model (Figure 10) and the saturable model (Figure 11) have the same tissue levels. However, as the highest dose is approached, we see that the rate of entry of chemical in the tissue with saturable membrane transport is much lower than that in Figure 10. If the plasma concentration were maintained at this level for sufficient time, then eventually the tissue concentration in the upper curve Figure 11 would reach 10 μg/ml as in Figure 10. However, if exposure were intermittent, then the intracellular tissue concentration might not achieve the same levels (10 μg/ml) as those in Figure 10. It is worth noting, however, that if the influx and efflux are symmetrical, then the smaller amounts of chemical that had entered the intracellular compartment in Figure 11, would be now slow to exit, and the exposure of intracellular components would be prolonged. This may have significant implication to toxicity, depending on the pharmacodynamics of the system.

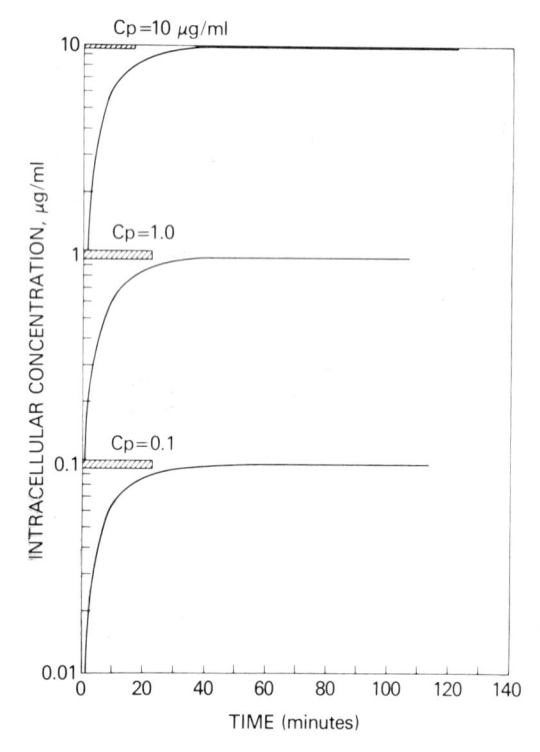

FIGURE 10: Simulations for a membrane-limited compartment exposed to several levels of constant plasma concentration for a linear cell permeability model.

PHYSIOLOGICAL PHARMACOKINETICS 143

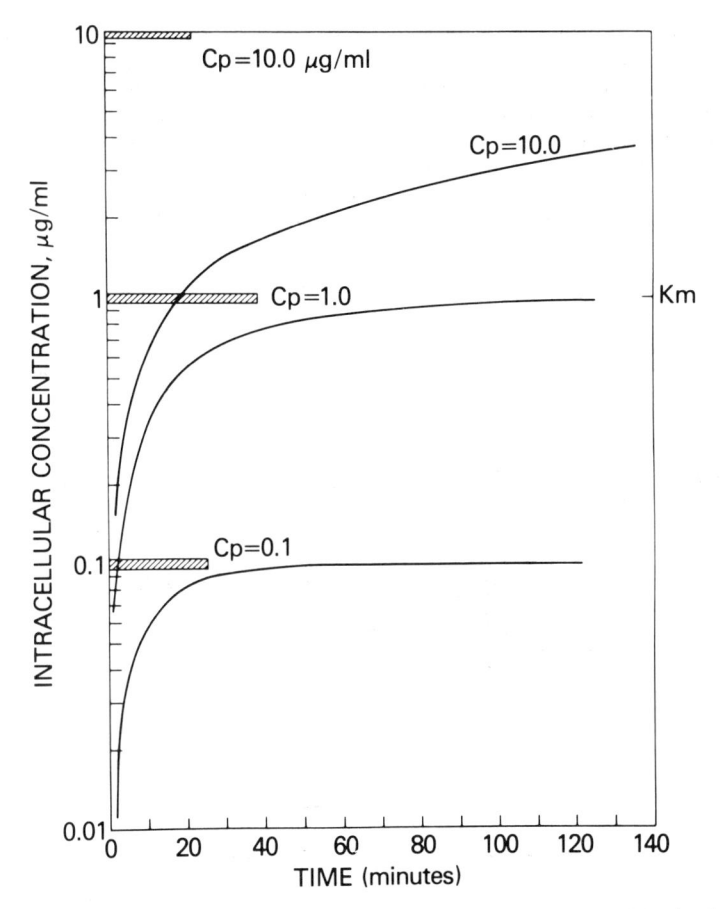

FIGURE 11: Simulations for a membrane-limited compartment exposed to several levels of constant plasma concentration showing intracellular concentration for a non-linear, saturable membrane permeability.

ROUTE OF ADMINISTRATION

An important consideration in toxicity studies is the route of administration of the chemical. Much of the environmental exposure to humans and animals occurs by oral ingestion, inhalation, or skin permeation. Since these modes of entry to the body are complex enough to entail significant pharmacokinetic studies unto themselves, most distribution studies are perfomed after simple intravenous administration of the chemical. However, the importance of these other routes of exposure on bioavailability has not been ignored, and physiological pharmacokinetic models become useful when considering non-parental routes of administration.

Bungay et al., (26) developed an enteric model for chlordecone (Kepone) transport in the rat. The full model is illustrated in Figure 12 showing the provision for oral dosing. The residence time for material in the stomach and other sections of the gastrointestinal tract were calculated from previous studies with nonabsorbable tracers. The gastrointestinal (GI) tract was subdivided into segments such as the small intestine, cecum, and large intestine. Each segment was further compartmentalized into a blood space, tissue space, and lumenal space with permeable membranes separating each. The model was used to analyze the experimental data for Kepone in the rat and resulted in an estimate of the permeability-gut surface area product (PA). The authors concluded that enteric transport in the rat was fecal-flow limited since the permeability of the mucosal membrane was high. The PA product for humans was estimated by assuming that the intrinsic permeability (P) for human mucosal membrane was the same as for the rat, and the surface area (A) for human gut scaled as the 2/3 power of body weight.

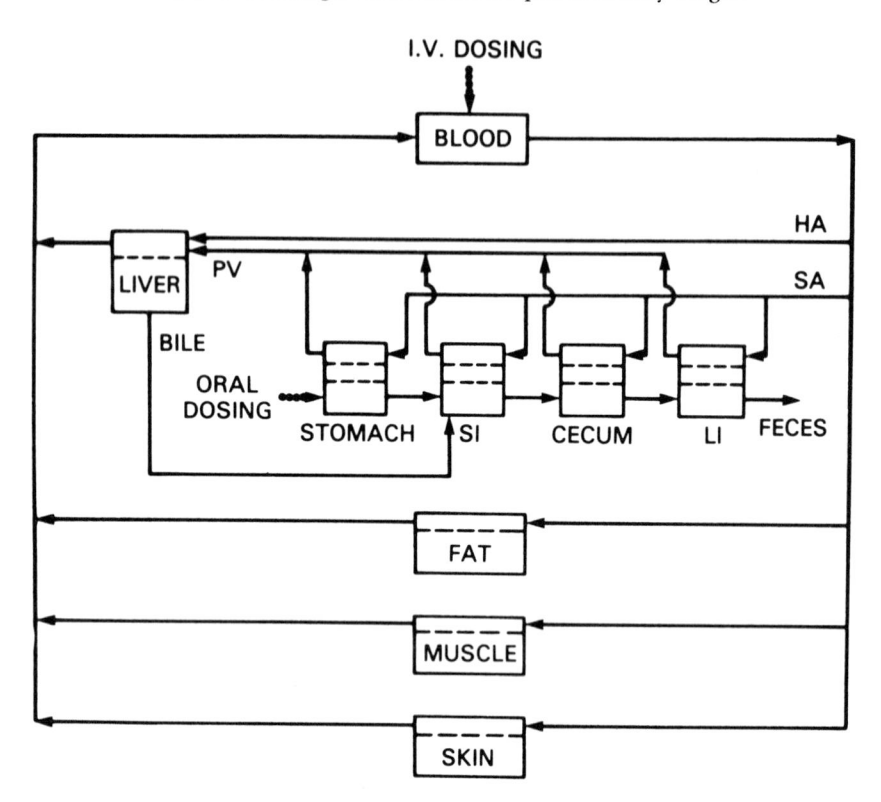

FIGURE 12: Schematic diagram for whole-body physiological pharmacokinetic model for chlordecone showing provision for oral dosing in gastrointestinal compartments (26).

Anderson et al., (27) have used physiological pharmacokinetic models to predict the concentration of inhaled gas and vapors at target tissues. The model includes transport across the alveolar membrane. The authors note that for inert gases that are poorly soluble in blood, blood flow limits the tissue uptake; while for inert gases highly soluble in blood, then alveolar ventilation and solubility regulate the uptake. Many inhaled vapors are metabolized in the liver by capacity limited enzyme systems, therefore, steady state arterial blood concentrations will not be a linear function of inhaled concentration but will increase disproportionately at high inhaled concentrations. The authors show examples of this effect with inhaled styrene in rats.

Dermal entry of some toxic chemicals may also be important. Complex mathematical models of drug permeation through the skin have been developed, such as that of

Michaelis et al., (28) for human skin. Their model includes processes of dissolution and molecular diffusion through a composite, multilayer membrane. Permeability was correlated with water solubility and oil/water partition coefficients of the penetrating molecule by *in vitro* experiments. Cooper (29) studied the pharmacokinetics of skin penetration and proposed a method that included diffusion theory coupled with a pharmacokinetic model of elimination for calculating skin permeabilities *in vivo* using excretion data.

In the models just described for oral, pulmonary, and dermal entry of chemicals into the body, the respective organs or tissues (i.e. GI tract, lung, and skin) were treated as inert membranes. In reality, each of these three tissues can be quite metabolically active. The ability of these tissues to interact biochemically with exposed chemical before they enter the body can greatly influence their toxic reponse, either enhancing it or diminishing it. However, these effects, too, can be incorporated into pharmacokinetic models to permit better predictability of reponse.

USE OF PHARMACOKINETICS IN RISK ASSESSMENT

There has been a growing acceptance of a role of pharmacokinetics in risk estimation; however, the means to accomplish this have not been fully elaborated. Pharmacokinetics is concerned with a description of the physical and chemical interactions of a foreign chemical in the body. Physiological pharmacokinetic principles offer the opportunity to extrapolate these interactions from one biological system to another or from one dose (or concentration) to another. These principles also provide an operational framework for examining temporal variation in dose and various routes of exposure. Changes in the host such as growth, enzyme induction, and altered physiological states can be incorporated quite naturally.

The application of pharmacokinetic theory to risk estimation requires a model of the toxic effect, and such "pharmacodynamic" models have been studied relatively little. Most risk models remain rooted in the concept of "dose-reponse" in which the dose schedule is usually quite simple such as a single administration or continuous exposure. Correlations are generally empirical and offer little guidance in how to account for varying temporal patterns of administration, species, sex and age variations, or extrapolation to low dose at which any response may be statistically inaccessible.

The range of pharmacodynamic models available may be illustrated with a few examples. Levy and his colleagues (30) have explored the relationship between the pharmacokinetics of warfarin enantiomers and anticoagulant effect. Jusko (31) has applied pharmacodynamic principles to chemical teratology. Cell killing or inhibition is of concern in cancer chemotherapy and has been approached by biochemical (32), compartmental (33,34), and population balance (35) methods. The importance of metabolic activation of the antimetabolite, Ara-C, has been stressed by Morrison et al., (36), and the kinetic implications of metabolic activation have been discussed by Gillette (37,38).

Cancer risk assessment has incorporated pharmacokinetic models only indirectly. Saturation of metabolic activation appears to account for the plateau in hepatic angiosarcoma induced by vinyl chloride in the rat, and it has been suggested that cancer risk assessments can be strengthened through examination of the amount of chemical metabolized (24), covalent binding to macromolecules (24,39,40), or specific levels of DNA adduct formation. (41).

It would appear that the rigorous application of pharmacokinetics to cancer risk assessment will require the use of biologically plausible mechanistic pharmacodynamic models which possess operational definitions of all parameters and permit incorporation of pharmacokinetic principles through their effect on model parameters. One such model might be the modification of the two-stage model of Armitage and Doll (42) described by Moolgavkar and his colleagues (43,44). Temporal effects of exposure can be incorporated naturally and, thus, can vary significantly with mechanism as shown by Day and Brown (45) by their application of a multistage model.

In conclusion, physiological pharmacokinetic models can provide a valuable tool in risk assessment because of their usefulness in interspecies extrapolation and dose extrapolation. Their utility is greatly strengthened when suitable pharmacodynamic models of biological effect are available.

REFERENCES

1. *Guess, H.; Crump, K.; Peto, R.*: Uncertainty Estimates for Low-Dose-Rate Extrapolations of Animal Carcinogenicity Data. *Cancer Research, 37* :3475-3483, 1977.

2. *Gibaldi, M. and Perrier, D.*: *Pharmacokinetics,* Marcel Dekker, New York, 1982.

3. *Lutz, R. J.; Dedrick, R. L.; Zaharko, D. S.*: Physiological Pharmacokinetics: An *In Vivo* Approach to Membrane Transport. *Pharmac Ther, 11*:559-592, 1980.

4. *Adolph, E. F.*: Quantitative Relations in the Physiological Constitutions of Mammals. *Science, 109*:579-585, 1949.

5. *Bischoff, K. B.; Dedrick, R. L.; Zaharoko, D. S.; and Longstreth, J. A.*: Methotrexate Pharmacokinetics, *J. Pharm. Sci., 60*:1128-1133, 1971.

6. *Biology Data Book,* edited by Atltman, P. L. and Dittmer, D.S.: Federation of American Societies for Experimental Biology, Washington, DC, 1964.

7. *Bungay, P.M.; Dedrick, R. L.; Guarino, A.M.*: Pharmacokinetic Modeling of the Dogfish Shark (Squalus Acanthias): Distribution and Urinary and Biliary Excretion of Phenol Red and Its Glucuronide. *J. Pharmacokin. Biopharm. 4* :377-388, 1976.

8. *Zaharko, D. S.; Dedrick, R. L.; Oliverio, V. T.*: Prediction of the Distribution of Methotrexate in the Sting Rays Dasyatide Savina and Sayi by Use of a Model Developed in Mice, *Comp. Biochem. Physiol., 42A*:183-194, 1972.

9. *Bischoff, K. B.; Dedrick, R. L.*: Thiopental Pharmacokinetcs, *J. Pharm. Sci., 57,* 1436-1351, 1968.

10. *Dedrick, R. L.; Forrester, D. D.; Ho, D. H. W.*: *In Vitro - In Vivo* Correlation of Drug Metabolism - Deamination of 1-D-Arabinofuranosylcytosine. *Biochem. Pharmacol., 21*:1-16, 1972.

11. *Lutz, R. J.; Dedrick, R. L.; Matthews, H. B.; Eling, T. E.; Anderson, M. W.*: A Preliminary Pharmacokinetic Model for Several Chlorinated Biphenyls in the Rat. *Drug Metab. Dispos., 5*:386-396, 1977.

12. *Lindstrom, F. T.; Gillette, J. W.; Rodecap, S. E.*: Distribution of HEOD (Dieldrin) in Mammals: I. Preliminary Model. *Arch. Environ. Contam. Toxicology, 2*:9-42, 1974.

13. Lin, J. H.; Suguyama, Y.; Awazu, S.; Hanano, M.: In Vitro and In Vivo Evaluation for the Tissue-to-Blood Partition Coefficients for Physiological Pharmacokinetic Models. *J. Pharmacokin. Biopharm.*, 10:637-647, 1982.

14. Terasaki, T.; Iga, T.; Sugiyama, Y.; Hanano, M.: Experimental Evidence of Characteristic Tissue Distribution of Adriamycin. Tissue DNA Concentration as a Determinant. *J. Pharm. Pharmacol.* 34:597-600, 1982.

15. Werkheiser, W. C.: Specific binding of 4-Amino Folic Acid Analogues by Folic Acid Reductase. *J. Biol. Chem.*, 236:888-893, 1961.

16. Bungay, P. M.; Dedrick, R. L.; Matthews, H. B.: Pharmacokinetics of Halogenated Hydrocarbon, *Ann. N. Y. Acad. Sci.*, 320:257-270, 1979.

17. Dedrick, R. L.; Forrester, D. D.; Cannon, J. N.; El Dareer, S. M.; Mellet, L. B.: Pharmacokinetics of 1-β-D-Arabinofuranosylcytosine (Ara-C) Deamination in Several Species. *Biochem. Pharmacol.*, 22:2405-2417, 1973.

18. Dedrick, R. L.; Bischoff, K. B.; Zaharko, D. S.: Interspecies Correlation of Plasma Concentration History of Methotrexate, *Cancer Chemother. Rep. Part I*, 54:95-101; 1970.

19. Bourne, G. R.; Barber, H. E.: The Pharmacokinetics of Inulin and Urea: A Comparison of the Dose Eliminated from the Compartmental Model and that Eliminated in Urine. *J. Pharm. Pharmacol.*, 24:532-537, 1972.

20. Dedrick, R. L.; Forrester, D. D.: Blood Flow Limitations in Interpreting Michaelis Constants for Ethanol Oxidation In Vivo, *Biochem. Pharmacol.*, 22:1133-1140, 1973.

21. Collins, J. M.; Blake, D. A.; Egner, P. G.: Phenytoin Metabolism in the Rat - Pharmacokinetic Correlation Between *in vitro* Hepatic Microsomal Enzyme Activity in *in vivo* Elimination Kinetics, *Drug Metab. Dispos.*, 6:251-257, 1978.

22. Lin, J. H.; Sugiyama, Y.; Awazu, S.; Manabu, H.: Physiological Pharmacokinetics of Ethoxybenzamide Based on Biochemical Data Obtained *in vitro* as well as on Physiological Data. *J. Pharmacokin. Biopharm.* 10:649-661, 1982.

23. McManus, M. E., Monks, A.; Collins, J. M.; White, R.; Strong, J. M.: Nonlinear Pharmacokinetics of Misonidazole and Desmethylmisonidazole in the Isolated Perfused Rat Liver, *J. Pharmacol. Exp. Ther.*, 219:669-674, 1981.

24. Gehring, P. J., P. G. Watanabe, and C. N. Park: "Risk of Angiosarcoma in Workers Exposed to Vinyl Chloride as Predicted from Studies in Rats, *"Toxicol. Appl. Pharmacol.* 49:15-24, 1979.

25. Anderson, M. W.; Eling, T. E.; Lutz, R. J.; Dedrick, R. L.; Matthews, H. B.: The Construction of a Pharmacokinetic Model for the Distribution of Polychlorinated Biphenyls in the Rat. *Clinical Pharmacol. Ther.*, 22:765-773, 1977.

26. Bungay, P. M.; Dedrick, R. L.; Matthews, H. B.: Enteric Transport of Chlordecone (Kepone) in the Rat, *J. Pharmacokin. Biopharm.*, 9:309-341, 1981.

27. Anderson, M. E.: Pharmacokinetics of Inhaled Gases and Vapors; *Neurobehavioral Toxicology and Teratology*, 3:383-389, 1981.

28. *Michaels, A. S.; Chadrasekaran, S. K.; Shaw, J. E.*: Drug Permeation Through Human Skin. Theory and *In Vivo* Experimental Measurement. *AIChE Journal, 21*:985-996, 1975.

29. *Cooper, E. R.*: Pharmacokinetics of Skin Penetration, J. Pharm. Sci., 65:1396-1397, 1976.

30. *Levy, G.; O'Reilly, R. A., and Wingard, Jr., L. B.*: Relationship Between the Kinetics of the Anticoaguoant Effects of Racemic Warfarin and Its Individual Enantiomers in Man. *Research Communication in Chem. Pathology and Pharmacology,* 7:359-365, 1974.

31. *Jusko, W. J.*: Pharmacodynamic Principles in Chemical Teratology: Dose-Effect Relationships. *Journal of Pharmacology and Experimental Therapeutics, 183* :469-480, 1972.

32. *Werkhesier, W. C.*: Mathematical Simulation in Chemotherapy. *Ann. N. Y. Acad. Sci., 186*:343-358, 1971.

33. *Jusko, W. J.*: Pharmacodynamics of Chemotherapeutic Effects: Dose-Time-Response Relationships for Phase-Nonspecific Agents. *Journal of Pharmaceutical Sciences, 60*:892-895, 1971.

34. *Jusko, W. J.*: A Pharmacodynamic Model for Cell-Cycle-Specific Chemotherapeutic Agents. *Journal of Pharmacokinetics and Biopharmaceutics, 1*:175-200, 1973.

35. *Bischoff, K. B.; Himmelstein, K. J.; Dedrick, R. L.; Zaharko, D. S.*: Pharmacokinetics and Cell Population Growth Models. In *Cancer Chemotherapy, Advances in Chemistry Series, No. 118, Chemical Engineering in Medicine,* pp. 46-64, 1973.

36. *Morrison, P. F.; Lincoln, R. L.; and Aroesty, J.*: Disposition of Cytosine Arabinoside (NSC-63878) and Its Metabolites: A Pharmacokinetic Simulation, *Cancer Chemotherapy Reports,* 59:861-876, 1975.

37. *Gillette, J. R.*: Application of Pharmacokinetic Principles in the Extrapolation of Animal Data to Humans. *Clin. Toxicol.,* 9:709-722, 1976.

38. *Gillette, J. R.*: Kinetics of Reactive Metabolites and Covalent Binding *In vivo* and *In Vitro.* In: *Biologically Reactive Intermediates,* D. J. Jallow, et al., Eds., Plenum Press, New York, pp. 25-41, 1977.

39. *Dedrick, R. L.*: Letters to the Editor, *Environmental Health Perspectives, 28:* 311-314, 1979.

40. *Anderson, M. W., Hoel, D. G. and Kaplan, N. L.*: A General Scheme for the Incorporation of Pharmacokinetics in Low-Dose Risk Estimation for Chemical Carcinogenesis: Example - Vinyl Chloride, *Toxicol. Appl. Pharmacol., 55*:154 (1980).

41. *Hoel, D. G.; Kaplan, N. L.; Anderson, M. W.*: Implication of Nonlinear Kinetics on Risk Estimation in Carcinogenesis, *Science, 219*:1032-1037, 1983.

42. *Armitage, P. and Doll, R.*: "A Two-Stage Theory of Carcinogenesis in Relation to the Age Distribution of Human Cancer", *British J. Cancer, 11*:161-169, 1957.

43. *Moolgavkar, S. H. and Venzon, D. J.*: "Two-Event Model for Carcinogenesis: Incidence Curves for Childhood and Adult Tumors", *Math. Biosci.*, 47:55-77, 1979.

44. *Moolgavkar, S. H., Day, N. E. and Stevens, R. G.*: Two-Stage Model for Carcinogenesis: Epidemiology of Breast Cancer in Females, *J. Nat. Cancer Inst.* 65:559-569, 1980.

45. *Day, N. E. and Brown, C. C.*: Multistage Models and Primary Prevention of Cancer. *JNCI*, 64:977-989, 1980.

New Approaches in Toxicity Testing and Their
Application in Human Risk Assessment, edited by
A. P. Li. Raven Press, New York © 1985.

Pharmacokinetics of Inhaled Chlorobenzene in the Rat

†Timothy M. Sullivan, *Gordon S. Born, *Gary P. Carlson, and *Wayne V. Kessler

*Schools of Pharmacy and Health Sciences, Purdue University, West Lafayette, Indiana 47907; †College of Medicine, University of South Florida, Saint Petersburg, Florida 33701

The Environmental Protection Agency (EPA), as required by the Toxic Substances Control Act (TSCA), has published proposed rules which would require specific health effects testing by manufacturers and processors of certain chemical substances (1). Chlorobenzene (CB) was included in the proposal. Basic to the interpretation of the required studies is an understanding of the pharmacokinetics of inhaled CB. The toxicity of CB is mediated by a metabolic product, presumably an epoxide (2,3). The detoxification of the epoxide in the rat is predominantly by conjugation with reduced glutathione (GSH), leading to excretion in the urine as a mercapturic acid (4). GSH conjugation has, however, been shown to be a dose dependent reaction, due to depletion of the GSH cofactor (5). Impairment of GSH conjugation has direct effects on the amount of covalent binding to proteins (2-4). Pharmacokinetic data have been applied to low dose risk assessments for various metabolically-activated xenobiotics. Few studies, however, have been published regarding the pharmacokinetics of CB. The present study was designed to measure tissue burdens, metabolism, and excretion of CB in rats following inhalation exposures similar to those mandated under TSCA.

METHODS

Male Sprague-Dawley rats were used. A recirculating exposure chamber was constructed from a 40-liter glass chromatography jar (5). ^{14}C-CB vapor was generated by passing a portion of the total air flow through a heated flask containing glass beads. The ^{14}C-CB was infused through a septum immediately upstream from the flask using a gas-tight syringe and variable speed syringe pump. The vapor passed through a mixing chamber before re-entering the main air flow. Total air flow was 14 liters/min. CB vapor concentrations were monitored with a Wilkes Miran Model 1A-CVF infrared gas analyzer at 9.25 μm. The IR absorbances recorded during all exposure periods remained within ± 20% of the desired level, and usually within ± 10%.

Treatment Groups

Fifteen animals were exposed at 100, 400, or 700 ppm for 8 hr. Six of each group were exposed for 5 consecutive days (multiple exposure regimen). Another three rats were exposed for the first 4 days of the multiple exposure regimen, but were sacrificed by decapitation on the morning of the fifth day, 16 hr after their final exposure. The other six rats were exposed only on the fifth day of each exposure block (single exposure regimen). Another group of 12 rats was exposed in a 1-day repeat study at 400 ppm to account for the statistical significance of the blocking effect.

Immediately after the fifth day of exposure, six of the 12 remaining rats (three singly exposed and three multiply exposed) were placed in metabolism cages for collection of urine and expired material. The other six rats were sacrificed for analysis of tissue ^{14}C burdens. The rats maintained in the metabolism cages were sacrificed 48 hr after exposure for assessment of remaining tissue burdens.

Excretion

Preliminary studies indicated that ^{14}C-labeled material excreted in the urine and expired air after 48 hr post-exposure amounted to no more than 2% of the total excreted from 0-48 hr. Elimination of labeled material in the expired air was measured by drawing laboratory air through each metabolism cage at 1 ft^3/hr, exiting through individual charcoal tubes. The charcoal tubes were changed at 0.5, 2, 4, 12, 24, 36, and 48 hr post-exposure. Urine was collected at 12, 24, and 48 hr post exposure.

Glass tubes for collection of expired ^{14}C contained 1 g of activated bituminous charcoal separated into a 0.75-g primary section and a 0.25-g backup section. Analysis of the trapped ^{14}C activity was direct liquid scintillation counting in 15 ml of toluene-PPO (2,5-diphenyloxazole, 4 g/liter). The efficiency of recovery of trapped ^{14}C activity from the charcoal was established to be 78 ± 5% (mean ± SD). The amount of ^{14}C breakthrough into the backup section was never more than a few percent of the primary section activity.

Urinary Metabolite Profile

Urine collected in the first 24 hr after exposure was examined for CB metaboite profile (4). An aliquot was first extracted three times with three volumes of ethyl ether. The pH of the urine was then adjusted to 4.5-5.0 with sodium acetate. Glucuronidase-sulfatase enzyme was added, and the urine was incubated overnight at 37°C. The urine was then adjusted to pH 7 with NaOH and extracted four times with three volumes of ether. Finally, the urine was acidified to pH 1 with HCl and again extracted four times with three volumes of either. The CB metabolite categories generated in this procedure are referred to as intitial, glucuronide/sulfate (G/S), mercapturic acid, and unextracted.

RESULTS

The design of the treatment procedure allowed only one exposure concentration to be used in any given exposure block. The significance of the blocking factor was estimated in an analysis of variance (ANOVA) using the two groups of singly exposed rats exposed to 400 ppm. The magnitude of all other treatment effects was estimated by performing ANOVA on the data from the 100, 700 and the first 400-ppm exposure blocks. The data from the repeat 400-ppm block are not presented for reasons of clarity.

Tissue Burdens

Table 1 presents the ^{14}C burdens of adipose, liver, and kidney. Lung and blood burdens were 25-50% and 10-30%, respectively, of liver burdens and followed the same patterns over exposure concentration and sacrifice time. There was no evidence of accumulation in the rats sacrified immediatley after exposure, except in the kidney (single exposure 0-hr vs multiple exposure 0-hr). There was a tendency at the 48-hr sacrifice time, however, for multiply exposed rats to exhibit higher tissue burdens than rats exposed only once. The ^{14}C burden of adipose tissue increased about 8- to 10-fold when the concentration was increased from 100 to 400 ppm and about 3- to 5-fold from 400 to 700 ppm.

TABLE 1

TISSUE ^{14}C BURDENS IN RATS EXPOSED TO ^{14}C-CHLOROBENZENE VAPOR.[a]

Hours after exposure	Exposure regimen	Exposure concentration, ppm		
		100	400	700
A. Liver				
0	single	75 ± 17	429 ± 46	806 ± 94
	multiple	69 ± 17	578 ± 49	814 ± 106
16	multiple	41 ± 3	143 ± 35	336 ± 16
48	single	ND	88 ± 9	184 ± 18
	multiple	ND	154 ± 14	213 ± 8
B. Kidney				
0	single	51 ± 5	277 ± 20	439 ± 18
	multiple	96 ± 9	486 ± 28	538 ± 137
16	multiple	33 ± 7	174 ± 25	258 ± 11
48	single	ND	17 ± 5	88 ± 23
	multiple	ND	100 ± 12	159 ± 2
C. Adipose				
0	single	449 ± 139	4,540 ± 230	15,800 ± 4,400
	multiple	415 ± 123	2,920 ± 580	15,300 ± 1,100
16	multiple	15 ± 5	275 ± 116	2,370 ± 410
48	single	13 ± 8	47 ± 14	119 ± 14
	multiple	ND	74 ± 10	142 ± 14

[a] nmoles chlorobenzene equivalents per gram, Xh ± SE, N = 3.
ND = not detectable.

Excretion

Figure 1 shows the amounts of label excreted in the urine (open portions of the bars) and expired breath (shaded portions). The entire heights represent the total excreted. Asterisks within the bars represent decreased respiratory elimination among the multiply exposed rats, significant at all three exposure levels (although respiratory elimination is too small to be represented at 100 ppm). The asterisk above the bar for rats multiply exposed to 700 ppm indicates a significant decrease in the total amount eliminated. There are no differences due to dosing regimen in the amount of material excreted in the urine. Table 2 indicates the dose-dependent increase in the percentage of the eliminated total which was excreted in expired air.

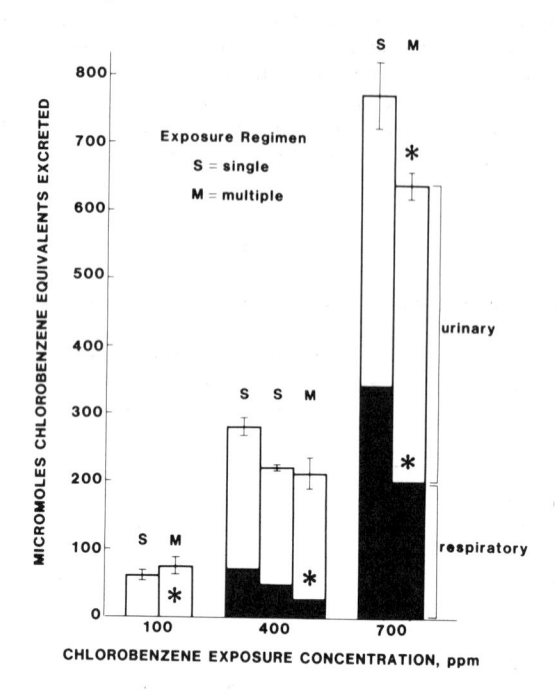

FIGURE 1. Elimination of ^{14}C following inhalation exposure of rats to ^{14}C-Chlorobenzene. The shaded portions of the bars represent the amount expired in exhaled breath, the open portions represent urinary excretion, and the entire heights represent the total amount eliminated, expressed as micromoles of chlorobenzene equivalents. Asterisks indicate significant (p<0.05) differences between multiple and single exposure results.

TABLE 2

PERCENTAGE OF TOTAL ELIMINATED LABEL EXCRETED IN RESPIRATION[a]

Exposure regimen	Exposure concentration, ppm		
	100	400	700
single	5.1 ± 0.4	21.3 ± 2.3†	44.3 ± 4.1†
multiple	2.9 ± 0.3*	13.1 ± 0.4*†	31.7 ± 0.5*†

[a]Means ± SE, N = 3. Asterisks indicate significant differences compared to single exposure results. Daggers indicate significant differences compared to results at lower exposure concentrations.

Elimination Kinetics

The rate of respiratory elimination, expressed as the percentage remaining to be exhaled at t hours post-exposure, is best represented by a two term model $Ae^{\alpha t} + Be^{\beta t}$. Analysis of treatment effects was performed by examining the apparent half-lives ($T_{1/2}$) derived from the "fast" and "slow" phase rate constants (α and $\beta\Pi$ respectively) calculated for each rat (Table 3). The exposure regimen effect was significant only at the 700-ppm concentration, with multiply exposed rats yielding a shorter phase $T_{1/2}$ than singly exposed rats. There was no significant effect of exposure concentration between the 100- and 400-ppm groups. However, the fast phase half-lives of the 700-ppm rats were longer than those observed at the lower concentrations. The analysis procedure correlates the rate constants α and β, and thus differences in the fast phase are accompanied by opposing changes in the slow phase.

Analysis of the rates of urinary excretion was conducted in a similar manner, but only one term was used. Neither the number of exposures nor exposure concentration had any effect on the rate of urinary excretion, and one regression equation was computed to describe the common rate of urinary elimination:

$$\text{percentage remaining} = 94.8\, e^{-0.133t}$$

with $r^2 = 0.92$. According to this equation, the half-life of urinary excretion of radioactivity derived from inhaled ^{14}C-CB was 5.2 hr.

TABLE 3

APPARENT HALF-LIVES OF RESPIRATORY ELIMINATION FOLLOWING INHALATION EXPOSURE OF RATS TO ^{14}C-CHLOROBENZENE

Exposure conc. (ppm)	Exposure regimen	Apparent $T_{1/2}$ (hr) fast phase	slow phase
100	single	0.81	8.77
100	multiple	0.60	9.24
400	single	1.13	7.62
400	multiple	0.83	8.56
700	single	3.65[a]	5.73[a]
700	multiple	1.62[a,b]	6.60[a,b]

[a]Significant difference due to exposure concentration ($p<0.05$).

[b]Significant difference due to exposure regimen ($p<0.05$).

Urinary Metabolites

Analysis of treatment effects on the metabolite profile was based on the percentage of mercaputric acid, since this is the parameter most relevant to toxicity (Table 4). Differences between singly and multiply exposed groups were not significant. The three concentrations resulted in significantly different mercapturic acid percentages among the singly exposed groups. In the multiply exposed groups, the difference between the 400-ppm and the 700-ppm results was not significant, although both were significantly decreased from the 100-ppm results. When the exposure concentration was increased from 100 to 700 ppm, the mercapturic acid percentage of the total was reduced by 27% for the singly exposed group and 24% for the multiply exposed group.

TABLE 4

MERCAPTURIC ACID PERCENTAGE OF URINARY METABOLITES FOLLOWING INHALATION EXPOSURE OF RATS TO CHLOROBENZENE

Exposure conc. (ppm)	Exposure regimen	Percentage mercapturic acid[a]
100	single	69.7 ± 0.6
100	multiple	67.8 ± 1.9
400	single	61.0 ± 0.2*
400	multiple	54.8 ± 3.5*
700	single	51.0 ± 0.9*
700	multiple	51.9 ± 0.9*

[a]Means ± standard errors, N = 3. Astericks indicate significant difference compared to 100 ppm results ($p < 0.05$).

DISCUSSION

Adipose tissue accumulated large amounts of ^{14}C, assumed to represent unchanged CB since the parent compound is much more lipophilic than any of the metabolites. The data suggest that the amount accumulated in adipose increased at a greater rate than increases in exposure concentration. Other tissues did not demonstrate this tendency. The ^{14}C label excreted in exhaled breath also represents primarily unmetabolized CB. The four-fold increase in exposure concentration from 100 to 400 ppm caused an increase of over 10-fold in the CB expired. The further 75% increase to 700 ppm caused a 7-fold increase in expired CB.

The change in the apparent half-lives of the respiratory excretion curve between 100 and 700 ppm is also of biological significance. The observed kinetics of CB expiration should be reflective of blood CB levels after exposure. Release of unchanged CB from the adipose tissue serves to maintain high blood CB concentrations after cessation of exposure. The loss of distinction between the fast and slow phases of respiratory excretion following exposure to 700 ppm indicates that the efflux of CB from adipose prolonged the duration of maximal respiratory elimination rates.

The pharmacokinetic changes are consistent with saturation of CB metabolism. The decrease in the fraction of blood CB which would be removed by metabolism under these conditions would allow alternative mechanisms of CB elimination to increase in proportion. The uptake of CB into tissue, most specifically adipose, would therefore be greater, since blood CB is increased disproportionately. Similarly, exhalation of unchanged CB after exposure would occur in a greater percentage.

Evidence of metabolic saturation is found after exposure to 400 ppm, as compared to 100 ppm, and is more pronounced following exposure to 700 ppm. The results of the urinary metabolite profiles, however, describe a dose dependent change in another aspect of CB pharmacokinetics. The dose dependent decrease observed in the relative abundance of mercapturic acid following inhalation exposure of rats to CB vapor was similar to previous results following *i.p.* administration of bromobenzene (4). The decrease in mercapturic acid formation has been correlated with decreased GSH availability and increased toxicity (2-4).

Pharmacokinetic changes due to multiple versus single exposure regimen were less dramatic than the dose dependent changes. The minor differences seen between the two exposure regimens may be due to some stimulation of metabolism in the multiply exposed rats, at least among the 700-ppm groups, although this was not demonstrated directly. It has been reported that rat liver GSH rebounds to greater than control levels within 24 hr of a toxic ip dose of bromobenzene. However, no evidence was found in the present study that any increase in the ability to form the mercapturic acid from inhaled CB occurred after five exposures.

The present data lead to the conclusion that the pharmacokinetics of inhaled CB in the rat are dose dependent in two different respects. Tissue burden and excretion data indicate the metabolic clearance of CB from the blood becomes saturated at exposure concentrations as low as 400 ppm for 8 hr. The same concentration also caused changes in the urinary metabolite profile, manifested by reduced predominance of the mercaputuric acid. The dose dependent pharmacokinetics of these two metabolic functions might affect the incidence and severity of toxic response because the toxicity of CB is mediated by a reactive metabolite. The fact that evidence of important pharmacokinetic alterations in rats was observed at 8-hr exposure concentrations of 400 ppm should be considered in the design and assessment of health effects studies such a proposed by the EPA.

ACKNOWLEDGMENT

This study was supported by Training Grant 5-T32-ES 07039 from the U.S. Public Health Service, National Institute of Environmental Health Science.

REFERENCES

1. *Environmental Protection Agency*: Chloromethane and chlorinated benzenes proposed test rule: amendment to proposed health effects standards. *Federal Register, 45*:48524-48566, 1980.

2. Brodie, B. B.; Reid, W. D., Cho, A. K., Sipes, G., Krishna, G., and Gillette, J. R.: Possible mechanism of liver necrosis caused by aromatic organic compounds. *Proc. Natl. Acad. Sci. USA, 68*:160-164, 1971.

3. Reid, W. D.; and Krishna, G.: Centrolobular necrosis related to covalent binding of metabolites of halogenated acromatic hydrocarbons. *Exp. Mol. Pathol., 18*:80-99, 1973.

4. Zampaglione, N.; Jollow, D. J., Mitchell, J. R., Stripp, B., Hamrick, M., and Gillette, J. R.: Role of detoxifying enzymes in bromobenzene-induced liver necrosis. *J. Pharmacol. Exp. Ther., 187*:218-227, 1973.

5. Paustenbach, D. J.; Carlson, G. P., Christian, J. E., Born, G. S., and Rausch, J. E.: A dynamic closed-loop recirculating inhalation chamber for conducting pharmacokinetic and short-term toxicity studies. *Fundam. Appl. Toxicol.,* (in press)

New Approaches in Toxicity Testing and Their Application in Human Risk Assessment, edited by A. P. Li. Raven Press, New York © 1985.

Discussion

Will Ridley: I'm wondering if you see nasal olfactory damage when the compound (3-methylfuran) is administered by a route other than inhalation.

Mike Boyd: We do.

Alan Wilson: Mike, do you think you're looking at a specific isozyme of cytochrome P450 in the clara cell that may not be there in some other cell type, such as the pulmonary type II cell.

Mike Boyd: We can't answer that question completely. But as you know from the studies that we've done with 4-ipomeanol in isolated clara cell preparations, and with purified preparations of cytochrome P450 isozymes that we've done in collaboration with the group at Research Triangle Park, there definitely seems to be marked differences in the ability of the various isozymes to mediate the production of the reactive metabolite of 4-ipomeanol. Whether or not these things are differentially distributed among the different cell types is, in our present state of knowledge, difficult to say definitively, although that is the suggestion that we have based on the patterns of cell damage that we have. For example, clearly 4-ipomeanol is preferentially destructive to clara cells, although we know that type II cells in fact have quote "a cytochrome P450 pool" that mediates the metabolism of other substrates very nicely, but 4-ipomeanol was not a particularly good substrate. So, I think we have a lot to learn, but we're beginning to figure out just what kind of questions that we need to be asking.

Vincent St. Omer: What is the possibility of protecting such effects with N-acetylcysteine?

Mike Boyd: We've not done the experiment with 3-methylfuran *in vivo.* However we've attempted to protect animals against a similar type of toxicity produced by 4-ipomeanol by pre-treating them heavily with N-acetylcysteine, which didn't work particularly well. Cysteine itself will give you a little bit of a protective effect, although whether or not those effects are mediated through the trapping of a reactive intermediate is something we can't answer. In the case of cysteine, we know that cysteine changes the total pattern of metabolism *in vivo* in a way other than through formation of a conjugate type material. It in fact decreases the overall rate of metabolism. You can demonstrate that *in vitro.* Other sulfhydryl reagents that we've tried to use to modify the toxicity have similar properties, even more so than cysteine. Some of the mercaptan compounds, for example, are extremely potent inhibitors of the activation pathway. So, the experiment is difficult to interpret in terms of the protective effect; are you either protecting by trapping the reactive intermediate, intercepting it before it can do damage to the tissue or are you actually preventing it's formation. In fact, you're doing both and with a particular inhibitor how the balance falls is a rather complex question to answer with an *in vivo* study.

Bill Broddle: How does the concentration of the 3-methylfuran present in an environmentally polluted area, like the Washington D.C. area, compare with some of the no effect and effect levels that you've seen.

Mike Boyd: The critical information we don't have is the human exposure concentrations. The only study that I've quoted, the only study that I know of, was not a quantitative one, it was purely a qualitative study. So over the past six or seven years we've been hoping that someone would get sufficiently interested and do some careful quantitative studies. At least we would be that step further ahead. Now what we could make of that is yet another question entirely, but we don't have the first step done yet. As far as the experimental concentrations we've used, they're very high. But, in our particular setting the kinds of studies that we can do are limited to rather short term experiments. That's why we became involved with the group at Oak Ridge, but even then the ability to study very low concentrations over a greatly extended period of time is not within the range of the facility.

Bill Broddle: So you've not gone down those low concentrations in your animal studies.

Mike Boyd: There are lower doses in these studies and we can define within the limits of the experiments we've done, doses that don't produce any gross effect like you see there. More subtle perturbations we really can't answer. You need to look at this thing at an ultrastructural level if you really want to get a real fine picture of what's going on. That was not really the purpose of our studies. I might mention that it's interesting that we did attempt to determine if this compound is carcinogenic. At least it is very carcinogenic? It doesn't appear to be very carcinogenic in the studies that we have done in hamsters, rats and mice, which is quite interesting because it really is a potent alkylator of pulmonary bronchioles and a potent cytotoxin, but it doesn't appear to be particularly carcinogenic even at the very high doses that we've used. Fortunately, I might add, because I've probably breathed a lot of it!

Al Li: I have a question for Dr. Sipes. There was a cliché used for those of us that work with cell free homogenate preparations that our findings may never represent what is really happening because of the disruption of the actual subcellular distribution of the enzymes. I am just wondering, since Dr. Sipes is using cell-free preparation to reach great goals like species extrapolation and health-risk analysis, how would he deal with such an accusation?

Glen Sipes: I think it is the age old question of can you take data from an *in vitro* cell free type of preparation and really extrapolate. I think this is a question that can be argued and I guess the most important thing here is what is the question that is being asked. For example, in the case of the PCB's we knew that the metabolism relates to the microsomal membranes and we therefore felt very comfortable looking at reaction rates. If this is relationship of a phase I to a phase II system, where you break down the normal integrity, the maintenance between the microsomal membranes and the cytosolic enzyme, then the question of predictability is more difficult. So the question we were asking was a very simple question. I think it is legitimate for these highly lipophilic compounds that have to go through phase I metabolism, to use these systems as a basis to predict species differences. I appreciate what you are saying and I think the field is going to try to develop various types of cell culture systems. I must stress that you always have to keep in mind, if you are doing disposition work, that you have to maintain the viability of the enzyme systems. There are alot of early papers which used enzyme systems in which the enzyme activity was falling. Everyone was trying to do the right thing by using cells in culture, but did not focus on maintaining the P450 levels. Fortunately that is now realized and there is a tremendous effort to maintain both P450 levels, and glutathione levels and I think that would be a really good system. Whether or not you are going to be able to use cells in culture on a routine basis, is another question. For example, if we got a call at 3:00 in the afternoon that a human liver would be available at about 9:00 at night, it would be difficult to isolate cells and carry out everything. Now we have a pool of enzymes in the freezer and you can ask specific questions with those preparations, but I heartily agree with the comment you made on cell free preparations; that they can also lead to inaccuracies and artifacts so it is very critical to know the question that you are asking.

DISCUSSION

Leon Golberg: This question is directed to Dr. Lutz. I am reminded of the expression "always a bridesmaid and never a bride" with regard to the system that he has described. It makes such sense, and it has its disciples, but it really hasn't been adopted to the degree which I would have anticipated. It hasn't totally displaced the old classical pharmacokinetics with regard to drugs for instance, as distinct from anti-cancer agents. Do you think this is just prejudice or is it that the classical system is better adapted at resolving some of the issues that arise, let's say in clinical pharmacokinetics.

Bob Lutz: When you refer to classical systems I assume you mean the classical methods of pharmacokinetic analysis, even compartmental analysis. You didn't hear it from me, but I would say yes. I think it is a question of inertia or of bias. The physiological type models that I have just described are relatively new on the time scale of the other types of models that have been around. To show that perhaps it has arrived, Milo Gibaldi just recently published a revised issue of his book on pharmacokinetics where he has now devoted a whole chapter to the use of physiological pharmacoknetics. So I hope soon that we will be a bride, and also hope that more and more people will catch on to the use of the systems. I see it more and more in the literature. Naturally it is a biased opinion, but I think it makes more sense because, as I mentioned before, the key issue is that the parameters that are involved in our models have physiological meaning. So you can think of them in the right way and you can find measurements for them, methods of measuring them, you can find these parameters in the literature, they have anatomical and physical significance. They are not just arbitrary numbers pulled out by a computer. They represent flow, they represent volume, they represent enzyme kinetics. I think the time is coming when there will be a greater use of these models.

Toxicity to the Immune System and the Fetus

Section Editor: D. K. Flaherty

Assessment of the Effects of Chemicals on the Immune System

Peter H. Bick, Michael P. Holsapple, and Kimber L. White, Jr.

Immunotoxicology Program, Department of Microbiology and Immunology, and Department of Pharmacology and Toxicology, Virginia Commonwealth University, Richmond, Virginia 23298

IMMUNE SYSTEM AS A TARGET ORGAN

The immune system is comprised of a complex network of specialized cells that interact to mount a response following recognition of foreign materials termed antigens. The potential responses of the system range from the production of antibody or cell-mediated reactions to the induction and modulation of inflammatory reactions (1). The response to antigens and the mechanisms of many cellular interactions is under genetic control. The complexity of the immune response is increased by the fact that a given antigen may stimulate several simultaneous reactions, each of which contributes to the overall response. In reponse to a virus, for example, cytolytic killer cells may be elicited as well as an antibody response. While the killer cells may remove virally-infected cells, the antibody may remove free virus reducing virus spread. An alteration in one of these reponses may not result in the host becoming totally susceptible to infection by the virus. The existence of complimentary and compensating alternative response pathways is of great selective advantage to the host but confounds the study of immune alteration. Because of this complexity and interrelated functions it is necessary to appreciate the organization of the immune system and its reponse mechanisms in order to rationally evaluate the effect of a potential immunotoxin on the system.

The immune system is depicted in Figure 1. Stem cells follow one of two major pathways during differentiation into mature lymphocytes. One pathway utilizes the thymus as a site of differentiation of 'T' lymphocytes. Mature T cells are classified into several functional subpopulations, also identified by surface antigens, and carry out the functions of cell-mediated immunity and immunoregulation. A second major pathway results in the development of immunocompetent cells that are the progenitors of antibody-forming cells. These bone-marrow derived or 'B' cells also reside in several subpopulations definable by functional and cell-surface characteristics.

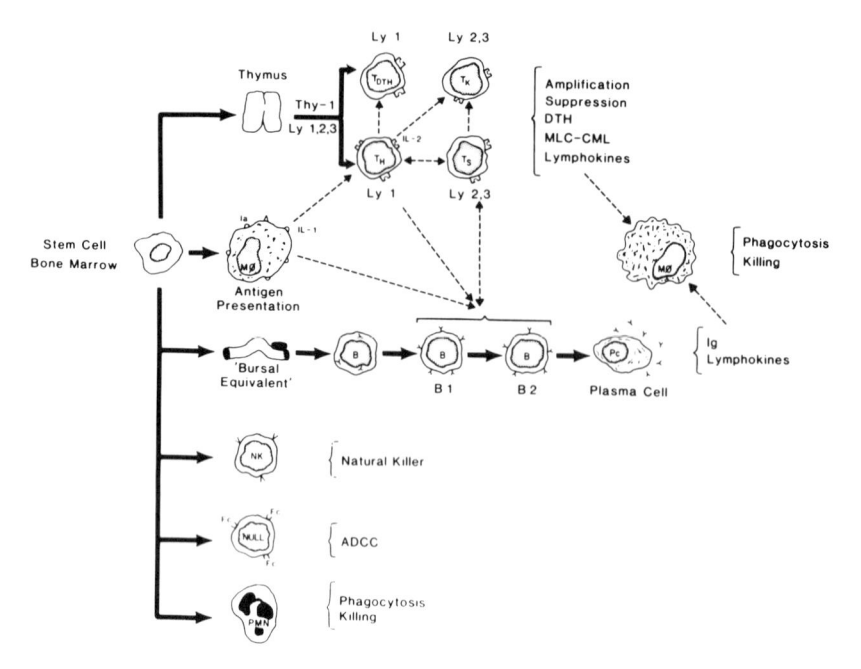

FIGURE 1: Cellular Components of the Immnune System (reprinted with permission from "The Immune System: Structure and Function", In: Toxicology of the Immune System J. H. Dean, A. E. Munson. M. I. Luster and H. E. Amos, eds. Raven Press, New York, 1984).

The third major cell that is central to the induction and regulation of immune responses is the monocyte-macrophage. These cells ingest and process antigen into a form that is recognizable to the T lymphocytes and is necessary for the induction of the majority of immunological responses. These cells also carry out effector functions in inflammatory reponses and as killer cells.

The Natural Killer (NK) cells represent a population of lymphoid cells that are not derived from the 2 major developmental pathways and do not bear characteristic cell-surface markers of T or B cells. These cells bear receptors for the Fc portion of immunoglobulin heavy chain and receptors for antigen. The NK cells are capable of killing certain malignant cells without prior sensitization and are the best candidate for carrying out immune surveillance. In addition, these cells are active in defending against certain infectious organisms. Null cells are a second family of lymphoid cells whose lineage is uncertain. These cells bear Fc receptors and are capable of killing target cells that are coated with antibody. The Null cell is also active in host defense.

The polymorphononuclear leukocyte (PMN) is included in this description because of its importance in host defense through its particpation in inflammatory responses and its role as a phagocytic cell. The reponse of the PMN can be significantly modulated by T lymphocytes.

Not depicted in this representation of the immune system is the complement cascade or the 5 classes of immunoglobulin. Activation and/or binding of these components may profoundly alter the course of an immune reponse. The numerous potential sites for alteration of immunocompetence and the inherent complexity of the system necessitates careful design of comprehensive studies to detect and define immunotoxic events.

Introduction of a chemical into a host may elicit a variety of reactions (Figure 2). Many chemicals, or their metabolites, may be recognized as antigens. This response may be directed at the native molecule or metabolite or may result from the chemical group binding to host protein creating new antigenic determinants. Foreign chemicals may enhance or suppress immune competence. It is possible for these interactions to occur at the same time in various combinations. Lastly, a chemical may have no affect on the immune system at doses that produce toxicity in other organ systems.

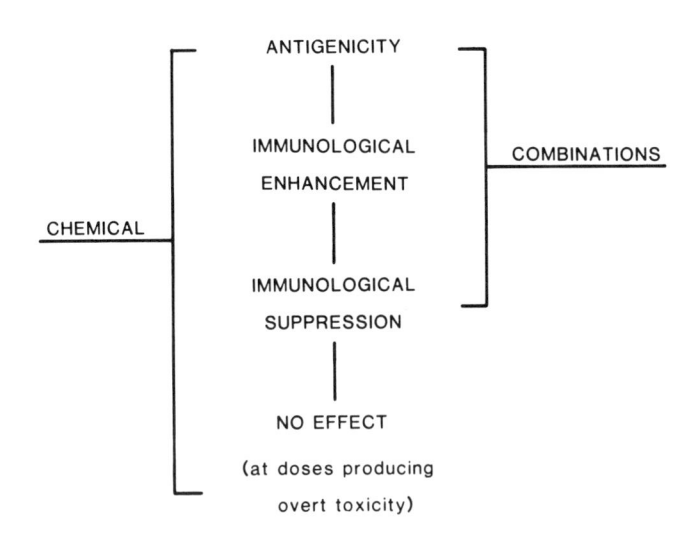

```
                      ┌─  ANTIGENICITY           ─┐
                      │        │                  │
                      │   IMMUNOLOGICAL           │    COMBINATIONS
                      │   ENHANCEMENT             │
          CHEMICAL    │        │                  │
                      │   IMMUNOLOGICAL           │
                      │   SUPPRESSION             │
                      │        │                  │
                      │    NO EFFECT              │
                      │  (at doses producing      │
                      └─   overt toxicity)       ─┘
```

FIGURE 2: Potential Effects of Chemicals Interacting with the Immune System.

ASSESSMENT OF IMMUNOLOGIC ALTERATION

The development of protocols for the detection of immunotoxicologic effects should make use of multiple assay systems in order to assess several functional pathways. As described in the previous section, the immune system relies on diverse populations of immunocompetent cells to interact and carry out responses to antigen. There is no single assay that is capable of detecting alterations in immunity. It is necessary to use a panel of assay systems for an initial canvassing of the lymphoid compartment followed by assays that allow definitive probing of selected populations which may be at risk. Several immunotoxicology laboratories utilize a 'Tier System' to approach this problem. One such Tier System is presented later in this chapter.

The choice of a model system for testing is of principal concern. Cellular immune systems are best described for the mouse. Elegant *in vivo* and *in vitro* systems are available to dissect the immune system at the functional lymphoid population and at the single cell level. The availability of numerous genetically defined inbred mouse strains and characterized monoclonal antibody reagents afford the investigator wide latitude in study design. The rat is a useful system for limited immunotoxicological testing at the present time. This is due to our lack of developed methodology, reagents and inbred strains of rats as compared to the mouse. One advantage of the rat is the ready availability of tissue and biopsy specimens over time. Clearly, standardized toxicological assays for other target organ systems are established for the rat allowing comparisons between organ systems.

In our program we have chosen to use the (C57B1/6xC3H)F1 mouse (B6C3F1) as our standard animal. This strain has been designated by the National Toxicology Progam as the standard for NTP immunotoxicological assays. We have developed standard toxicological assays for non-immunological target organs to establish non-immune toxicologic effects.

The choice of route of exposure and duration of the exposure are important factors in designing informative studies of immune function. The route of chemical exposure in the ideal situation should not be the same as the route to be used for antigen or challenge with an infectious agent. This avoids potential interactions between the study chemical and antigen. The relative timing of chemical exposure and antigenic challenge is important in determining the immunologic mechanisms to be tested. Immune responses are composed of induction and effector phases. The operative cellular subpopulations and regulatory mechanisms differ in these phases. In order to test both phases it may be necessary to overlap chemical exposure and antigenic challenge. For many chemicals a 14 day subchronic exposure is sufficient to induce immunotoxic events. By administering antigen at various time points during chemical exposure, it is possible to determine the chemical-induced alteration of induction as well as expression of immune responses. The immune system has the capability for recovery from insult. Depending on which cellular subpopulations are involved, recovery may be rapid or may be prolonged. Exposure to chemicals during neonatal development may lead to long lasting alteration of immunocompetence whereas exposure to the same chemical in adulthood may cause only transient effects (2-7). In risk assessment, it is important to examine the duration of the immunotoxic effect.

In the following sections experimental data will be presented that have been obtained using assay systems that probe defined immunological responses. These assays utilize the mouse as an experimental animal and while some of the systems may be adapted to other species, several have not been developed outside the mouse system. The rationale for the use of each assay is presented and a structured Tier System of analysis is presented as a summary.

Antibody Response to a Thymic-Dependent Antigen

Antibody responses to Thymic-Dependent (TD) antigens require the participation of monocytes to present antigen to T lymphocytes which then interact with B lymphocytes in the presence of antigen to stimulate antibody production. This response is regulated by T-helper and T-suppressor cells. The complex nature of this reponse makes it a good candidate for initial analysis of potential toxic compounds as it will test the integrity of a number of critical reactive sites. Routinely this response may be assessed by challenging a chemically-exposed animal with Sheep red blood cells (SRBC) and measuring the number of antibody-forming cells in a Jerne plaque assay (plaque-forming cells, PFC). Other T-dependent antigens may be used and antibody production may be detected by several methods (8-10).

In our studies, mice are exposed to chemical for 14 days. On day 11 the mice are sensitized with SRBC. The chemical exposure continues through day 14 and the animals are sacrificed and spleens harvested on day 15. Splenic lymphocytes are analyzed for antibody-forming cells in a Jerne plaque assay. Routinely IgM responses are measured initially and IgG responses measured in a follow-up experiment if effects are found. It is also possible to use these animals for determining changes in serum chemistries, serum immunoglobulins or liver enzymes as this immunization does not alter these levels.

Typical data for 3 chemicals is shown in Figure 3. Diethylstilbestrol (DES) had little effect on the antibody response in this experiment where the antigen was administered intraperitoneally (7). Benzo-(a)-pyrene (BaP) and Dimethylnitrosamine (DMN) had profound effects on the antibody response. These positive results would require further studies to define the cellular site and mechanism of alteration. Several *in vitro* methods are available that may be used to dissect the immune system and pinpoint the cellular target of toxic effects. Despite the complex nature of this response and the possibility for compensation of a minor defect in responsiveness, the *in vivo* antibody response to thymic-dependent antigens is a reproducible and powerful assay system.

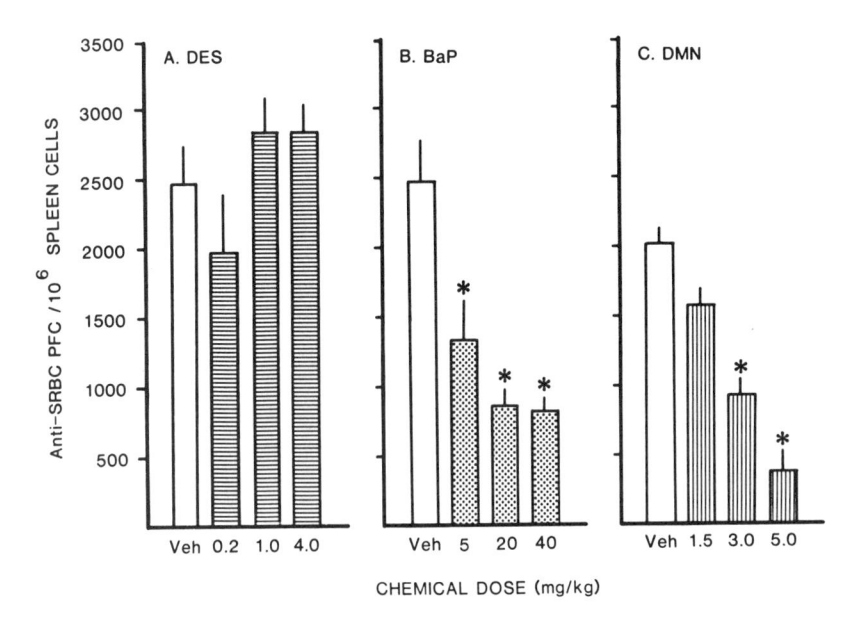

FIGURE 3: Assessment of Antibody Responses to the Thymic-Dependent Antigen Sheep Erythrocytes. Groups of B6C3F1 mice were exposed to chemical or vehicle for 14 consecutive days. On day 11, 5×10^8 SRBC were injected intraperitoneally. On day 15 the animals were sacrificed and the spleen cells assayed for IgM antibody-producing plaque forming cells in a Jerne plaque assay. Data are expressed as the mean ± S.E. of the response of each animal. Results of the different groups were analyzed using Dunnett's t test and significant differences as compared to the vehicle group are denoted by an asterisk ($p<0.05$).

Assessment of Cell-Mediated Immunocompetence

The T lymphocyte compartment is responsible for initiating cell-mediated immunity and T cells act as effector cells in the responses. As a result it is necessary to assess cell-mediated immunocompetence in several systems in order to probe the various functional populations. Delayed-type hypersensitivity (DTH) is mediated by populations of T lymphocytes in response to antigenic challenge and results in the induction of an inflammatory response. The mixed lymphocyte response (MLR) results from the recognition of foreign class II (Ia) histocompatibility antigens by T lymphocytes causing proliferation of the responding T cells. This reaction represents the induction stage of a response that may amplify the activation of cytolytic T cells. T lymphocytes that are capable of killing virally-infected target cells or malignant cells are members of a subpopulation of T cells that do not function in the above systems. The function of T killer cells may be measured in cell-mediated lympholysis assays.

Measurement of Delayed Hypersensitivity

Several methods are available for the assessment of DTH responsiveness. These methods vary in the regimen of antigen sensitization, elicitation of the inflammatory response and the method of measuring the response. It is important to critically analyze the methodology employed in order to understand exactly which cellular interactions are being measured. Many methods employ adjuvants in the immunization process which adds a complicating factor of additional stimulation above and beyond the antigen alone. Since all DTH methods rely on measuring the inflammatory response after antigen challenge, it is important to realize that anti-inflammatory effects may affect the results. Such a reduction in inflammation should not be confused with a central lymphoid defect. The chemical under test should be evaluated for anti-inflammatory activity.

Among the methods employed in immunotoxicologic studies of DTH are; a) the determination of extravasation of radio-iodinated-serum albumin following antigen challenge as described by Paranjpe and Boone and modified by Dean, et al., (8). b) the multiple sensitization method of Lefford as modified by Dean, et al., in which the animal is sensitized prior to chemical exposure and receives a booster immunization during chemical treatment (5). This method only measures the effect of chemical exposure on the elicitation phase of the response since the inductive phase of primary antigen sensitization takes place before exposure to chemical. c) the adjuvant independent method of Holsapple et al., (7). In this method mice are sensitized and boosted during chemical exposure with Keyhole Limpet hemocyanin (KLH) which is administered in saline. This method results in a strong DTH response and is sensitive to chemical perturbation during the inductive as well as challenge phases of the response. The absence of adjuvant avoids the potential complications of the added stimulation caused by the adjuvant.

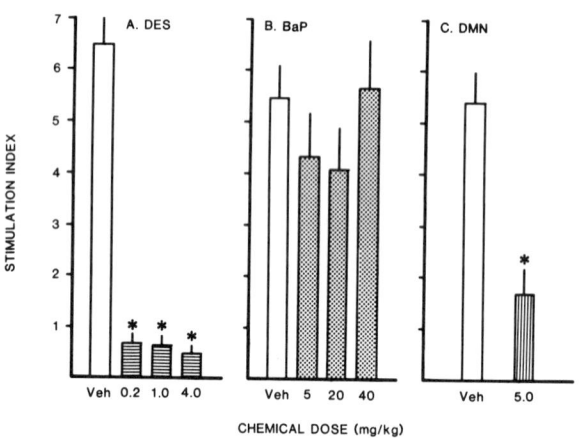

FIGURE 4: Delayed Hypersensitivity to Keyhole Limpet Hemocyanin Following Chemical Exposure. Groups of B6C3F1 mice were exposed to chemical for 14 consecutive days. On days 2 and 9 of exposure the animals were sensitized with 100 ug of KLH in saline. On day 15, all animals received 40 uCi of ^{125}I-IUDR. On day 16, the animals were challenged in one ear with 30 ug KLH in saline and in the contralateral ear with saline alone. On day 17, the animals were sacrificed and the central portion of the ear removed for gamma scintillation counting. Data are expressed as the mean ± S. E. of the stimulation index of all animals in a group comparing the antigen challenged and control ear. The data from the experimental groups were compared to the vehicle group using Dunnett's t test and significant differences ($p<0.05$) denoted by an asterisk.

The effects of 3 chemicals on the DTH response are compared in Figure 4. In these experiments animals were exposed to chemical or vehicle for 14 consecutive days. Using the method of Holsapple *et al.*, the animals were sensitized to KLH on day 2 and received a booster injection of KLH on day 9. On day 16, the animals received an antigenic challenge in the pinna of one ear and a saline challenge in the contralateral ear. The inflammatory response is measured by prelabelling immature monocytes in the bone marrow 24 hours prior to challenge (day 15) with ^{125}I-IUDR. The central part of the ear is removed 24 hours after antigen challenge (day 17) and the radioactivity in the inflamed ear counted by gamma scintillation counting. Stimulation indices are determined by calculating the ratio of radioactivity in the antigen-challenged ear versus the control ear after values for unsensitized control animals are subtracted. As shown in Figure 4, DES caused a dramatic reduction in the DTH response (7). This is in contrast to the lack of effect DES had on the antibody response.

Benzo-(a)-pyrene had little effect on the DTH response but caused a significant suppression on the antibody response. Dimethylnitrosamine caused significant suppression of the DTH response. Using the standard KLH-DTH method described above it was observed that DMN stimulated DTH responsiveness. This was due to a stimulation of production of immature bone-marrow cells which resulted in an elevated DTH response and compensated for reduced T lymphocyte function. To accurately assess the effects of DMN, the method was modified to take the bone marrow stimulation into account (Figure 4C). Rather than label monocytes *in situ* in the DMN-treated animal, exogenously labelled monocytes were adoptively transferred to the experimental animal prior to assay. In this case, the ability of the T lymphocyte to induce an inflammatory response was measured independent of the effects of DMN on the bone marrow and the results showed DMN to suppress DTH function. This example serves to emphasize the necessity of utilizing multiple systems to assess function and to be aware of the pitfalls of each assay system.

Mixed Lymphocyte Response

Foreign Immune Response-associated (Ia) antigens, class II products of the major histocompatibility complex, are recognized by T lymphocytes. Responder T cells proliferate and differentiate in response to the foreign antigens. T cells stimulated in this response are capable of enhancing the generation of cytolytic T killer cells and, therefore, represent an important effector cell population. In order to assess the functional capability of this population, spleen cells of chemically-exposed mice are placed in culture with inactivated foreign spleen cells from a genetically suitable stimulator strain. If the cells are capable of responding they will differentiate and proliferate. By adding radiolabelled thymidine as a precursor of DNA, uptake of radiolabel into proliferating cells can be measured (5,7,11). Such a method was used to evaluate the effects of DES and DMN on the generation of an MLR (Figure 5). Both DES and DMN suppressed the MLR response. These results correlate with the reduction of DTH caused by these chemicals. Since it is not clear that DTH and MLR responses are mediated by the same population of T lymphocytes (despite the fact that T cells operative in both responses express identical cell-surface phenotypes) both assays are used to detect deficits in cell-mediated immunity.

Assessment of Cytolytic Killer Cell Activity

Cytolytic T killer cells are distinct from the T cells involved in DTH and MLR reactions. These T cells bear different cell-surface markers and respond to different antigens than do the DTH and MLR responsive cells. Standard methodologies exist to analyze the functional capacity of these cells. Briefly, chemical exposed or control animals are immunized with cells of a foreign histocompatibility type and allowed to respond. After priming, spleen cells from responder animals are used as a source of effector killer cells and are incubated with radiolabelled target cells at various ratios. The target cells must share antigens with the immunizing cells. As the T cells kill the targets, radiolabel is released into the culture medium. Following incubation, the medium is removed and the released radiolabel is counted. Cytotoxic activity is calculated as the percentage of cell lysis as determined by the percent of radiolabel release (12,13). This method is sensitive and accurately assesses the ability of the host to generate killer T cells (8,14). As mentioned before, T cells active in MLR reactions can augment the generation of T killer activity even though the MLR reactive T cells do not participate in the killing process. A reduction in T cell-mediated cytotoxicity does not necessarily reflect a lesion at the T killer cell level.

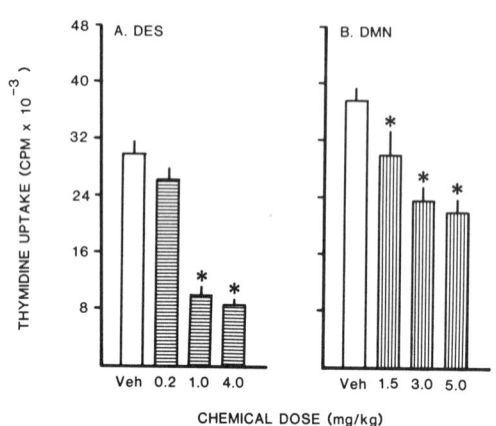

FIGURE 5: Mixed Lymphocyte Responsiveness Following Chemical Exposure. Groups of B6C3F1 mice were treated with chemical for 14 consecutive days. On day 15 the animals were sacrificed and spleen cells from each animal cultured (1 x 10^5) with mitomycin C treated DBA/2 stimulator cells (4 x 10^5) in microtiter wells for 4-6 days. Twenty-four hours prior to harvest each culture received 1.0 uCi of ^{3}H-thymidine. Cultures were harvested and assayed for thymidine uptake using liquid scintillation counting. The data are expressed as the mean ± S. E. of the counts incorporated by cultures obtained for each individual mouse. The data from the experimental groups were compared to the vehicle control using Dunnett's t test and significance (p<0.05) denoted by an asterisk.

Assessment of Natural Killer and Null cell killing activity is performed in a similar fashion using radiolabeled target cells (15). For the expression of NK and Null cell activity no preliminary immunization is necessary. To estimate Null cell activity, antibody-coated targets must be used.

Lymphocyte Proliferation in Response to Mitogens

Lymphocyte proliferation may be stimulated in a polyclonal fashion by a variety of non-specific stimulating agents known collectively as mitogens. This stimulation results in the differentiation of a high percentage of clones within the T and/or B cell compartment. Mitogens have been used as probes for the mechanisms of lymphocyte activation since lymphocytes stimulated by these agents carry out their preprogrammed functions. Lymphocyte responsiveness to mitogenic substances has been used clinically to evaluate the gross functional capacity of lymphocyte populations. A a diagnostic tool, this response can only be expected to yield an overall assessment of lymphocyte capacity. Since these are very powerful stimulants of lymphocyte division, they will not detect subtle changes in immunocompetence. Statistically significant alterations may be obtained when little change in responsiveness is observed because of tight experimental error. However, biologically relevant alterations may not be notice until a mitogen response is altered by

40% or more. Since different cell populations and different regulatory mechanisms are operative in response to different mitogen doses, it is imperative that mitogen responses be performed over a complete dose-response curve. This is particularly true for the T cell mitogens which display a very sharp dose-response. Studies in which only an optimal mitogen concentration is employed should be viewed with caution.

Typical data are shown in Figure 6 for splenic lymphocyte responses to the T cell mitogen Concanavalin A (Con A) and the B cell mitogen bacterial lipopolysaccharide (LPS) following DES treatment. Exposure to DES caused a reduction in the T cell response to Con A but did not affect the B cell reponse to LPS (5,7). These results agree with the functional assessment of these cells in antibody production and cell-mediated immunity.

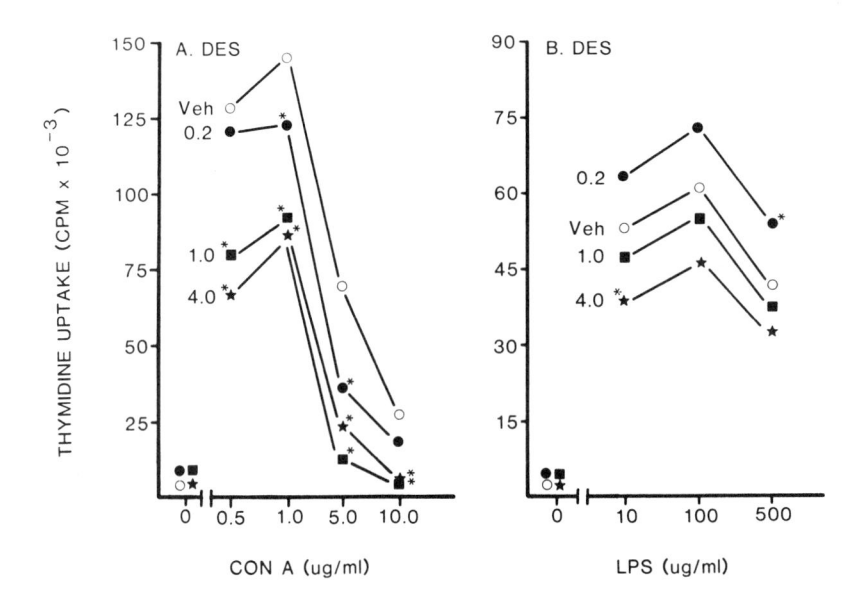

FIGURE 6: Lymphocyte Blastogenesis Following Exposure to Diethylstilbestrol. Groups of B6C3F1 mice were treated with DES for 14 consecutive days. On day 15 the mice were sacrificed and isolated spleen cells cultured with various concentrations of Concanavalin A or LPS for 2 days. Eighteen hours prior to harvest the cultures were pulsed with ^{3}H-thymidine. Cultures were harvested and the incorporated thymidine determined by liquid scintillation counting. The results of individual animal responses at each mitogen dose are presented as mean ± S.E. and compared to responses of the vehicle group using Dunnett's t test. Standard error bars are omitted for clarity. In these experiments, the standard errors did not exceed 15% of the mean value. Significant differences are denoted by an asterisk ($p<0.05$). Background responses ranged from 3-8,000 CPM.

Antigen Distribution and Monocyte-Macrophage Phagocytosis

Immunological responses rely on contact with antigen for initiation of the reponse. Antigen is processed by the macrophage and presented in recognizable form to lymphocytes. Without this interaction most immunological responses will not occur. Therefore, any alteration in macrophage function resulting in altered antigen handling or availability may result in suppression of responsiveness. Such a suppression may be mistaken for a defect in lymphocyte function. Chemicals that stimulate the mononuclear phagocyte system may cause altered distribution of antigen within the host resulting in reduced antibody or cell-mediated responses. This may be more pronounced when antigen is given intravenously than it would be when antigen is given intraperitoneally or subcutaneously. To determine if chemical exposure has caused a stimulation of phagocytic function, chemical-exposed and control animals may be injected intravenously with ^{51}Cr-labelled Sheep erythrocytes and the organ clearance from the blood followed with time (10,16,17). Altered blood clearance and organ distribution will indicate whether the phagocytes are activated. Antigen distribution is affected following DES exposure resulting in reduced antigen availability when antigen is administered by the intravenous route (6,18). To assess the phagocytic capacity of host cells, normal peritoneal or elicited peritoneal cells can be assayed for phagocytic activity *in vitro* using a number of experimental systems (16,19).

Serum Immunoglobulin and Complement Levels

Levels of serum immunoglobulins can be determined using radial immunodiffusion or turbidometric techniques (21, K. L. White unpublished data). It appears from the available data that these assays do not improve on or add to the functional antibody response information obtainable from the systems described above. Alterations in serum immunoglobulin levels may reflect the general health of the animal colony and are not as sensitive as indicator of alteration as the systems previously discussed.

Serum complement is an important component of defense against infectious agents. Alterations in complement levels can be determined in hemolytic assays and correlate with a increased susceptibility to infection with certain agents following chemical alteration (K. L. White, unpublished data).

Dissecting the Mechanisms of Immune Alteration

The use of the experimental systems described in the preceeding sections will detect alterations of immunologic function but will not define the cellular locus or mechanism of the lesion. To further define immunotoxic events, *in vitro* systems provide the best approach. Analysis of distinct cell populations can be made by purifying lymphocyte populations or subpopulations from chemically-exposed and control animals and admixing them in culture to test the capability of a given cell type in an environment of normal cells. Antibody responses can be analyzed by using a battery of polyclonal B cell activators or Thymus-Independent (TI) antigens to test defined B cell populations. Antibody responses to the TD antigen Sheep erythrocytes can be dissected using the primary *in vitro* antibody response system described by Mishell and Dutton (21). Generation and function of cytotoxic T cells can be analyzed in culture. The production of lymphokines and the ability of target cells to react appropriately may be defined. These systems are all currently available in the mouse system while only a few exist for other species. The availability of these powerful techniques supports the use of the mouse for routine immunotoxicological studies.

The *in vitro* systems allow the direct effects of chemicals on lymphocytes to be studied. Direct effects may be tested by adding the chemical directly to lymphocyte cultures. Suitable controls must be employed if non-aqueous solvents are used. In cases where a chemical must be metabolized at a site other than the lymphocyte, lymphoid tissue can be obtained from chemical-exposed animals and added to cultures of normal or vehicle-treated cells. These methodologies will allow the direct effects of a chemical on the lymphocyte to be separated from the effects of a secondary metabolite.

A Tier System of Immunological Assessment

In order to approach a complete assessment of chemical induced alteration and yet cover the potential sites of immunotoxic alteration, it is reasonable to begin by using experimental systems that assess multiple critical sites of cellular interaction. Subsequent experiments may then be aimed at further defining the underlying mechanism of the toxic effect. To achieve this goal several laboratories have found it useful to construct a tiered system of assays from which they can draw specific protocols to test defined immunological functions (20,22).

One possible Tier system is presented in Table 1. This system is not meant to include all possible assay systems but is intended to present the important considerations in organizing such an approach. In Tier I are presented assay systems that require complex cellular interactions in the response process or assays that address an important point concerning host resistance. The *in vivo* antibody response to a thymic-dependent antigen, DTH and MLR responses all require the participation of multiple cellular components of the immune system (macrophages, helper and suppressor T cells and, additionally, B cells in the antibody response). Antigen distribution is included because alterations at this level could be mistaken for primary lymphoid defects.

Table I. TIER SYSTEM OF IMMUNOLOGICAL ASSAYS

Tier	Experimental System
Tier I	Assessment of Complex Cellular Interactions *In Vivo* Antibody Response to a Thymic-Dependent Antigen. Delayed-Type Hypersensitivity Response Antigen Distribution; RES Clearance
Tier II	Assessment of Interactions of Restricted Complexity *In Vivo* Response to a Panel of Thymic-Independent Antigens *In Vitro* Polyclonal Antibody Response to *E. coli* Lipopolysaccharide *In Vitro* Primary Antibody Response to T-Dependent Antigen: Cellular Reconstitution Lymphocyte Proliferation to Mitogens *In Vitro*
Tier III	Assessment of Direct Cellular Capability Enumeration of T and B lymphocyte Populations and Subpopulations Estimation of Peritoneal Exudate Cells and Phagocytic Potential Estimation of Bone Marrow Precursor Cells Determination of Natural Killer and ADCC Potential Assessment of Cytotoxic and Cytostatic Capability of Adherent Normal and Activated Resident Peritoneal Exudate Cells Against Malignant Target Cells

The experimental systems in Tier II involve responses in which the cellular interactions are less complex than found in Tier I or allow a discrete cellular population to be examined. In many cases these reponses only require the interaction of macrophages and T or B cells. In Tier III are assays that examine the functions of discrete populations at the single cell level. By localizing an immunotoxic event to a major limb of the immune system using Tier I assays and then utilizing selected asssays from Tiers II and III, it is possible to rapidly define the cellular site of alteration and approach the mechanism of the toxic effect.

ASSESSING HUMAN RISK USING THE MOUSE MODEL SYSTEM

The immune system is described in the greatest detail in the mouse. For this reason alone, more information regarding the site(s) and mechanisms(s) of chemically induced alterations in function will be obtained using this model than in any other system. As our understanding of the human immune system evolves it is becoming clear that, apart from minor differences, the mouse and human systems are very similar. It is to be expected that differences between the systems should exist due to evolutionary distance alone. However, as the major response pathways are defined in the human, remarkable similarities arise in the mechanisms of interaction and regulation. Indeed, the mouse immune system has been an excellent model upon which to organize experimental probing of human immune function. It is reasonable, therefore, to utilize the mouse as an immunotoxicological model. While absolute parallels to the human situation may not be drawn, a chemical found to induce significant change in the immune function of the mouse should be regarded as potentially dangerous to humans.

A few points of consideration need to be kept in mind when using the mouse as a model system. The effective doses of a chemical may not be directly translated to the human. In certain cases the mouse may utilize different pathways of metabolism to degrade a compound resulting in a different array of products than are found in the human. It is important to establish if these differences affect the applicability of data obtained in the mouse to an assessment of risk for humans.

Information concerning the effects of immunotoxic drugs and chemicals gathered in animals correlates well with available human data in several systems. Studies of the immunosuppressive effects of cyclophosphamide in the mouse correlate with the observed immunnosuppression in humans (23,24). Similarly, studies of the effects of polybrominated and polychlorinated biphenyls in animals have yielded data similar to the epidemiological findings in man (25-29). These examples serve to illustrate the utility of the animal systems and particularly the mouse as a model of chemically-induced alterations of immune function.

REFERENCES

1. *Bick, P. H.*: The immune system: Organization and function. In: *Toxicology of the Immune System.* Dean, J. H.; Munson, A. E., Luster, M. I., and Amos, H. E. New York, Raven Press, In Press.

2. *Luster, M. I.; Faith, R. E., and McLachlan, J. A.*: Alterations of the antibody response following in utero exposure to diethylstilbestrol. *Bull. Environm. Contamin. Toxicol.* 20:433-437, 1978.

3. *Kalland, T., Strand, O., and Forsberg, J. G.*: long-term effects of neonatal estrogen treatment on mitogen responsiveness of mouse spleen lymphocytes. *J.N.C.I.* 63:413-415, 1979.

4. *Kalland, T.*: Alterations of antibody response in female mice after neonatal exposure to diethylstilbestrol. *J. Immunol,* 124:194-198, 1980.

5. *Luster, M. I.: Boorman, G. A., Dean, J. H., Leubke, R. W. and Lawson, L. A.*: The effect of adult exposure to diethylstilbestrol in the mouse: Alterations in immuncological functions. *J. Reticuloendothelial. Soc.* 28:561-569, 1980.

6. Bick, P. H.; Tucker, A. N., White, K. L., Jr. and Holsapple, M. P.: Effects of subchronic exposure to diethylstilbestrol on humoral immune function in adult female (B6C3)F1 mice. *Immunopharmacology, 7*:27-39, 1984.

7. Holsapple, M. P.; Munson, A. E., Munson, J. A. and Bick, P. H.: Suppression of cell-mediated immunocompetence following subchronic exposure to diethylstilbestrol in female B6C3F1 mice. *J. Pharmacol. Exp. Therap., 227*: 130-138, 1983.

8. Dean, J. H.; Padarathsingh, M. L., and Jerrells, T. R.: Application of immunocompetence assays for defining immunosuppression. *Ann. N. Y. Acad. Sci. 320*:579-590, 1979.

9. Baecher-Steppan, L., and Kerkvliet, N. I.: The haemolytic antibody isotope release (HAIR) assay: An efficient alternative technique to conventional plaque assays. *Clin. Exp. Immunol. 44*:440-444, 1981.

10. Munson, E. A.; Sanders, V. M. Douglas, K. A., Sain, L. E., Kaufmann, B. M., and White, K. L. Jr.: In vivo assessment of immunotoxicity. *Environ. Health Persp. 43*:41-52, 1982.

11. Lawrence, D. A.: In vivo and in vitro effects of lead on humoral and cell-mediated immunity. *Infect. and Immun., 31*:136-143, 1981.

12. Brunner, K. T.; Mauel, J., Cerottini, J. T., and Chapius, B.: Quantitative assay of the lytic action of immune lymphoid cells on ^{51}Cr-labelled allogeneic target cells *in vitro*; inhibition by isoantibody and by drugs. *Immunology, 14*:181-196, 1968.

13. Cerottini, J. C.; and Brunner, K. T.: Cell-mediated cytotoxicity, allograft rejection, and tumor immunity. *Adv. Immunol. 18*:67-132, 1974.

14. Kervliet, N. I.; Baecher-Steppan, L., and Schmitz, J. A.: Immunotoxicity of pentachlorophenol (PCP): Increased susceptibility to tumor growth in adult mice fed technical PCP-contaminated diets. *Toxicol. and App. Pharmacol. 62*:55-64, 1982.

15. Herberman, R. B.: editor: *NK cells and other natural effector cells.* New York, Academic Press, 1982.

16. Sanders, V. M.; Tucker, A. N., White, K. L. Jr., Kaufmann, B. M., Hallet, P. Carchman, R. A., Borzelleca, J. F., and Munson, A. E.: Humoral and cell-mediated immune status in mice exposed to trichloroethylene in the drinking water. *Toxicol. App. Pharmacol. 62*:358-368, 1982.

17. Munson, A. E.; Regelson, W., and Wooles, W. R.: Tissue localization studies in evaluating the functional role of the RES. *J. Reticuloendothelial Soc. 7*:366-374, 1974.

18. Warr, G. W. and Sljivic, V. S.: Activity of the reticuloendothelial system and the antibody response. I. Effect of stilboestrol on RES activity and localization of sheep erythrocytes in the mouse. *Br. J. Exp. Path. 54*:56-68, 1973.

19. Boorman, G. A.; Luster, M. I., Dean, J. H., and Wilson, R. E.: The effect of adult exposure to diethylstilbestrol in the mouse on macrophage function and numbers. *J. Reticuloendothelial. Soc. 28*:547-560, 1980.

20. Dean, J. H.: Luster, M. I., Boorman, G. A., and Lauer, L. A.: Procedures available to examine the immunotoxicity of chemicals and drugs. *Pharmacol. Revs. 34*:137-148, 1982.

21. Mishell, R. I. and Dutton, R. W.: Immunization of dissociated spleen cell cultures from normal mice. *J. Exp. Med.* 126:423-442, 1967.

22. Bick, P. H.: Immune system as a target organ for toxicity. *Environ. Health Persp.* 43:3-7, 1982.

23. Turk, J. L.; and Parker, D.: The effect of cyclophosphamide on the immune response. *J. Immunopharmacol.* 1:127-137, 1979.

24. Dean, J. H.; Padarathsingh, M. L., Jerrells, T. R.: Assessment of immunobiological effects induced by chemicals, drugs, and food additives. I. Tier testing and screening approach. *Drug and Chemical Toxicol.* 2:5-17, 1979.

25. Luster, M. I.; Faith, R. E., and Moore, J. A.: Effects of polybrominated biphenyls (PBB) on immune response in rodents. *Environ. Health Persp.* 23:227-232, 1978.

26. Bekesi, J. G.; Holland, J. F., Anderson, H. A., Fischbein, A. S., Rom, W., Wolff, M. S., and Selikoff, I. J.: Lymphocyte function of Michigan dairy farmers exposed to polybrominated biphenyls. *Science* 199:1207-1209, 1978.

27. Vos, J. G. Faith, R. E., and Luster, M. I.: Immune alterations. In: *Halogenated Biphenyls, Terphenyls, Napthalenes, Dibenzodioxins and Related Products.* Kimbrough, R. D. ed. pp 241-266. Elsevier, Amsterdam, 1980.

28. Chung, K. J.; Ching, J. S., Huang, P. C., and Tung, T. C.: Study of patients with PCB poisoning. *J. Mormosan Med. Assoc.* 79:304-312, 1979.

29. Shigematsu, N.; Ishmaru, S., Saito, R., Ikeda, T., Matsuba, K., Sugiyams, K., and Masuda, Y.: Respiratory in involvement in PCB poisoning. *Environ. Res.* 16:92-100, 1978.

Risk Assessment for Transplacental Carcinogenesis

Lucy M. Anderson, Paul J. Donovan, and Jerry M. Rice

Laboratory of Comparative Carcinogenesis, National Institutes of Health, National Cancer Institute, Frederick Cancer Research Facility, Frederick, Maryland 21701

RISK ASSESSMENT FOR TRANSPLACENTAL CARCINOGENESIS

In this era of expanding availability of useful synthetic chemicals in the market place, the pharmacy, and industry, and of increased penetration of women into all types of employment situations, the possibility of transplacental chemical carcinogenic effects on human fetuses has become a focus for concern. This chapter will review three general topics pertinent to this concern: the possibility that transplacental carcinogenesis is a significant contributor to human cancer risk; characteristics of the transplacental carcinogenesis process, as deduced from animal models, that might apply to the human situation; and methods for determining whether a chemical may act as a transplacental carcinogen.

POSSIBILITY OF HUMAN TRANSPLACENTAL CARCINOGENESIS

Direct Evidence from Epidemiological Studies

In 1971, Herbst, *et al.,* provided the first direct evidence of a human transplacental carcinogenic effect, with their finding that seven of eight young women with vaginal carcinoma had been exposed *in utero* to diethylstilbestrol (DES). In a recent review, Herbst (1981) reported that 429 cases of adenocarcinoma of the vagina and cervix had been registered, and that 63% of those with maternal histories available were associated

---

The views expressed are those of the authors and do not represent an official statement of policy by the National Cancer Institute.

with prenatal exposure to DES or related chemicals. In some cases, as little as one week of treatment was sufficient to result in later appearance of a tumor in the daughter, whereas no cancers have been seen in the mothers at risk, even after extensive DES treatment. This difference suggests a special sensitivity of the developing female reproductive tract. However, the relative risk of exposed female offspring for cancer development has thus far proved to be low, estimated at 0.14 to 1.4 per thousand (Herbst, *et al.,* 1977). Several prospective studies of young women known to have encountered DES prenatally did not uncover new cancers, though numerous genital abnormalities were observed (Lanier, *et al.,* 1973; Herbst, *et al.,* 1975; Fowler and Edelman, 1978). In fact, discovery of the transplacental carcinogenic effect of DES was made possible only by the previous rarity of the type of tumor caused by it, leading to retrospective investigation. Transplacental carcinogenesis by DES confirms that such a process can occur in humans; it does not shed much light on the question of which and how many more common cancers of children and adults arise as the result of transplacental exposure to chemicals.

Although DES is the only chemical firmly established at present as having a transplacental carcinogenic effect, evidence is starting to accumulate from epidemiological studies implicating other chemicals and exposure situations. Gold, *et al.* (1978) reported a possible association between brain tumors in children, one of the common forms of childhood cancer, and maternal use of barbiturates. These data were indicated to be suggestive rather than definitive by the authors (Gold, *et al.,* 1979) and others (Annegers, *et al.,* 1979). Nevertheless, brain tumors in children have been found to be correlated with a variety of chemical exposure situations in another recent study. Peters, *et al.* (1981) found that mothers of children with brain tumors were twice as likely to have worked during the year before pregnancy than the mothers of matched controls (a significant difference); a significant association was found between brain tumor occurrence and occupational exposure of the mothers to chemicals, paternal exposure to solvents, and paternal employment in the aircraft industry. These epidemiologists further noted apparent associations between childhood brain tumors and maternal contact with or consumption of burning incense, sidestream cigarette smoke, face make-up, diuretics, antihistamines, pesticides and cured meats (Preston-Martin, *et al.,* 1982). The authors proposed that each of these exposure situations has the potential of engendering nitroso compounds, some of which are potent transplacental inducers of brain tumors in experimental animals (see below).

Other recent reports of association between childhood cancers and maternal exposure include a review of four cases of neuroblastoma in children exposed *in utero* to phenytoin and phenobarbitone (Fabro, 1982), and a study of rhabdomyosarcoma in childhood, in which a significant increase in relative risk was found to be correlated with paternal smoking, exposure to a variety of chemicals, consumption of organ meats, antibiotics, and family history of asthma (Grufferman, *et al.,* 1982).

Each of these putative associations will require confirmation in several independent epidemiological studies before real effects can be considered established, and even then the actual chemical(s) responsible will probably remain elusive in many cases. It should also be noted that in many of these situations the child and the father as well as the pregnant mother were exposed to the agent or condition in question, so that paternal and postnatal as well as prenatal effects were possible. Nevertheless, these investigations clearly indicate that determination of the etiological factors in childhood cancer is a fruitful objective for epidemiological study and that a much fuller understanding of this subject may be forthcoming.

Negative findings should also be mentioned. A number of factors were found to be unassociated with the childhood cancers investigated in the studies described above, including beer drinking, cigarette smoking, and use of hair dyes, aspirin, sedatives, amphetamines, and vitamins by the pregnant mothers in the brain tumor study (Preston-Martin, *et al.,* 1982) and, for rhabdomyosarcoma, use of cigarettes, alcohol, aspirin, cold remedies, and tranquilizers by the mother, and family consumption of milk, cured meats, and saccharin. Jensen and Kamby (1982) addressed specifically the question of whether individuals exposed *in utero* to saccharin during the sugar shortage of World War II have experienced an increased risk of bladder cancer, since bladder carcinogenicity of saccharin in rats was greater when perinatal exposure was combined with adult treatment (Arnold, *et al.,* 1980; Taylor, *et al.,* 1980). Thus far, 30-35 years after prenatal exposure, no increased risk of bladder cancer has developed. These negative findings, like the positive ones, cannot yet be considered conclusive; but it is interesting that maternal cigarette smoking, aspirin, and saccharin were each found to be unassociated with the progeny's cancer risk in two separate studies. Maternal smoking was also exonerated in an earlier report (Neutel and Buck, 1971). Childhood cancer was found to be associated with hydrocarbon-related occupations of the parents in one study (Fabia and Thuu, 1974), but this was not confirmed in two other investigations (Hakulinen, *et al.,* 1976; Zack, *et al.,* 1980). A sorting out of causative from noncausative factors for various childhood cancers may be feasible when enough information is available, and this will be of much help in designing preventive measures.

A question which has not been addressed in epidemiological studies is whether human cancers of middle and old age, which are of course much more common than childhood tumors, originate from transplacental exposure. Experiments with animal models indicate that this is a real possibility, since tumors caused transplacentally in rodents are usually of adult type, and may appear at any time after birth up to the old age of the animal. Frequently a given carcinogen elicits the same types of tumor from both fetus and adult, as is the case, for example, for lung tumors in mice, mammary tumors in rats, and tracheal tumors in hamsters. Effects that are qualitatively unique to the fetus, similar to the action of DES in the human, are unusual in rodents. Thus it appears possible if not indeed likely that some of the common human cancers appearing during middle and late adulthood originate during early life. Such phenomena will be difficult to establish epidemiologically. Nevertheless studies of emigrant groups provide suggestive evidence: individuals who emigrate as adults, usually young adults, have cancer risk patterns for some organ sites which are different from those of their children, the latter being more similar to the natives of the adopted country. For example, in a recent updating of the study of native and foreign-born Japanese in the United States begun by Haenszel and Kurihara (1968), many differences were noted, among them, that leukemias, which are often suspected to be of prenatal origin, had an incidence in U.S.-born Japanese similar to that of U.S. whites, whereas foreign-born Japanese exhibited significantly fewer cases (about one half) of this cancer, at a rate identical to that of Japanese living in Japan (Locke and King, 1980). While such observations may simply reflect differences in habits or in lengths of time of exposure to cancer risk-modifying exogenous factors, they may also indicate an important determining role of exposure situations during early life with regard to later cancer risk.

Indirect Evidence from Animal Models

Responsiveness of the human fetus to the carcinogenic actions of chemicals is expected from the fact that all mammals tested thus far, including rats, mice, hamsters, rabbits, dogs, gerbils, guinea pigs, and notably, primates, are susceptible to transplacental carcinogenesis. Members of most classes of organic chemical carcinogens are effective to some degree, including the nitrosamines, mycotoxins, aromatic amines, and polycyclic aromatic hydrocarbons often mentioned as potential human carcinogens. There are several systematic compilations of references on transplacental actions of chemicals (Tomatis, *et al.,* 1972, Rice, 1973a, 1976, 1981; Tomatis, 1979; Napalkov, 1979; Anderson,

1980; Mohr, *et al.,* 1980; Kleihues, 1982). References to pertinent new reports appearing since 1980 are included here in the bibliography, in addition to those discussed specifically in this review.

High sensitivity of fetal tissues to chemical carcinogens might be predicted from their high rate of cell division, incomplete state of differentiation, and immaturity of detoxification and surveillance systems. On the other hand, responsive target cells in sufficient number or necessary enzyme systems for metabolic activation of carcinogens might be absent, and absorption and metabolism in the body of the mother as well as in the placenta provide significant protection against chemical insults to the fetus. It is, therefore, not surprising that there is a wide range in quantitative degrees of effectiveness of transplacental carcinogens. Ethylnitrosourea (ENU), a low molecular weight, rapidly-diffusing chemical that does not require metabolic activation caused neuroectodermal tumors in 100% of transplacentally-exposed rats, at doses having no effect on their mothers (Swenberg, *et al.,* 1972). Dimethylnitrosamine (DMN), also of low molecular weight but requiring metabolic activation, was not an especially effective transplacental carcinogen in the rat, even when given throughout pregnancy at the highest tolerable dose: tumors developed in only 4% of the offspring, compared with 88% of the mothers (Alexandrov, 1968). Low levels of nitrosamine-activating enzymes in the fetus may explain this difference. Similar transplacental ineffectiveness of diethylnitrosamine (DEN) in the rat, and lack of fetal rat dealkylating activity toward DEN, were reported by Ivankovic (1973). However, urethane, which also requires metabolic activation, was estimated to be four times more effective in lung cells of mouse fetuses at 15 days of gestation, compared with adults (Nomura, 1976), and the tumors resulting from exposure of mouse fetal lung were more malignant in type than those induced in adults (Rice, 1973b). Furthermore, if urethane was administered just before birth and was thus present in the newborn, with low capacity for metabolic clearance, the incidence of lung tumors increased tenfold, in part because the newborns metabolized the urethane only slowly and thus experienced a prolonged exposure period (Mirvish, *et al.,* 1964; Nomura, 1973, 1974).

From findings such as these one might predict that in the human case carcinogens would vary from highly effective to inconsequential as transplacental tumorigens. Penetrating chemical carcinogens of low molecular weight such as ENU, which interact directly and efficiently with biological molecules, may be expected to cause tumors transplacentally in high yields and have been found to do so in every animal model in which they have been tested. These chemicals are also likely to be human transplacental carcinogens. Assessment of risk due to other types of chemical carcinogens is less simple, as the examples cited above indicate. In fact, as is elaborated in the review and discussion below, it is not possible at present to make quantitative predictions about human transplacental carcinogenic risk based on data from animal model experiments.

MODULATING FACTORS IN TRANSPLACENTAL CHEMICAL CARCINOGENESIS

What determines whether a given chemical carcinogen will be a highly, moderately, or poorly effective agent in transplacental initiation of neoplasms, and whether these will grow after birth? If general principles providing answers to these questions could be formulated, then human risk assessment would be greatly facilitated. However, at present few such general principles can be derived from the complexity of modulating factors governing susceptibility to transplacental carcinogenesis.

Organ, Species and Time-Specific Effects

Species effects are prominent in transplacental carcinogenesis, as in chemical carcinogenesis experiments in general, and constitute a major limitation in extrapolation of data from animal models to humans. Transplacental ENU, for example, initiates primarily neurogenic tumors in rats and hamsters (e.g. Ivankovic and Druckrey, 1968), liver and lung tumors in mice (Rice, 1969), renal tumors in rabbits (Fox, et al., 1975), and tumors of the blood vessels and other connective tissues in Patas monkeys (Rice, et al., 1978). Representatives of other classes of chemical carcinogens induce tumors in these same targets: mouse lung tumors can be initiated transplacentally by urethane (e.g. Larsen, 1947; the first demonstration of a transplacental carcinogenic effect); polycyclic aromatic hydrocarbons (e.g. Tomatis, et al., 1971; Bulay and Wattenberg, 1971); and DEN (Mohr and Althoff, 1965; Diwan and Meier, 1976). In the rat, transplacental dimethylbenzanthracene (DMBA), like ENU, caused neurogenic tumors (Napalkov and Alexandrov, 1974), but DEN, even though it led to an assortment of other tumors, was not effective transplacentally in the rat as a carcinogen for the nervous system (Pielsticker, et al., 1967; Thomas and Bollmann, 1968). Thus, the sensitivity of particular target organs in transplacental carcinogenesis is a species characteristic, but not every chemical carcinogen elicits a response from the species' most sensitive target tissue. It is noteworthy, however, that ENU-induced neurogenic tumors of fetal origin can be coaxed from the mouse and rabbit by appropriate choice of strain and time of administration: thirty percent of C3HeB/Fe mice showed brain tumors after transplacental exposure to enu (Denlinger, et al., 1974), and rabbits treated with this chemical very early in gestation developed brain or peripheral nerve tumors (Stavrou, et al., 1977). Chinchilla rabbits given ENU late in gestation developed a mixture of kidney and peripheral nerve tumors (Dimant and Beniashvili, 1978). Furthermore, while DMN is not an effective transplacental carcinogen in rats, its activated form, DMN acetate, induced a variety of tumors in rat fetuses, including tumors of brain and both spinal and cranial nerves (Rice, et al., in preparation). These findings are of some interest in light of the commonness of brain tumors among childhood cancers and their possible association with chemical exposure (see above).

The histological types of tumor induced transplacentally in animal models are usually similar to those found in adults. Examples of histologically embryonic tumors are occasionally reported, for example, cerebellar medulloblastomas in mice treated with ENU as neonates (Searle and Jones, 1972). Primary renal tumors caused by transplacental action of ENU in rabbits are nephroblastomas and appear early in postnatal life (Fox, et al., 1975), but kidney tumors which arise in adult rabbits are also nephroblastomas. There are no animal models for major embryonal tumors associated exclusively with early human life, such as the neuroblastomas and medulloblastomas, so that experimental study of etiology of such neoplasms is not possible at present. A variety of embryonal tumors were induced in opossums by postnatal treatment with ENU; embryonic and fetal development is completed after birth in this species (Jurgelski, et al., 1976, 1979). Although the embryonic opossum is an unusual model, requiring special facilities and skills, it should receive further attention for study of direct interaction of carcinogens with tissues in early stages of development to cause embryonal neoplasms.

The time of gestation during which a carcinogen is administered has an important quantitative and sometimes qualitative effect on the carcinogen's action, as noted above for ENU in rabbits. In general, acute doses of chemicals are most likely to have a carcinogenic effect if administered after the end of organogenesis, approximately days 10-12 in most rodents. Earlier treatment is likely to result in abortion or teratogenesis. However, few experiments have been reported in which subtoxic doses of carcinogens were administered chronically during early gestation. In mice exposed transplacentally to DMBA, significant numbers of tumors were caused in four of the seven responsive target organs as early as day six of gestation (Goerttler, et al., 1981). Spatz and Laqueur (1967) found jejunal tumors in rats whose mothers had been fed a diet containing 3% cycad meal (a source of the carcinogen methylazoxymethanol) only during the first 5 days of pregnancy. Furthermore, recent studies have confirmed that exposure of either parent to chemical carcinogens prior to mating can result in increased incidence of tumors in the offspring (Tomatis, et al., 1981; Nomura, 1982). These findings substantiate the possibility of a genetic mutation basis for increased tumor incidence in the descendants of transplacentally-treated animals (e.g. Tanaka, 1973; Tomatis, et al., 1975; Tomatis and Goodall, 1969; Nomura, 1975; Rao, 1982). It would seem that not only the entire gestational period, but also the time before conception, must be regarded as potentially sensitive, but variably so.

Changes in fetal organ sensitivity to carcinogens during the course of gestation have been described (e. g. Vesselinovitch, et al., 1977). A particularly complete and illustrative study was recently reported by Goerttler, et al. (1981), in which single intragastric doses of DMBA were given to mice on successive days of pregnancy. Tumors were initiated in seven organs, and all differed with regard to period of any or maximum sensitivity. Liver and lung tumors could be induced throughout gestation, but susceptibility was greatest and more or less constant through the last week. Incidence of skin papillomas increased dramatically on days 18-19, Harderian gland tumors were inducible only near the end of gestation, but leukemias and granulosa cell tumors were most likely to be seen in mice exposed on gestational days 6-13.

In contrast to the rodent, where sensitivity of most fetal organs to carcinogens is greatest in mid to late gestation, fetuses of the nonhuman primate *Erythrocebus patas* exhibited susceptibility to transplacental carcinogenesis by ENU only early in gestation: tumors appeared in high frequency and relatively shortly after birth if treatment was initiated on day 30 of gestation, but not if it was begun on day 50 or 70 (Rice, et al., 1978). This sensitivity period in the patas corresponds to the first trimester of human pregnancy. Similarly, the carcinogenic effects of DES in human fetuses occurred only if treatment was begun before the 18th week of gestation (Herbst, et al., 1979). These findings do not necessarily indicate that primates are qualitatively different from rodents in fetal responsiveness to carcinogens, since primates at the end of the first trimester are comparable developmentally to late-gestation rodents. In the context of human risk assessment it will clearly be useful to establish, through further experiments with primates and by epidemiological studies, the relative human fetal sensitivities to carcinogens at various gestational ages.

Postnatal Effects

Transplacentally-induced tumors can appear at a variety of times after birth, ranging from a few weeks to the old age of the animal. For example, lung tumors in BALB/c mice exposed transplacentally to urethane appeared in two crops, an initial small group which occurred prior to 10 weeks of age and did not increase in number between 10 and 36 weeks, and a later, larger crop which started to become evident at about 9 months (Anderson, 1978). Factors which modulate the appearance and development of transplacentally caused tumors have received relatively little attention. Postnatal treatment with the same or different chemicals can enhance the yield of tumors initiated in the fetus. Promotion of such tumors can occur, as has been demonstrated by postnatal application of promoting agents to skin; indeed such treatment is needed for transplacentally-initiated skin tumors to be expressed (Bulay and Wattenberg, 1971; Armuth and Berenblum, 1979, 1982; Goerttler and Loehrke, 1976, 1977; Goerttler, et al., 1980, 1981). In mice, a subthreshold transplacental dose of urethane combined with a subthreshold postnatal exposure of the same chemical resulted in tumor appearance in three organs, including a high incidence of liver tumors (Vesselinovitch, 1973). Modification of hormonal environment by gonadal ablation in Syrian golden hamsters resulted in an increased incidence of peripheral nervous system tumors (Rustia, 1976).

In other cases postnatal chemical exposure reduces the effect of the transplacental treatment. Postnatal treatment with methylnitrosourea (MNU) following transplacental exposure of chinchilla rabbits to ENU resulted in a reduction of tumors, presumably because of a chemotherapeutic action (Dimant and Beniashvili, 1978). This interpretation is supported by the similar results of Schiffer, et al. (1976). N-Butylbiguanidine administered to adult rats that had been treated transplacentally with MNU caused a significant reduction in incidence of neurogenic tumors (Alexandrov, et al., 1980), as did nerve growth factor (Vinores and Koestner, 1982). In contrast to the effect of gonadal ablation on ENU-initiated neurogenic tumors in hamsters, the same treatment in male mice after transplacental ENU, coupled with administration of estrogenic hormones, effectively prevented hepatoma development (Rice, 1973). Postnatal treatment of rats with human serum albumin, hydrocortisone, cyclophosphamide, nicotine, or Bacille Calmette-Guerin after fetal exposure to ENU had no effect on incidence of any tumor (Habs and Schmähl, 1976).

In this context the effect of prenatal chemical exposures on susceptibility to postnatal carcinogens should be mentioned. Chemical treatment of fetuses and newborns may have many long-lasting effects, among them alterations in the biochemical interactions of carcinogens. Transplacental or transmammary exposure of mice or rats to barbiturates and polychlorinated biphenyls resulted in alteration of microsomal enzyme activities and/or carcinogen binding to DNA in these animals as adults (Dieringer, et al., 1979; Yanai, 1979; Faris and Campbell, 1981, 1983). Transplacental plus transmammary exposure of mice to a mixture of polychlorinated biphenyls resulted in induction of fewer tumors when DMN was given to the sucklings, presumably as a result of induction of detoxification enzymes, but there were indications of promotion of liver tumors later in life (Anderson, et al., 1983). Transplacental exposure of hamsters or rats to DES rendered them more susceptible to postnatal causation by DMBA of tumors in the reproductive tract, mammary glands, and elsewhere (Rustia and Shubik, 1979; Boyland and Calhoon, 1981). Such findings are important in consideration of human risk assessment because in human epidemiological studies, noncarcinogenic prenatal exposure situations could sometimes appear as carcinogenic if coupled with particular postnatal chemical encounters.

Cellular Determinants of Risk

Reasons for the species-, organ-, and time-specific effects of transplacental carcinogens have been sought in numbers of target cells and in variations in rates of cell division, of carcinogen activation by enzymes, and of repair of DNA damage. In the first place, in the developing fetuses the risk of tumor initation increases in proportion to the number of cells at risk, if all other factors are equal (Vesselinovitch, 1973; Muller and Rajewsky, 1983). Frequency of cell division is undoubtedly also important. Kauffman (1976) observed a close correlation between percentage of fetal mouse lung cells in division and sensitivity of the lung to tumor initiation by ENU. It would be worthwhile to extend such determinations of cell numbers and cell turnover time, as related to tumor initiation, to other species, organs, and carcinogens. If the correlation were to prove to be a general one, it might be applied to the human risk situation to identify periods of particular sensitivity for various fetal target cells.

Chemically-stable carcinogens, including most of those likely to be encountered from exogenous sources by humans, are detoxified in the body by enzyme action. In the course of this process reactive intermediates may be generated which modify or damage cellular molecules, leading in some cases to tumor initiation. Thus there is a complex relationship between metabolism and carcinogenesis, since both detoxification and activation result from the same set of processes. Rodent, primate, and human fetal tissues have been found to have the capacity to metabolize carcinogens, to catalyze mutagenesis in the process of this metabolism, and in the case of rodents, to respond to exogenous inducers with an increased level of fetal tissue carcinogen metabolism (for review and references, see Lucier, et al., 1979; Pelkonen, 1980a,b, 1982). For example, in a large study of metabolism of benzo[a]pyrene (BP) by homogenates of tissues in human fetuses of less than 22 weeks of gestational age, Rifkind, et al. (1978) found a wide range of enzyme activities, including a sevenfold variation in the case of liver, which did not correlate with gestational age. In spite of this variation, there was a clear difference between organs: BP hydroxylase activity was highest in the adrenal gland, threefold lower on the average in liver, testis, and uterus, with activities of decreasing magnitude in ovary, intestine, kidney, and lung. All of these values were much lower than those for BP hydroxylase in corresponding adult tissues. Other reactions, including demethylation, various hydroxylations, and some conjugations were most prominent in fetal liver and displayed activity levels of up to 50% or more of adult values (Pelkonen, 1980a). Furthermore, homogenates of human fetal hepatic, pulmonary, adrenal, and renal tissue catalyzed the formation of bacterial mutagens from BP, DMBA, and N-2-fluorenylaceamide (Jones, et al., 1977). The possibility must also be considered that maternal organs and the placenta generate activated carcinogenic intermediates of sufficiently long half-life to reach the fetus and cause neoplastic change, even in the absence of fetal capacity to carry out such necessary activation.

Although wide variations have been observed between human fetuses with regard to carcinogen-metabolizing capabilities, there is no clear evidence that these activities may be induced transplacentally in humans, as is the case for rodents. No consistent differences have been found in fetal enzyme activities from smoking vs non-smoking mothers, even though placental enzymes are clearly induced by smoking (reviewed by Pelkonen, et al., 1980). Results from fetuses of phenobarbital-treated mothers were equivocal.

An important question then is the nature of the relationship between carcinogen-metabolizing enzymes in human maternal, placental, and fetal tissues and tumorigenesis, since these enzyme activities vary greatly between organs and between individuals. There is indirect evidence supporting a positive correlation between level of carcinogen metabolism in the fetus and tumorigenic effect. In the case of transplacental nitrosamine carcinogenesis in rodents, development of sensitivity of the fetus to the carcinogen coincides with appearance of capacity to metabolize these agents and to catalyze their tissue binding (Druckrey, 1973; Ivankovic, 1973; Diwan and Meier, 1976; Emura, et al., 1980; Reznik-Schuller and Hague, 1981; Jannetti and Anderson, 1981). Metabolism of BP and causation of chromosomal damage by this chemical was detected in mouse embryos during the first week of gestation (Galloway, et al., 1980; Filler and Lew, 1980), an observation that is consistent with transplacental carcinogenic effects of polycyclic aromatic hydrocarbons as early as gestational day six in the mouse (Goerttler, et al., 1981). The capacity of rat and mouse fetal organs to catalyze formation of mutagenic metabolites from various carcinogens correlated reasonably well with susceptibility of the organ to tumorigenesis by these agents (Juchau, et al., 1979).

On the other hand, pretreatment of pregnant mice with the enzyme inducer β-naphthoflavone, which caused an increase in both maternal and fetal levels of aryl hydrocarbon metabolism, resulted in significant protection of the fetuses from subsequent transplacental lung tumorigenesis by methylcholanthrene (Anderson and Priest, 1980). Possibly the increase in maternal detoxifying metabolism overrode the effects of metabolism increase in the fetus, as is the case for transplacental BP toxicity (Shum, et al.,

1979). In general, however, increased carcinogen metabolism through enzyme induction results in protection against the action of systemically administered carcinogens (Wattenberg, 1978). The role of metabolism in determining fetal risk remains an open question. Efforts have been initiated to compare human fetal and maternal carcinogen-metabolizing characteristics by utilization of cultures of lymphocytes from cord and maternal blood (Pelkonen, *et al.,* 1980, 1981; Karki, *et al.,* 1981). Such studies could shed light on relationships between maternal and fetal carcinogen metabolism and cancer risk, particularly if coupled with epidemiological follow-up.

Formation and removal of DNA sites damaged by transplacental carcinogens have also been considered as factors in target specificity. Fetal rat brain is a sensitive target in transplacental carcinogenesis whereas fetal liver is resistant in this species. Such livers were found to be able to repair the carcinogen-caused promutagenic lesions, O^6-ethyl- and O^6-methylguanine whereas the fetal brains lacked this capacity and retained the modified base for a long period (Goth and Rajewsky, 1974; Kleihues, *et al.,* 1979; Chang, *et al.,* 1980; Muller and Rajewsky, 1983). A repair enzyme activity for depurinated DNA regions, apurinic endonuclease, was likewise found to be plentiful in fetal rat liver but absent from brain (Chen, *et al.,* 1982). However, similar differences between levels of DNA repair enzymes were found when mouse liver and brain were studied, and in this species the liver is more likely to be a target than brain. In rats, the retention of O^6-ethylguanine was similar in adult and fetal brains, even though only the animals exposed as fetuses were highly susceptible to brain tumorigenesis. Thus, while alterations of fetal DNA may be necessary and important steps in transplacental carcinogenesis, this is clearly not the only determinant, and persistence of DNA binding products may or may not be a reliable indicator of tissue risk for carcinogenesis.

In sum, a number of factors have been implicated as possible determinants of fetal risk for carcinogenesis, but in all cases the evidence is mainly of the indirect-correlation type and not conclusive, and should be used only with much circumspection in specific human risk assessment situations.

IDENTIFICATION OF TRANSPLACENTAL CARCINOGENS

Assay Systems

From the above discussion, it may be concluded that quantitative assessment of human transplacental carcinogenic risk is not possible from animal model bioassay data, because of the large differences observed among organs and species and the complexity of potential prenatal and postnatal modifying factors. Qualitative extrapolations are more feasible, since a carcinogen which is effective transplacentally in one or more animal species is likely to have the same general potential in humans. Methods for detection of transplacental carcinogenic effects are summarized below.

In Vivo Assays

Inclusion of early-life exposure (preconceptional, gestational, and neonatal) in chronic life-time tests for carcinogenicity of chemicals is sometimes advocated, because of the possible special sensitivities of the immature animal. For example, DES affects the human fetus but apparently not the adult, and the tumorigenic effects of saccharin in rats were most marked in two generation studies (Arnold, *et al.,* 1980). Methods and problems associated with such total-life exposure assays have recently been reviewed (Swenberg, 1979; Rice, 1980).

There are several circumstances in which a chemical might be tested specifically for transplacental (or transplacental plus lactational) effects. Such tests might be indicated for chemicals that give highly positive results in short-term tests for transplacental action (see below), that induce embryonal tumors or neoplasms at an unusually young age in chronic total-life exposure assays, that are implicated by epidemiological studies as carcinogens for human fetuses or children, or that pregnant women and children are particularly likely to contact. Some of the special features that must be considered in the design of a bioassay including perinatal effects have been discussed recently (Rice, 1980). In particular, many chemicals given to pregnant mothers are retained in their bodies to some degree and secreted in the milk, so the offspring must be foster-nursed if exposure is to be limited to the gestational period. The possibility of litter effects must be considered, so that either all but two pups of each litter must be discarded, or treatment group sizes must be large enough to allow for statistical tests of litter effects. With regard to choice of species, rats are less likely to experience nonspecific teratogenic effects. Mice are less costly in terms of space and funds, and an additional advantage is that almost every transplacental carcinogen tested thus far in mice has induced lung tumors, which have a short latency. Thus sacrifice of a portion of the test mice 8-12 months after birth would give a reasonably reliable preliminary indication as to the chemical's transplacental effectiveness. Noninbred Swiss mice exhibit considerable but not exquisite sensitivity to lung and liver tumor induction, and are easy to breed and maintain; these might often be the animal of choice for transplacental assays.

In a qualitative assay for transplacental effect, the dose should be chronic and may include preconception treatment of both parents. Choice of dose is a complicated matter, since toxicity may change as a function of gestational and postnatal age and in the pregnant vs. lactating mother. The maximum tolerated dose permitting conception and finally survival of a high percentage of offspring to weaning would seem to be a reasonable choice, unless this is so low as to be unconvincing in case of a negative result. In this instance, the developmental periods of particular sensitivity to toxicity would have to be discovered experimentally and the dose reduced during these periods.

The transplacental carcinogenesis literature has been searched for information pertaining to application and outcome of transplacental assays involving chronic exposure. Remarkably few experiments of this type have been reported, and in general no or only small effects were seen. Sydow (1970) exposed rats before and during pregnancy to DEN (1 mg/rat/day); no tumorigenic effects were observed in the offspring or in several successive generations. In rats exposed throughout gestation to diet containing 1-3% crude cycad material, none of six progeny developed tumors, whereas about 25% of a larger group exposed in the same way during one-week intervals of pregnancy were found to be tumor-bearing (Spatz and Laqueur, 1967). Daily oral doses of 0.5 mg DMN given to rats throughout pregnancy resulted in kidney tumors in 4% of the offspring (Alexandrov, 1968). In a test of hexamethylenetetraamine in rats, females were exposed to the chemical in drinking water before conception and throughout pregnancy and lactation, and half of their progeny received additional exposure. No tumors were found (Della Porta, et al., 1970).

Chronic or repeated-dose exposures during the last third of pregnancy have been much more commonly employed, no doubt because of 1) the apparent lack of effectiveness of total pregnancy exposure in experiments such as those cited above, 2) the likelihood of toxic and teratogenic effects earlier, and 3) a presumed limitation of sensitivity to tumorigenesis to the late gestational period. However, as recent findings have shown, preconceptional and early gestational events may have a significant effect on tumor incidence in the progeny. The effect of chronic exposure during these periods with putative carcinogens is a matter that deserves attention, and model studies should be carried out with known transplacental carcinogens of varying potency to establish appropriate methodologies. Stepwise modification of doses may well be necessary to avoid early toxic and teratogenic effects while providing the late fetus with maximum tolerated dose.

A simplified approach for *in vivo* testing of carcinogenic effects in the immature mammal has been proposed by Clayson (1981), who suggested that much time and expense could be spared by starting treatment at birth. Most of the factors confering sensitivity to carcinogenesis on the fetus still pertain in the newborn, and problems associated with reproductive toxicity and litter effects *in utero* would thus be spared. While this procedure should not replace preconception and transplacental testing, it would have merit in certain situations where tests for perinatal effects are indicated but could not include the prenatal period because of practical limitations.

Ogawa, *et al.* (1982) recently investigated the possibility of causing early appearance of transplacentally-initiated liver tumors in rats by using the Solt-Farber (1976) method for stimulating the growth of hepatic hyperplastic nodules, a procedure which could be completed ten weeks after birth. Significant numbers of hepatic foci of cellular alteration, identified by positive staining for γ-glutamyltranspeptidase, were found after transplacental exposure to DEN or DMBA. This method may have utility as a relatively short *in vivo* test for transplacental carcinogenicity, if further trials confirm its validity.

Short-Term Assays

Considerable effort has been invested recently in the design and testing of short *in vitro* tests for detecting carcinogens, and some of these have been utilized in transplacental carcinogenesis, with interesting results. In a pioneering study DiPaolo, *et al.* (1973) exposed Syrian hamsters to carcinogens transplacentally and then demonstrated transformation in cell cultures derived from the treated fetuses. This approach is conceptually appealing, since the fetuses were exposed to the carcinogen in their natural environment, and the endpoint observed was neoplastic transformation. It has been used with some success by subsequent investigators (e.g., Quarles, *et al.*, 1979), but in general has proved to be methodologically intractable, with high variability depending in part on the particular hamster and the batch of fetal calf serum used in the culture medium and other unknown factors. Negative results with known carcinogens or flat dose-response curves are also frequently encountered. Furthermore, rats and mice are usually not suitable subjects for such experiments, because of the high rate of spontaneous transformation of their fetal cells in culture. Brain cells from fetal rats treated transplacentally with ENU underwent malignant transformation in culture, but only after latencies similar to those observed in the intact animal (Laerum and Rajewsky, 1975; Yoshida, *et al.*, 1980), so that the procedure has little value as a short-term assay.

Tests of genetic damage caused by transplacental carcinogens have been technically more successful (recently reviewed by Cole and Henderson, 1982). Both sister chromatid exchanges and clastogenic (micronucleus) effects have been demonstrated in fetal rodent tissues after transplacental carcinogen exposure (Kram, *et al.*, 1980; Allen, *et al.*, 1981; Pereira, *et al.*, 1982; Cole, *et al.*, 1979; 1980, 1982a,b,). In a comparison of these two methods for a number of genotoxic agents, the results were found to be sufficiently different that complementary use of both was recommended (Cole, *et al.*, 1983). Application of these techniques to human cord blood lymphocytes has begun (Cole and Henderson, 1982) and should provide interesting information on genetic damage sustained by human fetal cells by the time of birth.

These morphological tests do not, of course, allow conclusions as to functional genetic damage, such as is presumed to precede cancer development. The *in vivo-in vitro* transplacental mutagenesis assay bridges the gap between the *in vivo-in vitro* transformation procedure of DiPaolo and the morphological demonstrations of chromosomal impact. This assay was originally developed by Dean for adult animals (Dean and Senner, 1977; Dean and Hodson-Walker, 1979) and applied transplacentally by Inui and co-workers (recently reviewed in Inui and Nishi, 1981). Following transplacental exposure of Syrian golden hamsters to chemicals, the fetal cells were cultured and tested for resistance to 8-azaguanine or 6-thioguanine. The method was used successfully to detect transplacental mutagenesis by oral or intraperitoneal administration of the food additive furylfuramide and of the nitrosation products of morpholine and sulfanilamide (Inui, *et al.,* 1976; 1978; 1979; Endo, *et al.,* 1980). Cells from individual fetal organs were cultured after transplacental exposure to BP, DMN, and MNU, and differences were observed, with BP being a particularly effective mutagen for lung, DMN for liver, and NMU for brain. These findings correlated only partially with tumorigenic potential, and in any case the cells established in the cultures were fibroblastic, whereas most transplacentally-caused tumors are epithelial.

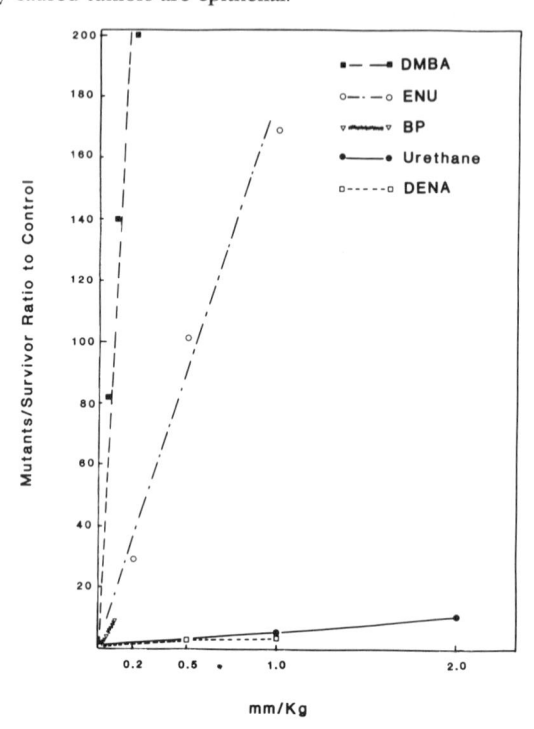

FIGURE 1. Pregnant Syrian hamsters were injected intraperitoneally on the twelfth day of gestation with the carcinogen indicated dissolved in dimethylsulfoxide, except for ENU, which was prepared in citrate buffer at pH 3.0. After twenty-four hours the fetuses were removed, and dissociated into single cells by trypsinization. Pooled cells from the fetuses of individual mothers were suspended in Dulbecco's minimal essential medium (DMEM) and frozen in liquid nitrogen. For determination of number of mutants the cells were thawed, grown in DMEM for an expression time of five days and then plated at 10^6 cells per plate, or cloned to determine survival rate, on twenty-four hour-old feeder layers of rat fetal fibroblasts. After forty-eight hours diphtheria toxin (Cannaught Research Laboratories, Toronto) was added to the plated cells at a concentration of 0.1 liquid flocculating units per ml and incubation continued for forty-eight hours. The number of diphtheria toxin resistant mutant colonies was determined after staining with giemsa. The spontaneous mutation rate was 0.2 to 0.5 x 10^{-6} mutant per surviving cell. Each point represents cells from fetuses of one mother (average of twenty plates).

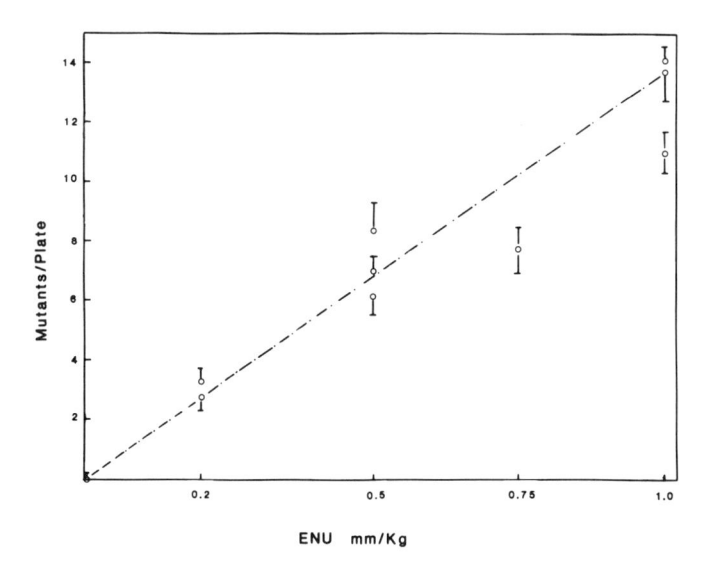

FIGURE 2. Pregnant Syrian hamsters were treated with ENU and the fetal cells were processed and selected for diphtheria-toxin resistant mutants as indicated in the legend for Fig. 1. Each point represents cells from fetuses of one mother (average of twenty plates). The bars indicate the standard error of the mean number of mutant colonies on plates of the same cell preparation.

In our laboratory we have extended this approach to several additional carcinogens with resistance to diptheria toxin as the genetic marker. Number of mutants per surviving cells were determined for transplacentally-exposed and control fetuses. This value for treated fetuses was divided by the control value and plotted as a function of dose (Fig. 1). DMBA and ENU were very effective transplacental mutagens, causing an increase in mutant colonies 100- to 200- fold over background, comparable to the results of Inui (1981). Benzo[a]pyrene and urethane caused a tenfold increase relative to background, and DEN was marginally mutagenic, giving a threefold elevation in number of mutants. These relative degrees of effectiveness of the five mutagens correlate well with their potency as transplacental carcinogens in rodents. Data showing the reproducibility of the assay for different mothers given ENU are plotted in Figure 2. A clear dose-response was seen without any correction for toxicity.

These data establish the *in vivo-in vitro* mutagenesis assay as a particularly attractive short-term test for transplacental effects. Positive results have been obtained with eight known chemical carcinogens, with at least some correspondence between the known mutagenic activity and their quantitative effectiveness and favored target organs in tumorigenesis. The data is dose-responsive and reproducible. The test is thus practical and reliable for detecting functional genetic damage by transplacental carcinogens. Further applications will reveal the extent of its fidelity in implicating new transplacental carcinogens, or indeed carcinogens in general.

SUMMARY

Expanding epidemiological data indicate the possibility that some cancers of childhood may result from transplacental exposure to chemicals. Experiments with laboratory rodents and primates demonstrate that most kinds of chemical carcinogens may act transplacentally, with varying degrees of effectiveness; that there is a high degree of species, organ, and time specificity in their transplacental effects; and that adult-type tumors appearing late in life are a usual result. Possible cellular determinants of fetal carcinogenic risk are number of responsive target cells present, percentage of dividing cells, capacity to activate carcinogens to mutagenic forms, and persistence of DNA damage. Further research is needed to establish which of these or other determinants are critical, so that animal findings can be extrapolated to estimations of human risk. At present, no such quantitative extrapolation can be made. Qualitative accessment of whether or not a chemical is or likely to be a human transplacental carcinogen, can be carried out in rodents or in short term tests. A new *in vivo - in vitro* mutagenesis assay appears to have particularly high potential in this regard.

REFERENCES

Alexandrov, V. A.: Blastomogenic effect of dimethylnitrosamine on pregnant rats and their offspring. *Nature, 218*:280, 1968

Alexandrov, V. A.; Anisimov, V. N., Belous, N. M., Vasilyeva, I. A., and Mazon, V. B.: The inhibition of the transplacental blastomogenic effect of nitrosomethylurea by postnatal administration of buformin to rats. *Carcinogenesis, 1*:975, 1980.

Allen, J. W.; El-Nahass, E., Sanyal, M. K., Dunn, R. L., Gladen, B., and Dixon, R. L.: Sister-chromatid exchange analysis in rodent maternal, embryonic and extra-embryonic tissues. Transplacental and direct mutagen exposures. *Mut. Res., 80*:297, 1981.

Anderson, L. M.: Two crops of primary lung tumors in BALB/c mice after a single transplacental exposure to urethane. *Cancer Lett., 5*:55, 1978.

Anderson, L. M.; and Priest, L. M.: Reduction in the transplacental carcinogenic effect of methylcholanthrene by prior treatment with β-naphthoflavone. *Res. Comm. Chem. Pathol. Pharmacol., 30*:431, 1980.

Anderson, L. M. (ed.).: *Oncology Overview: Selected Abstracts on Transplacental Carcinogenesis,* National Cancer Institute/International Cancer Research Data Bank, Washington, 1980.

Anderson, L. M.; and Budinger, J. M.: Qualitative histological differences between transplacentally-induced lung tumors in young and aging mice. *Cancer Lett., 11*:285, 1981.

Anderson, L. M.; Last-Barney, K., and Budinger, J. M.: Sensitivity to carcinogenesis in nude mice: skin tumors caused by transplacental exposure to ethylnitrosourea. *Science, 218*:682, 1982.

Anderson, L. M.; Van Havere, K., and Budinger, J. M.: Effects of polychlorinated biphenyls on lung and liver tumors initiated in suckling mice by N-nitrosodimethylamine. *JNCI, 71*:157, 1983.

Annegers, J. F.; Kurland, L. T., and Hauser, W. A.: Brain tumors in children exposed to barbiturates (Letter to the Editor). *JNCI, 63*:3, 1979.

Armuth, V.; and Berenblum, I.: Tritiated thymidine as a broad spectrum initiator in transplacental two-stage carcinogenesis with phorbol as promoter. *Int. J. Cancer, 24*:355, 1979.

Armuth, V.; and Berenblum, I.: A possible *in vivo* skin model for tumour promoter assays. *Cancer Lett., 15*:343, 1982.

Arnold, D. L.; Moodie, C. A., Grice, H. C., Charbonneau, S. M., Stavric, B., Collins, B. T., McGuire, P. F., Zawidzka, Z. Z., and Munro, I. C.: Long-term toxicity of ortho-toluenesulfonamide and sodium saccharin in the rat. *Toxicol. Appl. Pharmacol.*, 52:113, 1980.

Birch, J. M.; Marsden, H. B., and Swindell, R.: Pre-natal factors in the origin of germ cell tumors of childhood. *Carcinogenesis*, 3:75, 1982.

Borzsonyi, M.; Torok, G., Pinter, A., Surjan, A., Nadasdi, L., and Roller, P.: Carcinogenic effect of dinitrosopiperazine in adult Swiss mice and after transplacental or translactational exposure. *Cancer Res.*, 40:2925, 1980.

Boylan, E. S.; and Calhoon, R. E.: Prenatal exposure to diethylstilbestrol: ovarian-independent growth of mammary tumors induced by 7,12-dimethylbenz-[a]-anthracene. *JNCI*, 66:649, 1981.

Brandt, I., Darnerud, P. O., Bergman, A., and Larsson, Y.: Metabolism of 2,4',5-trichlorobiphenyl: enrichment of hydroxylated and methyl sulphone metabolites in the uterine luminal fluid of pregnant mice. *Chem. Biol. Interact.*, 40:45, 1982.

Bulay, O. M.; and Wattenberg, L. W.: Carcinogenic effects of polycyclic-hydrocarbon carcinogen administration to mice during pregnancy on the progeny. *JNCI*, 46:397, 1971.

Chang, M. J. W.; Hart, R. W., and Koestner, A.: Retention of promutagenic O^6-ethylguanine in the DNA of various rat tissues following transplacental inoculation with ethylnitrosourea. *Cancer Lett.*, 9:199, 1980.

Chen, B. P.; Feng, X., and Rice J. M.: Apurinic endonuclease (APE) activity in nuclear fractions from fetal rat liver and brain: inverse correlation with susceptibility to transplacental carcinogenesis by alkylating agents. *Proc. Am. Assoc. Cancer Res.*, 23:12, 1982.

Clayson, D. B.: Carcinogenesis in the developing organism: could protocols for testing be improved? *Biol. Res. Pregn.*, 2:150, 1981.

Cole, R. J.; Taylor, N. A., Cole, J., and Arlett, C. F.: Transplacental effects of chemical mutagens detected by the micronucleus test. *Nature*, 277:317, 1979.

Cole, R. J.; Taylor, N., Cole, J., and Arlett, C. F.: Short-term tests for transplacentally active carcinogens. I. Micronucleus formation in fetal and maternal mouse erythroblasts. *Mut. Res.*, 80:141, 1980.

Cole, R. J.; Aghamohammadi, Z., Cole, J., and Henderson, L.: Short-term tests for transplacentally active carcinogens. Multiple-dose regimes in the transplacental micronucleus test. *Mut. Res.*, 105:115, 1982.

Cole, R. J.; Taylor, N., Cole, J., Henderson, L., and Arlett, C. F.: Short-term tests for transplacentally active carcinogens. Sensitivity of the transplacental micronucleus test to diethylnitrosamine. *Mut. Res.*, 104:165, 1982.

Cole, R. J.; and Henderson, L.: Measuring prenatal genotoxic effect in mice and man. *Banbury Report 13: Indicators of Genotoxic Exposure*, Cold Spring Harbor Laboratory, New York, p. 355, 1982.

Cole, R. J.; Cole, J. Henderson, L., Taylor, N. A., Arlett, C. F., and Regan, T.: Short-term tests for transplacentally active carcinogens. A comparison of sister-chromatid exchange and the micronucleus test in mouse fetal liver erythroblasts. *Mut. Res.*, 113:61, 1983.

Dean, B. J.; and Senner, K. R.: Detection of chemically induced somatic mutation in Chinese hamsters. *Mut. Res.*, 46:403, 1977.

Dean, B. J.; and Hodson-Walker, G.: Organ-specific mutations in Chinese hamsters induced by chemical carcinogens. *Mut. Res.*, 64:407, 1979.

Della Porta, G.; Cabral, J. R., and Parmiani, G.: Transplacental toxicity and carcinogenicity of hexamethylenetetraamine in rats. *Tumori*, 56:325, 1970.

Denlinger, R. H.; Koestner, A., and Wechsler, W.: Induction of neurogenic tumors in C3HeB/FeJ mice by nitrosourea derivatives: observations by light microscopy, tissue culture, and electron microscopy. *Int. J. Cancer*, 13:559, 1974.

Dieringer, C. S.; Lamartiniere, C. A., Schiller, C. M., and Lucier, G. W.: Altered ontogeny of hepatic steroid-metabolizing enzymes by pure polychlorinated biphenyl congeners. *Biochem. Pharmacol.*, 28:2511, 1979.

Dimant, I. N.; and Beniashvili, D. S.: The significance of some modifying factors during transplacental blastomogenesis by ethylnitrosourea in rabbits. *Neoplasma*, 25:453, 1978.

DiPaolo, J. A.; Nelson, R. L., Donovan, P. J., and Evans, C. H.: Host mediated in vivo-in vitro assay for chemical carcinogens. *Arch. Pathol.*, 95:380, 1973.

Diwan, B. A.; and Meier, H.: Transplacental carcinogenic effects of diethylnitrosamine in mice. *Naturwissen.*, 63:487, 1976.

Druckrey, H.: Chemical structure and action in transplacental carcinogenesis and teratogenesis. *IARC Sci. Publ.*, 4:45, 1973.

Dvorchick, B. H.; and Hartman, R. D.: Hydroxylation of hexobarbital and benzo[a]-pyrene by hepatic microsomes isolated from the fetal stumptailed monkey (Macaca arctoides). A developmental study. *Biochem. Pharmacol.*, 31:1150, 1982.

Emura, M.; Richter-Reichhelm, H. B., and Mohr, U.: Some aspects of prenatal risk of N-nitrosodiethylamine carcinogenesis. *IARC Sci. Publ.*, 31:767, 1980.

Endo, H.; Noda, H., Kinoshita, N., Inui, N., and Nishi, Y.: Formation of transplacental mutagen, 1,3-di(4-sulfamoylphenyl)triazene, from sodium nitrite and sulfanilamide in human gastric juice and in the stomachs of hamsters. *JNCI*, 65:547, 1980.

Fabia, J.; and Thuy, T. D.: Occupation of father at time of birth of children dying of malignant diseases. *Br. J. Prev. Soc. Med.*, 28:98, 1974.

Fabro, S.: Anticonvulsant-induced transplacental carcinogenesis. *Reproduct. Toxicol. Lett.*, 1:1, 1982.

Faris, R. A.; and Campbell, T. C.: Exposure of newborn rats to pharmacologically active compounds may permanently alter carcinogen metabolism. *Science*, 211:719, 1981.

Faris, R. A.; and Campbell, T. C.: Long-term effects of neonatal phenobarbital exposure on aflatoxin B1 disposition in adult rats. *Cancer Res.*, 43:2576, 1983.

Filler, R.; and Lew, K. J.: Developmental onset of mixed-function oxidase activity in preimplantation mouse embryos. *Proc. Natl. Acad. Sci.*, 78:6991, 1981.

Fowler, W. C.; and Edelman, D. A.: In utero exposure to DES. Evaluation and followup of 199 women. *Obstet. Gynecol.*, 51:459, 1978.

Fox, R. R.; Diwan, B. A., and Meier, H.: Transplacental induction of primary retal tumors in rabbits treated with 1-ethyl-1-nitrosourea. *JNCI*, 54:1439, 1975.

Fox, R. R.; Meier, H., Pottathil, R., and Bedigian, H. G.: Transplacental teratogenic and carcinogenic effects in rabbits chronically treated with N-ethyl-N-nitrosourea. *JNCI*, 65:607, 1980.

Fujii, K.; and Watanabe, M.: Comparative study of tumorigenicity in mice administered transplacentally or neonatally with metabolites of tryptophan and its related compounds. *J. Cancer Res. Clin. Oncol.*, 96:163, 1980.

Fujii, K.: Induction of tumors in transplacental or neonatal mice administered 3'-methyl-4-dimethylaminoazobenzene or 4-aminoazobenzene. *Cancer Lett.*, 17:321, 1983.

Galloway, S. M.; Perry, P. E., Meneses, S. J., Nebert, D. W., and Pedersen, R. A.: Cultured mouse embryos metabolize benzo(a)pyrene during early gestation; genetic differences detectable by sister chromatid exchange. *Proc. Natl. Acad. Sci.*, 77:3524, 1980.

Goerttler, K., and Loehrke, H.: Diaplacental carcinogenesis: initiation with the carcinogens dimethylbenzanthracene (DMBA) and urethane during fetal life and postnatal promotion with the phorbol ester TPA in a modified 2-stage Berenblum-Mottram experiment. *Virchows Archiv.*, 372:29, 1976.

Goerttler, K.; and Loehrke, H.: Diaplacental carcinogenesis: tumor localization and tumor incidence in NMRI mice after diaplacental initiation with DMBA and urethane and postnatal promotion with the phorbol ester TPA in a modified 2-stage Berenblum-Mottram experiment. *Virchows Archiv.*, 376:117, 1977.

Goerttler, K.,; Loehrke, H., Schweizer, J., and Hesse, B.: Two-stage skin carcinogenesis by systemic initation of pregnant mice with 7,12-dimethylbenz[a]anthracene during gestation days 6-20 and postnatal promotion of the F1-generation with the phorbol ester 12-tetradecanoylphorbol-13-acetate. *J. Cancer Res. Clin. Oncol.*, 98:267, 1980.

Goerttler, K., Loehrke, H., Schweizer, J., and Hesse, B.: Effects of aflatoxin B_1 on pregnant inbred Sprague-Dawley rats and their F_1 generation. A contribution to transplacental carcinogenesis. *JNCI*, 64:1349, 1980.

Goerttler, K.; Loehrke, H., Hesse, B., Milz, A., and Schweizer, J.: Diaplacental initiation of NMRI mice with 7,12-dimethylbenz[a]anthracene during gestation days 6-20 and postnatal treatment of the F_1-generation with the phorbol ester 12-0-tetradecanoylphorbol-13-acetate: tumor incidence in organs other than skin. *Carcinogenesis*, 2:1087, 1981.

Gold, E. B.; Gordis L., Tonascia, J., and Szklo, M.: Increased risk of brain tumors in children exposed to barbiturates. *JNCI*, 61:1031, 1978.

Gold, E. B.; Gordis, L., Tonascia, J. A., and Szklo, M.: Brain tumors in children exposed to barbiturates. Letter to the editor. *JNCI*, 63:4, 1979.

Goth, R.; and Rajewsky, M. F.; Persistence of O^6-ethylguanine in rat brain DNA: correlation with nervous system-specific carcinogenesis by ethylnitrosourea. *Proc. Natl. Acad. Sci. USA*, 71:639, 1974.

Grufferman, S.; Wang, H. H., DeLong, E. R., Kimm, S. Y. S., Delzell, E. S., and Falletta, J. M.: Environmental factors in the etiology of rhabdomyosarcoma in childhood. *JNCI*, 68:107, 1982.

Habs, M., and Schmähl, D.: Influence of five different postnatal lifelong treatments on the transplacental carcinogenicity of ethylnitrosourea in Sprague-Dawley rats. *Cancer Lett.*, 2:93, 1976.

Haenszel, W.; and Kurihara, M.: Studies of Japanese migrants. I. Mortality from cancer and other diseases among Japanese in the United States. *JNCI*, 40:43, 1968.

Hakulinen, T.; Salonen, T., and Teppo, L.: Cancer in the offspring of fathers in hydrocarbon-related occupations. *Br. J. Prev. Soc. Med.*, 30:138, 1976.

Herbst, A. L.; Ulfelder, H., and Poskanzer, D. C.: Adenocarcinoma of the vagina: association of maternal stilbestrol therapy with appearance in young women. *N. Engl. J. Med.*, 284:878, 1971.

Herbst, A. L.; Poskanzer, D. C., Robboy, S. J., Friedlander, L., Scully, R. E.: Prenatal exposure to stilbestrol: a prospective comparison of exposed female offspring with unexposed controls. *N. Engl. J. Med.*, 292:334, 1975.

Herbst, A. L.; Cole, P., Colton, T., Robboy, S. J. and Scully, R. E.: Age-incidence of risk of diethylstilbestrol-related clear cell adenocarcinoma of the vagina and cervix. *Am. J. Obstet. Gynecol.*, 128:43, 1977.

Herbst, A. L.; Scully, R. E., and Robboy, S. J.: Prenatal diethylstilbestrol exposure and human genital tract abnormalities. *Nat. Cancer Inst. Mono.*, 51:25, 1979.

Herbst, A. L.: Clear cell adenocarcinoma and the current status of DES-exposed females. *Cancer*, 48:484, 1981.

Herd, J. E.; and Greene, F. E.: Effects of perinatal exposure to benzo(a) pyrene on the aryl hydrocarbon hydroxylase system of adult rat liver. *Biol. Neonate*, 38:291, 1980.

Hertzog, P. J.; Lawson, T. A., and Gingell, R.: The binding of 7,12-dimethylbenz[a]anthracene to mammary gland macromolecules in the hamster: effects of enovid feeding or transplacental exposure to diethylstilbestrol. *Chem. Biol. Interact.*, 37:199, 1981.

Inui, N.; Taketomi, M., and Nishi, Y.: Mutagenic effects of AF-2, a food additive, on embryonic cells of the Syrian golden hamster on transplacental application. *Mutat. Res.*, 41:351, 1976.

Inui, N.; Nishi, Y., and Taketomi, M.: Mutagenic effect of orally given AF-2 on embryonic cells in pregnant Syrian hamsters. *Mutat. Res.*, 57:69, 1978.

Inui, N.; Nishi, Y., Taketomi, M., Mori, M., Yamamoto, J., Yamada, T., and Tanimura, A.: Transplacental mutagenesis of products formed in the stomach of golden hamsters given sodium nitrite and morpholine. *Int. J. Cancer*, 24:365, 1979.

Inui, N.; and Nishi, Y.: Host-mediated mutagenesis for detection of mutagens/carcinogens. *Gann Mono. Cancer Res.*, 27:73, 1981.

Ivankovic, S.; and Druckrey, H.: Transplacentare Erzeugung maligner Tumoren des Nervensystems. I. Aethylnitrosoharnstoff (ANH) an BD IX-Ratten. *Z. Krebsforsch.*, 71:320, 1968.

Ivankovic, S.: Experimental prenatal carcinogenesis. *IARC Sci. Publ.*, 4:92, 1973.

Jannetti, R. A.; and Anderson, L. M.: Dimethylnitrosamine demethylase activity in fetal, suckling, and maternal mouse liver and its transplacental and transmammary induction by polychlorinated biphenyls. *JNCI*, 67:461, 1981.

Jensen, O. M.; and Kamby, C.: Intra-uterine exposure to saccharin and risk of bladder cancer in man. *Int. J. Cancer*, 29:507, 1982.

Jones, A. H.; Fantel, A. G., Kocan, R. A., and Juchau, M. R.: Bioactivation of procarcinogens to mutagens in human fetal and placental tissues. *Life Sci.*, 21:1831, 1977.

Juchau, M. T.; DiGiovanni, J., Namkung, M. J., and Jones, A. H.: A comparison of the capacity of fetal and adult liver, lung, and brain to convert polycyclic aromatic hydrocarbons to mutagenic and cytotoxic metabolites in mice and rats. *Toxicol. Appl. Pharmacol.*, 49:171, 1979.

Jurgelski, W.; Hudson, P. M., Falk, H. L., and Kotin, P.: Embryonal neoplasms in the opossum: a new model for solid tumors of infancy and childhood. *Science, 1983*:328, 1976.

Jurgelski, W.; Hudson, P., and Falk, H. L.: Tissue differentiation and susceptibility to embryonal tumor induction by ethylnitrosourea in the opossum. *Natl. Cancer Inst. Monogr., 51*:123, 1979

Kalter, H.; Mandybur, T. I., Ormsby, I., and Warkany, J.: Dose-related reduction by prenatal x-irradiation of the transplacental neurocarcinogencity of ethylnitrosourea in rats. *Cancer Res., 40*:3973, 1980.

Karki, N. T.; Pelkonen, O., Tuimala, R., Kauppila, A., and Koivisto, M.: Aryl hydrocarbon hydroxylase induction in maternal and cord blood mitogen-treated lymphocytes. *Dev. Pharmacol. Ther., 2*:32, 1981.

Kauffman, S. L.: Susceptibility of fetal lung to transplacental 1-ethyl-1nitrosourea: its relations to epithelial proliferation. *JNCI, 57*:821, 1976.

Kawade, N.; and Onishi, S.: The prenatal and postnatal development of UDP-glucuronyltransferase activity towards bilirubin and the effect of premature birth on this activity in the human liver. *Biochem. J., 196*:257, 1981.

Kleihues, P.; Cooper, H. K., Buecheler, J., Kolar, G. F., and Diessner, H.: Mechanism of perinatal tumor induction by neuro-oncogenic alkyl-nitrosoureas and dialkylaryltriazenes. *Natl. Cancer Inst. Mono., 51*:227, 1979.

Kleihues, P.: Developmental carcinogenicity. In: *Developmental Toxicology,* K. Snell, ed., Croome-Helm, London, p. 213, 1982.

Kram, D.; Bynum, G. D. Senula, G. C. Bickings, C. K, and Schneider, E. L.: *In utero* analysis of sister chromatid exchange: alterations in susceptibility to mutagenic damage as a function of fetal cell type and gestational age. *Proc. Natl. Acad. Sci. USA, 77*:4784, 1980.

Laerum, O.D.; and Rajewsky, M. F.: Neoplastic transformation of fetal rat brain cells in culture after exposure to ethylnitrosourea *in vivo. JNCI, 55*:1177, 1975.

Lanier, A. R.; Noller, K. L., Decker, D. G., Elveback, L. R., and Kurland, L. T.: Cancer and stilbestrol. A follow-up of 1,719 persons exposed to estrogens *in utero* and born 1943-1959. *Mayo Clin. Proc. 48*:793, 1973.

Larsen, C. O.: Pulmonary tumor induction by transplacental exposure to urethane. *JNCI, 8*:63, 1947.

Locke, F. B.; and King, H.: Cancer mortality risk among Japanese in the United States. *JNCI, 65*:1149, 1980.

Lucier, G. W., Lui, E. M. K., and Lamartineire, C. A.: Metabolic activation/deactivation reactions during perinatal development. *Environ. Health Perspect., 29*:7, 1979.

McLachlan, J. A.; Newbold, R. R., and Bullock, B. C.: Long-term effects on the female mouse genital tract associated with prenatal exposure to diethylstilbestrol. *Cancer Res., 40*:3988, 1980.

Mirvish, S.; Cividalli, G., and Berenblum, I.: Slow elimination of urethane in relation to its high carcinogenicity in newborn mice. *Proc. Soc. Expt. Biol. Med., 116*:265, 1964.

Mohr, U.; and Althoff, J.: Die diaplacentare Wirkung des Cancerogens Diäthylnitrosamin bei der Maus. *Z. Krebsforsch., 67*:152, 1965.

Mohr, U.; Emura, M., and Richter-Reichhelm, H. B.: Transplacental carcinogenesis. *Invest. Cell Pathol., 3*:209, 1980.

Muller, R.; and Rajewksy, M. F.: Elimination of O^6-ethylguanine from the DNA of brain, liver, and other rat tissues exposed to ethylnitrosourea at different stages of prenatal development. *Cancer Res., 43*:2897, 1983.

Naito, M.; Naito, Y., and Ito, A.: Effect of age at treatment on the incidence and location of neurogenic tumors induced in Wistar rats by a single dose of N-ethyl-N-nitrosourea. *Gann, 72:569, 1981.*

Napalkov, N. P.; and Alexandrov, V. A.: Neurotropic effect of 7,12-dimethylbenz-(a)anthracene in transplacental carcinogenesis. *JNCI, 52*:1365, 1974.

Napalkov, N. P.: Carcinogenic hazards from prenatal exposure to environmental chemicals. *Cancer Detect. Prevent., 2*:21, 1979.

Napalkov, N. P.; Alexandrov, V. A., and Anisimov, V. N.: Transplacental carcinogenic effect of N-nitrosoethylurea in dogs. *Cancer Lett., 12*:161, 1981.

Newbold, R. R.; and McLachlan, J. A.: Vaginal adenosis and adenocarcinoma in mice exposed prenatally or neonatally to diethylstilbestrol. *Cancer Res., 42*:2003, 1982.

Neutel, C. I.; and Buck, C.: Effect of smoking during pregnancy on the risk of cancer in children. *JNCI, 47*:59, 1971.

Nomura, T.; Takebe, H., and Okamoto, E.: Long retention of urethane transferred into newborn mice transplacentally, as a possible cause of high carcinogenesis. *Gann, 64:29,* 1973.

Nomura, T.: Sensitivity of a lung cell in the developing mouse embryo to tumor induction by urethane. *Cancer Res., 34*:3363, 1974.

Nomura, T.: Transmission of tumors and malformation to the next generation of mice subsequent to urethane treatment. *Cancer Res., 35*:264, 1975.

Nomura, T.: Comparison of tumor susceptibility among various organs of fetal, young, and adult ICR/JCL mice. *Br. J. Cancer, 33*:521, 1976.

Nomura, T.: Parental exposure to X rays and chemicals induces heritable tumors and anomalies in mice. *Nature, 296*:575, 1982.

Ogawa, K.; Yokokawa, K., Tomoyori, T., and Onoe, T.: Induction of γ-glutamyl-transpeptidase-positive altered hepatocyte lesions by combination of transplacental initiation and postnatal selection. *Int. J. Cancer, 29*:333, 1982.

Pacifici, G. M.; Norlin, A., and Rane, A.: Glutathione-S-transferase in human fetal liver. *Biochem. Pharmacol., 30*:3367, 1981.

Pelkonen, O.: Biotransformation of xenobiotics in the fetus. *Pharmac. Ther., 10*:261, 1980.

Pelkonen, O.: Environmental influences on human fetal and placental xenobiotic metabolism. *Eur. J. Clin. Pharmacol., 18*:17, 1980.

Pelkonen, O.; and Saarni, H.: Unusual patterns of benzo[a]pyrene metabolites and DNA-benzo(a)pyrene adducts produced by human placental microsomes *in vitro. Chem. Biol. Interact., 30*:287, 1980.

Pelkonen, O; Karki, N. T., and Sotaniemi, E. A.: Determination of carcinogen-activating enzymes in the monitoring of high risk groups. In: *Human Cancer. Its Characterization and Treatment.* W. Davis, R. R. Harrap, and G. Stathopoulos, eds. Excerpta Medica, Amsterdam, p. 48, 1980.

Pelkonen, O.; Karki, N. T., and Tuimala, R.: A relationship between cord blood and maternal blood lymphocytes and term placenta in the induction of aryl hydrocarbon hydroxylase activity. *Cancer Lett.*, *13*:103, 1981.

Pelkonen, O.: The differentiation of drug metabolism in relation to developmental toxicology. In: *Developmental Toxicology*, K. Snell, ed., Croome-Helm, London, p. 167, 1982.

Pereira, M. A.; McMillan, L., Kaur, P., Gulati, D. K., and Sabharwal, P. S.: Effect of benzo(a)pyrene on sister-chromatid exchange in fetal hamster liver exposed *in utero*. *Mut. Res.*, *105*:343, 1982.

Peters, J. M.; Preston-Martin, S., and Yu, M. C.: Brain tumors in children and occupational exposure of parents. *Science*, *213*:235, 1981.

Pielsticker, K.; Wieser, O., Mohr, U., and Wrba, H.: Diaplacentar induzierte Nierentumoren bei der Ratte. *Z. Krebsforsch.*, *69*:345, 1967.

Preston-Martin, S.; Yu, M. C., Benton, B., and Henderson, B. E.: N-nitroso compounds and childhood brain tumors: a case-control study. *Cancer Res.*, *42*:5240,1982.

Quarles, J. M.; Sega, M. W., Schenley, C. K., and Lijinsky, W.: Transformation of hamster fetal cells by nitrosated pesticides in a transplacental assay. *Cancer Res.*, *39*:4525, 1979.

Rády, P.; Arany, I., Uzvölogyi, É., and Boján, F.: Activity of pyruvate kinase and lactic acid dehydrogenase in mouse lung after transplacental exposure to carcinogenic and non-carcinogenic chemicals. *Toxicol. Lett.*, *8*:223, 1981.

Rády, P.; Arany, I., Uzvölgyi, É., Boján, F., and Kertai, P.: Transplacental effects of carcinogens and non-carcinogens on activities of pyruvate kinase and lactate dehydrogenase as well as isozymic pattern of LDH in mouse lung. *Toxicology*, *24*:251, 1982.

Rao, A. R.: Inhibitory action of BHA on carcinogenesis in F1 and F2 descendants of mice exposed to DMBA during pregnancy. *Int. J. Cancer*, *30*:121, 1982.

Reznik-Schüller, H. M.; and Hague, B. F.: Autoradiography in fetal Syrian golden hamsters treated with tritiated diethylnitrosamine. *JNCI*, *66*:773, 1981.

Reznik-Schüller, H. M.: Electron microscopic autoradiography of the trachea in fetal Syrian golden hamsters treated transplacentally with N-nitrosodiethylamine. *JNCI*, *69*:927, 1982.

Rice, J. M.: Transplacental carcinogenesis in mice by 1-ethyl-1-nitrosourea. *Ann. N. Y. Acad. Sci.*, *163*:813, 1969.

Rice, J. M.: An overview of transplacental chemical carcinogenesis. *Teratology*, *8*:113, 1973.

Rice, J. M.: The biological behavoir of transplacentally induced tumors in mice. *IARC Sci. Publ.*, *4*:71, 1973.

Rice, J. M.: Carcinogenesis: A late effect of irreversible toxic damage during development. *Environ. Health. Perspect.*, *18*:133, 1976.

Rice, J. M.; Palmer, A. E., London, W. T., Sly, D. L., and Williams, G. M.: Transplacental effects of ethylnitrosourea in the patas monkey. In: *Tumors of Early Life in Man and Animals*, L. Severi, ed., Perugia Quadrennial International Conferences on Cancer, Monteluce, Italy. p. 893, 1978.

Rice, J. M.: Incorporation of perinatal exposure into bioassays for carcinogenicity. In: *Proceedings of a Workshop on Methodologies for Assessing Reproductive Hazards in the Workplace*, P. F. Infante and M. S. Legator, eds., DHHS Publication No. 81-100, p. 247, 1980.

Rice, J. M.: Effects of prenatal exposure to chemical carcinogens and methods for their detection. In: *Developmental Toxicology*, C. A. Kimmel and J. Buelke-Sam, eds. Raven Press, N. Y., p. 191, 1981.

Rifkind, A. B.; Tseng, L., Hirsch, M. B., and Lauersen, N. H.: Aryl hydrocarbon hydroxylase activity and microsomal cytochrome content of human fetal tissues. *Cancer Res.*, 38:1572, 1978.

Romano, M.; Clos, V., Assael, B. M., and Salmona, M.: Perinatal development of cytochrome P-450, NADPH-cytochrome reductase and ethoxycoumarin deethylase in rat liver nuclear membranes. *Chem.-Biol. Interact.*, 42:225, 1982.

Rossi, L.; Barbieri, O., Sanguineti, M., Staccione, A., Santi, L. F., and Santi, L.: Carcinogenic activity of benzo[a]pyrene and some of its synthetic derivatives by direct injection into the mouse fetus. *Carcinogenesis*, 4:153, 1983.

Rouet, P.; Alexandrov, K., Markovits, P., Frayssinet, C., and Dansette, P. M.: Metabolism of benzo(a)pyrene by brain microsomes of fetal and adult rats and mice. Induction by 5,6-benzoflavone, comparison with liver and lung microsomal activities. *Carcinogenesis*, 2:919, 1981.

Rustia, M.: The effect of gonadal ablation on transplacentally-induced neurogenic tumors in hamsters. *Cancer Res.*, 36:240, 1976.

Rustia, M.; and Shubik, P.: Effects of transplacental exposure to diethylstilbestrol on carcinogenic susceptibility during postnatal life in hamster progeny. *Cancer Res.*, 39:4636, 1979.

Schiffer, D.; Giordana, M. T., Pezzotta, S., and Paoletti, P.: Chemotherapeutic effects of some alkylating derivatives of nitrosourea on the development of tumors transplacentally induced in rats by ENU. *Acta Neuropathol.*, 34:21, 1976.

Searle, C. E.; and Jones, E. L.: Tumors of the nervous system in mice treated neonatally with N-ethyl-N-nitrosourea. *Nature*, 240:559, 1972.

Shum, S.; Jensen, N. M., and Nebert, D. W.: The murine Ah locus: *In utero* toxicity and teratogenesis associated with genetic differences in benzo[a]pyrene metabolism. *Teratology*, 20:365, 1979.

Sinha, D. K.; and Pazik, J. E.: Tumorigenesis of mammary gland by 7,12-dimethylbenz[a]anthracene during pregnancy: relationship with DNA synthesis. *Int. J. Cancer*, 27:807, 1981.

Solt, D.; and Farber, E.: New principle for the analysis of chemical carcinogensis. *Nature*, 263:701, 1976.

Spatz, M.; and Laqueur, G. L.: Transplacental induction of tumors in Sprague-Dawley rats with crude cycad material. *JNCI*, 38:233, 1967.

Stavrou, D.; Dahme, E., and Schroder, B.: Transplacental induction of neurogenic tumors in rabbits. *Z. Krebsforsch.*, 89:331, 1977.

Sunderman, F. W.; McCully, K. S., and Rinehimer, L. A.: Negative test for transplacental carcinogenicity of nickel subsulfide in Fischer rats. *Res. Comm. Chem. Pathol. Pharmacol.*, 31:545, 1981.

Swenberg, J. A.; Koestner, A., Wechsler, W., and Denlinger, R. H.: Quantitative aspects of transplacental tumor induction with ethylnitrosourea in rats. *Cancer Res., 32*:2656, 1972.

Swenberg, J. A.: Incorporation of transplacental exposure into routine carcinogenicity testing. *Natl. Cancer Inst. Monograph, 51*:265, 1979.

Sydow, G.: Untersuchungen uber die diaplazentare teratogene, karzinogene, und mutagene Wirkung von Diäthylnitrosamin (DANA) nach oraler Applikation bei der Ratte. *Arch. Geschwulstforsch., 36*:331, 1970.

Tanaka, T.: Transplacental induction of tumors and malformations in rats treated with some chemical carcinogens. *IARC Sci. Publ., 4*:100, 1973.

Taylor, J. M.; Weinberger, M. A., and Friedman, L.: Chronic toxicity and carcinogenicity to the urinary bladder of sodium saccharin in the *in utero*-exposed rat. *Toxicol. Appl. Pharmacol, 54*:57, 1980.

Thomas, C.; and Bollmann, R.: Untersuchungen zur diaplacentaren krebserzeugenden Wirkung des Diäthylnitrosamin an Ratten. *Z. Krebsforsch., 71*:129, 1968.

Tomatis, L.; and Goodall, C. M.: The occurrence of tumours in F1, F2, and F3 descendants of pregnant mice injected with 7,12-dimethylbenz(a)anthracene. *Int. J. Cancer, 4*:219, 1969.

Tomatis, L.; Turusov, V., Guibbert, D., Dupperray, D., Malaveille, C., and Pacheco, H.: Transplacental carcinogenic effect of 3-methylcholanthrene in mice and its quantitation in fetal tissues. *JNCI, 47*:645, 1971.

Tomatis, L.; Turusov, V., and Guibbert, D.: Prenatal exposure to chemical carcinogens. In: *Topics in Chemical Carcinogenesis.* W. Nakahara, S. Takayama, and T. Sugimura, and S. Odashima, eds. University Park Press, Baltimore, p. 445, 1972.

Tomatis, L.; Hilfrich, J., and Turusov, V.: The occurrence of tumors in F_1, F_2, and F_3 descendants of BD rats exposed to N-nitrosomethylurea during pregnancy. *Int. J. Cancer, 15*:385, 1975.

Tomatis, L.: Prenatal exposure to chemical carcinogens and its effect on subsequent generations. *Natl. Cancer Inst. Mongr., 51*:159, 1979.

Tomatis, L.; Cabral, J. R. P., Likhachev, A. J., and Ponomarkov, V.: Increased cancer incidence in the progeny of male rats exposed to ethylnitrosourea before mating. *Int. J. Cancer, 28*:475, 1981.

Vesselinovitch, S. D.; Mihailovich, N., Rao, K. V. N., and Itze, L.: Perinatal carcinogenesis by urethane. *Cancer Res., 31*:2143, 1971.

Vesselinovitch, S. D.; Koka, M., Rao, K. V., Mihailovich, N., and Rice, J. M.: Prenatal multicarcinogenesis by ethylnitrosourea in mice. *Cancer Res., 37*:1822, 1977.

Vesselinovitch, S. D.: Comparative studies on perinatal carcinogenesis. *IARC Sci. Publ., 4*:14, 1973.

Vinores, S. A.; and Koestner, A.: Reduction of ethylnitrosourea-induced neoplastic proliferation in rat trigeminal nerves by nerve growth factor. *Cancer Res., 42*:1038, 1982.

Walker, B. E.: Uterine tumors in old female mice exposed prenatally to diethylstilbestrol. *JNCI, 70*:477, 1983.

Wattenberg, L. W.: Inhibition of chemical carcinogenesis. *JNCI, 60*:11, 1978.

Yanai, J.: Long-term induction of microsomal drug oxidizing system in mice following prenatal exposure to barbiturate. *Biochem. Pharmacol.,* 28:1429, 1979.

Yoshida, J.; Cravioto, H., and Ransohoff, J.: In vitro transformation of fetal brain cells from CDF rats exposed *in utero* to N-ethyl-N-nitrosourea: morphological and immunologic studies. *JNCI,* 64:1231, 1980.

Zack, M.; Cannon, S. Loyd, D., Heath, C. W., Falletta, J. M., Jones, B., Housworth, J., and Crowley, S.: Cancer in children of parents exposed to hydrocarbon-related industries and occupations. *Am. J. Epidemiol., 11*:329, 1980.

Validity of *In Vitro* Methods in Teratogenicity Testing

Allan R. Beaudoin

Department of Anatomy and Cell Biology, University of Michigan, Ann Arbor, Michigan 48109

The number of chemical compounds introduced into our environment since the year 1900 is staggering. Over 4 million distinct entities are listed in the Chemical Abstract Service of the American Chemical Society. A recent estimate suggests about 63,000 chemicals are in common use today (Maugh, 1978), and hundreds of new chemicals are introduced into the environment each year. How many of these chemicals become environmental contaminants is not known, nor is it known what effect, if any, they may have on the development of the human conceptus. The lack of a recognized epidemic in malformations, excepting thalidomide, of course, suggests that chemical compounds, by themselves, contribute little to the incidence of human malformations. The determination of the safety of all existing and new chemical compounds is a horrendous task and one that is probably impossible, at least with the current state of the art. Nonetheless, we must strive to perfect a system for the determination of risk to the human conceptus.

Current methodology for testing for potential teratogenicity with pregnant laboratory animals is elaborate, expensive, and time consuming. In 1976 Schardein estimated 2,000 compounds had been tested for teratogenicity. The figure now stands at 2900, of which 1/3 are teratogenic (Schardein, personal communication). The number of compounds to be tested far exceeds the capacity of the current testing system, using standard *in vivo* procedures. A rapid inexpensive test is needed to identify the teratogenic potential of compounds. But what test will satisfy the requirements of reliability and predictability?

There are many submammalian systems proposed for screening compounds for teratogenicity, e.g., hydra (Johnson, 1982), planaria (Best and Morita, 1982), brine shrimp (Kerster and Schaeffer, 1983), amphibia (Dumont, *et al.,* 1983), and the chick embryo (Fisher and Schoenwolf, 1983) to name a few. However, these are not strict *in vitro* systems (i.e., grown in an artificial environment) and, therefore, will not be discussed today. This is not to imply they lack merit, for in the future they may indeed prove to be valuable tools in the field of risk assessment.

Table 1 lists some criteria for an ideal test system for the prediction of teratogenic risk in humans. An analysis of this table reveals that the goal of an ideal test system for teratogenic risk assessment is unatainable with tests currently available. There is no *in vivo* animal test or *in vitro* culture system, no matter how sophisticated, that can fully duplicate the normal *in utero* conditions in the human female. As workable alternatives

Wilson (1973) proposed multilevel *in vivo* tests, and Moscona (1975) proposed a battery of *in vitro* tests. This in vitro approach, however, has been questioned as being as expensive and time consuming as an *in vivo* study (Brown and Fabro, 1982).

TABLE 1
SOME CRITERIA FOR AN IDEAL TEST SYSTEM FOR THE PREDICTION OF HUMAN TERATOGENIC RISK

1) Must predict teratogenic potential to the human conceptus in the absence of maternal toxicity.
2) Must have reproducible endpoint(s).
3) Must metabolize the compound the same as the human.
4) Must demonstrate a relevance between the *in vitro* dose and the dose used in humans.
5) Must exhibit the same developmental events as the human embryo.
6) Must be able to analyze all types of compounds without a change in protocol.
7) Must have no false negatives or false positives.
8) Must be rapid, easy to perform, and inexpensive.

Why all the current hoopla over the *in vitro* culture of mammalian cells, organs, and whole embryos? What advantages do *in vitro* systems have over *in vivo* systems for teratologic research and testing? Can *in vitro* systems be used to reliably predict teratogenic risk in humans? These are a few of the questions I hope to address in my talk today. First, what are the advantages and disadvantages of *in vitro* culture systems? Table 2 lists some of the perceived advantages of an *in vitro* system over an *in vivo* system. Not listed, but of current public interest, is the use of *in vitro* tests as alternatives to whole animal testing. Table 3 lists some of the perceived disadvantages of the *in vitro* culture system. A comparison of the two tables reveals a "catch-22" situation in which the major advantages are also the major disadvantages. Although it is advantageous to have the embryo and/or its parts to study in isolation for more precise experiments, the real world of embryo growth is *in utero* subjected to all the vagaries of the maternal-placental unit.

TABLE 2
PERCEIVED ADVANTAGES OF MAMMALIAN *IN VITRO* CULTURE SYSTEM

1) Cell, tissue, organ, whole embryo receives direct exposure to compound being tested.
2) Effects can be observed directly.
3) Conditions of exposure can be controlled precisely.
4) Under defined culture conditions, differentiation is consistent and reproducible.
5) Ultimate teratogen can be identified.
6) Confounding influence of the maternal-placental unit is eliminated.
7) Less expense
8) Less time

TABLE 3

PERCEIVED DISADVANTAGES OF MAMMALIAN IN VITRO TEST CULTURE SYSTEM

1) The contribution of the maternal-placental unit is absent
2) Only a limited period of embryogenesis can be studied
3) Drug metabolizing enzymes are usually absent
4) Development is not normal
5) Unknown compounds may be difficult to test
6) Extrapolation of results difficult
7) Chronic exposure is not possible
8) Cannot predict additive or synergistic effects
9) Limited route of administration

Cell Culture

Because the ultimate action of a teratogen is thought to be at the cell level, and because cells play a critical role in embryonic development, the use of *in vitro* cell culture methods has been proposed as a means to predict teratogenic risk in humans (review by Clayton and Zehir, 1982). In general, cells in culture grow as a monolayer of homogenous cells and as such they are far removed from the realities of *in vivo* development where they may have complex interrelationships with several types of cells. At best, cell culture can mimic only a limited number of developmental events, e.g., cell-cell recognition, cell replication, cell movement, cell differentiation. The *in vitro* cell culture system satisfies very few of the criteria of the ideal *in vitro* test system (table 1).

A variety of cells can be cultured, including human cells. I have selected two examples of cell cultures that have been proposed for use in the identification of teratogenic compounds. The first is the culture of neural crest cells (Wilk et al., 1980). In culture, cranial neural crest cells from early chick embryos can be induced to differentiate into pigment cells or neuron-like cells. For assay, the endpoints used were detachment of cells from the substrate, changes in cell morphology, and failure of cells to differentiate. Of nine teratogens tested (including two human teratogens) seven interfered with at least one developmental process and two (including thalidomide) had no effect. Three nonteratogens were tested without effect. The second proposed cell culture assay is reported to identify teratogens by their ability to inhibit attachment of ascitic mouse ovarian tumor cells to plastic surfaces coated with concanavalin A (Braun et al., 1982). Seventy-four teratogenic compounds were tested (including 4 human teratogens), 81% were inhibiting and 19%, including one human teratogen, were not (false negatives). Thalidomide was not active unless the standard protocol was altered. Twenty-eight nonteratogenic compounds were tested, 75% were noninhibitory, 25% were inhibitory (false positives). Overall the tumor cell attachment assay correctly assigned compounds 79% of the time.

When compared with the ideal test system (Table 1), I think it is obvious that cell culture assays cannot stand alone as teratogen predictors. To date there is an insufficient data base and validation is lacking. Even the proponents of cell culture assays suggest that cell culture can only be one component in the armamentarium for teratogen risk assessment. Cell culture, however, can provide valuable information about certain basic morphogenetic phenomena and teratogenic mechanisms, e.g., behavior of the test compound with respect to cell surface binding, cell penetration, and intracellular location.

Organ Culture

Organ culture possesses two major advantages over cell culture, (1) more than one cell type is involved, and (2) development is three dimensional. It is possible, therefore, to study basic biologic phenomena important in prenatal mammalian development, e.g., cell proliferation, cell differentiation, interaction between cells of the same and different types (inductions), cell movements, cell recognition, cell shape changes, natural (programmed) cell death, biosynthesis, and energy production. Very often an explanted organ primordium will exhibit progressive development in culture that closely resembles development of that organ in the intact organism.

Of the many different organs capable of successful culture (e.g., limb bud, palatal shelves, kidney, lung, liver, lens, teeth), the most thoroughly investigated is the mouse limb bud using the method pioneered in Kochhar's laboratory (Adelotte and Kochhar, 1972, Lessmollman et al., 1975; Kochhar, 1982). The method involves removal of limb buds from mouse embryos, usually at day 12 of gestation. The limb buds are placed on top of ultra thin Millipore filter and incubated in a nutrient medium to which test substances can be added. Culture usually lasts 6 days. The cultured limbs can be analysed morphologically and biochemically. Of 9 teratogens tested by Kochhar (1975), all induced malformations *in vitro*. Three agents which did not produce limb defects *in vivo* in the mouse did produce limb defects *in vitro* (including thalidominde). There have since been several reports of other teratogens inducing limb defects in culture, but no systematic study of teratogens and nonteratogens has been reported.

(Neubert, et al., 1974) pointed out several specific deficiencies in the *in vitro* culture of limb buds that limit its usefulness in teratogen prediction, e.g., unscheduled necrosis, changes in contact behavior, retarded development (6 days *in vitro* equivalent to 3 days *in vivo*), abnormal morphology because the limb bud is attached to the filter paper and cannot grow in three dimensions, lack of nerve and blood supply, incomplete differentation of muscle, lack of joint development, and an altered schedule of biochemical differentiation.

In spite of the considerable number of investigations performed with limb bud culture, it still lacks validation as a test system and has not been systematically studied as a test for risk assessment. As with cell culture, organ culture could perhaps be one component in a battery of tests for teratogenicity prediction. Certainly the technique is useful of obtaining valuable information about teratogenic mechanisms and basic morphogenetic phenomena.

Whole Embryo Culture

Perhaps the most attractive *in vitro* culture system, at least with respect to our ability to relate it to the *in vivo* condition, is whole embryo culture. Either the preimplantation embryo or the post-implantation embryo can be cultured.

The preimplantation embryo has been used extensively for biochemical characterization of early development (Biggers and Stern, 1973) and for the analysis of the nutritional requirements for growth during the preimplantation period (Brinster, 1974). *In vitro* culture of the preimplantation embryo has not been used extensively in teratological investigations, in large part because of the commonly held belief that the preimplantation embryo is not sensitive to the induction of malformations. However, Brinster (1975) has proposed that preimplantation embryos might be useful in teratogen screening because there is more similarity between preimplantation stages of mammalian embryos than postimplantation stages of mammalian embryos with respect to time spent in the preimplantation stages and in metabolic parameters (e.g., pyruvate as a central energy source, RNA and DNA metabolism). Therefore, difficulties with extrapolation from one species to another might be less. This method remains untested as a means to identify teratogens.

The modern use of the *in vitro* culture of postimplantation embryos began with New and Stein in 1964. Significant advances in technique have been made since then (New, 1978). Whole rodent embryos can be cultured successfully for 1 to 4 days at any stage during the period of organogenesis. At each stage the embryo has its own limitations and special requirements for growth. The younger the embryo at explant, the longer it will survive in culture. During *in vitro* culture, the rodent embryo undergoes considerable growth and development, comparable in many respects to that which occurs *in vivo* (Cockroft, 1976). Much hope has been placed on this
system. It has all the advantages of other *in vitro* systems and more. The embryo is complete when placed in culture, its development mimics development *in utero* during the same time span, the test substance has direct access to the embryo, the culture conditions can be controlled and monitored, and the effects are observable directly. The system also has the disadvantages of *in vitro* culture systems (Table 2) and it cannot satisfy the criteria for the ideal *in vitro* test system (Table 1). A disadvantage of unknown significance is that the embryo is hypoxic as soon as it is removed from the uterus. Hypoxia alone is teratogenic (Grabowski, 1977), and the hypoxic state may be able to potentiate the teratogenic action of other agents (Ugen and Scott, 1983). This might result in a proportionally lower effective dose *in vitro* compared with *in vivo*, or in an interaction between a nonteratogenic agent and the hypoxic state to produce a teratogenic effect *in vitro* when one is lacking *in vivo*. The effect of excess oxygen at normal pressures apparently has not been studied in the pregnant mammal (Grabowski, 1977), although, in culture excess oxygen resulted in abnormal morphogenesis of the neural folds (Morriss and New, 1979). The embryo in culture is known to have continually changing oxygen requirements and an imbalance could be suspected to lead to an abnormal outcome in culture.

There are other problems associated with whole embryo culture. It is not clear how much trauma the embryo suffers during its removal from the uterus, or what if any role this might play in subsequent development. There may be deleterious changes in osmolarity during culture. Strain differences may hold true in culture as they do in the intact animal. The duration of exposure in culture is relatively short whereas in the intact animal an effect may require several days of exposure. The culture system is in a delicate balance and a change in any one of a number of conditions could result in abnormal development, or influence the response to the added agent. Two methods have been used to try to circumvent problems associated with whole embryo culture. One method, to obviate the criticism of the lack of the dynamic relationship between the mother and embryo in culture, is to administer the agent to the mother at some time prior to removal of the embryo for culture (Beaudoin and Fisher, 1981). The major advantage with this procedure is that the maternal-placental-embryo unit is intact during exposure and during the time the agent is presumed to act. The agent, therefore, is processed by the maternal-placental-embryo unit, which is not possible when the agent is added to the culture medium. Another advantage is that the exposure of the pregnant animal to the test substance can be via the same route as human exposure (aerosol, diet, injection). It is not necessary that the agent be miscible with the culture media. Disadvantages with this procedure include a restricted exposure period and difficulty identifying the ultimate teratogen.

A second method receiving a great deal of attention and interest during the past three years is the system refined by Klein in which the whole rat embryo is cultured in human serum (Chatot, et al., 1980). The system is an attempt to combine *in vitro* procedures using the whole embryo with the metabolic capabilities and complexities of the human adult. The value of this system depends upon the ability of the human serum to accurately reflect the potential teratogenic state of the adult organism. This cannot be measured at present. A major disadvantage of this system is that serum from 10-20% of normal adults, not on drug therapy, is unable to support embryo growth. This observation may reflect a larger problem, because the full effect of the use of heterologous sera in culture is not known. The potential this system has to predict human teratogenesis is questionable. Its principle value may lie in its ability to monitor the condition of sera before and during pregnancy, and it may be able to contribute to our knowledge about habitual abortion among women. This technique is relatively new, lacks validation, and not all investigators have been able to successfully culture rat embryos in human serum (Reti, et al., 1982).

Metabolizing Enzymes

A major deficiency with all *in vitro* procedures is the lack of metabolizing enzymes. The metabolism of a chemical compound can be a prime factor in teratogenesis. Metabolism can influence a chemical's action either by inactivation or activation. Biotransformation usually results in the production of less active or inactive compounds. In some instances, however, the metabolite may be teratogenically more active than the parent compound, e.g., norchlorcylizine is the teratogenic metabolite of chlorcylizine (King et al., 1972). A related problem is that most *in vivo* testing for teratogenicity is chronic (i.e., day 6-15 in the rat) during the period of organogensis rather than acute (i.e. single treatment). In general, acute treatments have greater teratogenic effect than chronic treatments. The chronic administration of some compounds stimulate microsomal enzymes that enhance their own metabolism and sometimes the metabolism of the other compounds as well (Conney and Burns, 1972). The principal metablizing enzymes of exogenous chemicals are cytochrome P-450-linked monooxygenases in the endoplasmic reticulum of cells in the liver (Pelkonen, 1980). In the human conceptus, drug metabolism has been reported in the liver as early as week 8 of gestation (Pelkonen, 1973). In rats and rabbits, however, these enzymes are not reported active until the late prenatal or the neonatal period (Klinger, et al., 1981). Therefore, activation or detoxification of compounds may occur in the human conceptus late in the period of organogenesis whereas it presumably does not occur until after organogenesis in the common laboratory animals. Consequently maternal metabolism, not embryonic metabolism, may play the principal role in the teratogenic outcome in the laboratory.

Attempts have been made to circumvent the problem of the *in vivo* metabolism of compounds. Fantel *et al., 1979) were the first to demonstrate that the addition of an hepatic microsomal fraction together with cofactors for a monoxygenase system enabled cyclophosphamide to induce a teratogenic response in whole embryo culture. Without the added material, cyclophosphamide was innocuous. A similar technique utilizing mouse limb buds in culture with liver S9 or purified microsomal activating system failed to support the normal in vitro development of the limb buds* presumably because of diffusible noxious factors from the liver fractions (Manson and Simons, 1979). The system was capable of metabolizing cyclophosphamide, but the inherent cytotoxicity limited its use in limb bud culture. In the presence of hamster embryo cells, however, there was no abnormal development unless cyclophosphamide was added. Thus the hamster embryo cells contain a system capable of converting the drug to its active metabolite. This supports the observation that metabolic pathways exist other than in the liver which are used for the metabolism of naturally occurring metabolites, and which can be used to convert an inactive compound into an active compound (Krowke and Neubert, 1977).

The addition of liver-derived activating systems, therefore, may not be useful in all *in vitro* culture systems. If it becomes necessary to add a bioactivating system to each *in vitro* culture, the technique is no longer simple and may become too complex for routine testing. This will be especially true if several different bioactivating systems are required. Additional problems remain to be solved, e.g., are metabolic profiles the same *in vitro* and *in vivo*, will enzyme preparations from different species react the same, and how can one identify unknown compounds which require bioactivation?

Summary and Conclusions

The effect of an agent on the human conceptus depends, among other things, on its metabolic fate in the maternal organism, the permeability characteristics of the placenta, and the sensitivity of the conceptus itself, and each of these characters may vary from one species to another. In other words, the response of the conceptus is the result of complex maternal-placental-embryo interaction. This interaction cannot be duplicated in culture. It may be that agents which act through alterations in maternal or placental metabolism will not be testable by *in vitro* methods.

The focus of *in vitro* testing has been on the observation of induced malformations. There are, however, other aspects of the teratogenic reponse, e.g., death of the conceptus, growth retardation, and postnatal behavioral effects. These responses may be difficult to predict with *in vitro* tests. It is not clear, furthermore, that *in vitro* systems are able to detect agents that cause single, discreet, and isolated interference with differentiation rather than interference with developmental processes in general. There are conflicting reports about the similarites of malformations induced *in vitro* and *in vivo*. In a recent study (Beaudoin and Fisher, 1981) there was little or no correlation between the types of malformations induced in the rat *in vivo* with those induced by the same agents in whole embryo culture. The malformations seen *in vitro* were not predictive of the malformations seen *in vivo*. Other investigators using the mouse embryo report similarities in the patterns of malformations in embryos exposed to chemicals *in utero* and in embryos exposed to the same chemicals in culture (Warner et al., 1983).

Everyone in this audience is familiar with the admonitions accompanying the extrapolation of data from animal studies to the human. A species identical to the human in all relevent characteristics does not exist with respect to absorption, metabolism, elimination, and placental transmission of a compound nor does a conceptus exist with the same developmental schedule and metabolic pathways. Even among laboratory animals there are species differences. The extent and nature of the interaction of these many factors in teratogenesis is not understood. It appears to be a truism that animal studies cannot predict effects in human beings. With respect to teratogenicity the final test is still the pregnant woman.

What then is the value of *in vitro* testing and can it be used to predict human teratogenic response? Clearly, *in vitro* studies have great usefulness in the study of morphogenetic phenomena at the structural and biochemical level, and in the study of mechanisms of teratogenic action. The predictive value of *in vitro* tests is less clear. Almost every paper presenting an *in vitro* system for risk assessment contains the disclaimer that the test cannot stand alone. It appears that to be able to predict human risk with the greatest margin for safety a multiple overlapping system will be needed. Such a battery of tests may not be less expensive or less time consuming than current procedures. In the long run, it may not be possible to use an *in vitro* system to replace *in vivo* tests in routine testing of agents for teratogenic risk. The greatest value for *in vitro* testing may be its potential to establish a priority list of compounds for later testing by conventional means.

"This presentation today was not meant to be overly negative about the value of *in vitro* culture methods, however, problems exist with respect to the prediction of teratogenicity. In my mind, the problems are not receiving proper attention. The major problem is simply lack of information. We lack knowledge about the mechanisms of teratogenic action in the human conceptus, which makes the interpretation of *in vitro* studies more difficult. We lack a sufficient amount of data to have a base from which to interpret *in vitro* findings with new agents and from which to make predictions. We lack uniformity in the performance of *in vitro* tests, in the reporting of results, and in the interpretation of results. We lack the knowledge to select a group of *in vitro* tests to serve together in a complementary fashion to enhance our ability to predict risk. We lack sufficient information about many agents to know when bioactivating systems must be added to the culture. We lack the knowledge to determine if end points other than those seen in the human conceptus are relevant for risk assessment.

It seems to me that what we need now to overcome these deficiencies is a concerted effort toward validation of *in vitro* systems. Perhaps a well orchestrated attack with several laboratories committed to the use of identical methods to be used to test the same teratogens and nonteratogens might be a proper approach. Only after we obtain sufficient repoducible data from several sources will we have the confidence to decide if *in vitro* systems are reliable and to decide what role they may play in the prediction of teratogenic risk to the human conceptus".

REFERENCES

Aydelotte, M. D.; and Kochhar, D. M.: Development of mouse limb buds in organ culture: Chondrogenesis in the presence of proline analog, L-azetidine-2-carboxylic acid. *Develop. Biol.*, 28:191-201, 1972.

Beaudoin, A. R.; and Fisher, D. L.: An *in vivo/in vitro* evaluation of teratogenic action. *Teratology*, 23:57-61, 1981.

Best, J. B.; and Morita, M.: Planarians as a model system for in vitro teratogenesis studies. *Teratogen. Carcinogen. Mutagen.*, 2:277-291, 1982.

Biggers, J. D.; and Stern, S.: Metabolism of the preimplantation mammalian and embryo. *Adv. Reprod. Physiol.*, 6:1-59, 1973.

Braun, A. G.; Buckner, C. A., Emerson, D. J., and Nichinson, B. B.: Quantitative correspondence between the in vivo and in vitro activity of teratogenic agents. *Proc. Natl. Acad. Sci.*, 79:2056-2060, 1982.

Brinster, R. L.: Embryo development. *J. Anim. Sci.*, 38:1003-1012, 1974.

Brinster, R. L.: Teratogen testing using preimplantation mammalian embryos. In *"Methods for Detection of Environmental Agents that Produce Congenital Defects"* T. H. Shepard, J. R. Miller, M. Marois (eds.) pp. 113-124. Amsterdam, North Holland, 1975.

Brown, N. A.; and Fabro, S.: The *in vitro* approach to teratogenicity testing. In *"Developmental Toxicology"*, K. Snell (ed.), pp. 33-57, New York, Praeger, 1982.

Chatot, C. L.; Klein, N. W., Piatek, J., and Pierro, L. J.: Successful culture of rat embryos on human serum. Use in the detection of teratogens. *Science*, 207:1471-1473, 1980.

Clayton, R. M.; and Zehir, A.: The use of cell culture methods for exploring teratogenic susceptibility. In *"Developmental Toxicology"* K. Snell (ed), pp. 61-92. New York, Praeger, 1982.

Conney, A. H.; and Burns, J. J.: Metabolic interactions among environmental chemicals and drugs. *Science*, *178*:576-587, 1972.

Cockroft, D. L.: Comparison of *in vitro* and *in vivo* development of rat fetuses. *Dev. Biol.*, *48*:163-172, 1976.

Dumont, J. W.; Schultz, T. W., Buchanan, M. V., and Kao, G. L.: Frog embryo teratogenesis assay: Xenopus (fetax). A short term assay applicable to complex environemtal mixtures. In *"Short Term Bioassay in the Analysis of Complex Environmental Mixtures, III"*, Waters, Sandlu, Lewtas, Claxton, Chernoff, and Nesnow (eds) pp 393-405, Plenum, N.Y., 1983.

Fantel, A. G.; Greenway, J. C., Juchau, M. R., and Shepard, T. H.: Teratogenic bioactivation of cyclophosphamide *in vitro*. *Life Sci.*, *25*:67-72, 1979.

Fisher, M.; and Schoenwolf, G.: The use of early chick embryos in experimental embryology and teratology: Improvements in standard procedures. *Teratology*, *27*:65-72, 1983.

Grabowski, C. T.: Atmosphere Gases. In *"Handbook of Teratology"* J. G. Wilson and F. C. Fraser (eds.), pp. 405-420, New York, Plenum Press, 1977.

Johnson, E. M., Forman, R. M., Gabel, B. E. G., and George, M. E.: the hydra attenuata system for detection of teratogenic hazards. *Teratogen. Carcinogen. Mutagen.*, *2*:263-276, 1982.

Kerster, H. W.; and Schaeffer, D. J.: Brine shrimp (Artemia salina) Nauplii as a teratogen test system. *Toxicol. Environ. Safety*, *7*:342-349, 1983.

King, C. T. G.; Weaver, S. A., and Narrod, S. A.: Antihistamines and teratogenicity in the rat. *J. Pharmacol. Exp. Ther.*, *147*:391-398, 1965.

King, C. T. G.; Horigan, E., and Wilk, A. L.: Fetal outcome from prolonged versus acute drug administration in the pregnant rat. In *"Drugs and Fetal Development"* M. A. Klingbert, A. A. Abramovici, and J. Chemke (eds.), pp. 61-75, New York, Plenum Press, 1972.

Klein, N. W.; Vogler, M. A., Chatot, C. L., and Pierro, L.: The use of cultured rat embryos to evaluate the teratogenic activity of serum: Cadmium and cyclophosphamide. *Teratology*, *21*:199-208, 1980.

Klinger, W.; Muller, D., Kleeberg, U., and Barth, A.: Peri- and postnatal development of phase I reactions. In *"Developmental Toxicology"*, C. A. Kimmel and J. Buelke-Sam (eds.), pp. 83-100. New York, Raven Press, 1981.

Kochhar, D. M.: The use of *in vitro* procedures in teratology. *Teratology*, *11*:273-288, 1975.

Kochhar, D. M.: Embryonic limb bud organ culture in assessment of teratogenicity of environemtal agents. *Teratogen. Carcinogen. Mutagen.*, *2*:303-312, 1982.

Krowke, R.; and Neubert, D.: Embryonic intermediary metabolism under normal and pathological conditions. In *"Handbook of Teratology"*, J. G. Wilson and F. C. Fraser (eds.), pp. 117-151. New York, Plenum Press, 1977.

Lessmollman, U.; Neubert, D., and Merker, H. J.: Mammalian limb bud differentiating *in vitro* as a test system for the evaluation of embryotoxic effects. In *"New Approaches to the Evaluation of Abnormal Embryonic Development"*. D. Neubert and H. J. Merker (eds.), pp. 99-112. Stuttgart, Thieme, 1975.

Manson, J. M.; and Simons, R.: In vitro metabolism of cyclophosphamide in limb bud culture. *Teratology, 19*:149-158, 1979.

Maugh, T. H.: Chemicals. How many are there. *Science, 199*:162, 1978.

Morriss, G. M.; and New, D. A. T.: Effect of oxygen concentration on morphogenesis of cranial neural folds and neural crest in cultured rat embryos. *J. Embryol. Exp. Morphol., 54*:17-35, 1979.

Moscona, A. A.: Embryonic cells and tissue cultures as test systems for teratogenic agents. In *"Methods for Detection of Environmental Agents that Produce Congenital Defects"*. T. H. Shepard, J. R. Miller, and M. Marois (eds.), pp. 103-111. Amsterdam, North Holland, 1975.

Neubert, D.; Merker, H. J., and Tapken, S.: Comparactive studies on the prenatal development of mouse extremities *in vivo* and in organ culture. *Naunyn-Schmeideberg's Arch. Pharmacol., 286*:251-270, 1974.

New, D. A. T.; and Stein, K. F.: Cultivation of post implantation mouse and rat embryos and rat embryos on plasma clots. *J. Embryol. Exp. Morphol., 12*:101-111, 1964.

New, D. A. T.: Whole embryo culture and the study of mammalian embryos during oganogenesis. *Biol. Rev., 53*:81-122, 1978.

Pelkonen, O.: Drug metabolism in the human fetal liver relationship to fetal age. *Arch Int. Pharmacodyn. Ther., 202*:281-287, 1973.

Pelkonen, O.: Environmental influence on human foetal and placental xenobiotic metabolism. *Eur. J. Clin. Pharmacol., 18*:17-24, 1980.

Reti, L. L.; Beck, F., Bulman, S.: Culture of 9 1/2 day rat embryo in human serum supplemented and unsupplemented with rat serum. *J. Exp. Zool., 223*:197-199, 1982.

Schardein, J. L.: *Drugs as Teratogens*. Cleveland, CRC Press, 1976.

Ugen, K. E.; and and Scott, W. J.: Acetazolamide teratology: Enhancement by administration of uterine vasoconstrictive agents. *Teratology, 27*:81A, 1983.

Warner, C. W.; Sadler, T. W., Tulis, S. A., and Smith, M. K.: In vivo cadmium teratogenicity reproduced in whole embryo culture. *Teratology, 27*:82A, 1983.

Wilk, A. L.; Greenberg, J. H., Horigan, E. A., Pratt, R. M., and Martin, G. R.: Detection of teratogenic compounds using differentiating embryonic cells in culture. *In Vitro, 16*:269-276, 1980.

Wilson, J. G.: *Environment and Birth Defects*, New York, Academic Press, 1973.

New Approaches in Toxicity Testing and Their Application in Human Risk Assessment, edited by A. P. Li. Raven Press, New York © 1985.

Development and Validation of a Panel of Host Resistance and Immune Function Assays Designed to Detect Chemical-Induced Immunomodulation

Peter T. Thomas, Ruth A. Fugmann, Catherine Aranyi, and James D. Fenters

IIT Research Institute, Life Sciences Research, Chicago, Illinois 60616

Modulation of the immune response by drugs, chemicals or environmental toxicants recently has received considerable attention. This interest is due, in part, to both increased concern about the effects that environmental exposure to chemical contaminants have on the immune system and the increasing interest in drug-induced modulation of immunity as a novel treatment for certain diseases. Many studies have been performed evaluating the effects of chemical agents on host defenses and immunity (13, 16, 24). However, the results following exposure to a given compound may vary because of differences in dose and route of chemical exposure, methodologies used, analysis of the data, etc. In an attempt to standardize some of these variables, a series of studies designed to assess host resistance and immune function in mice exposed to known immunomodulating agents was initiated utilizing a variety of *in vivo* and *in vitro* models of infectious disease and immune function. The results presented here summarize studies performed using the known immunomodulating agents diethylstilbestrol (DES) and dimethylnitrosamine (DMN). The findings indicate the DES and DMN modulate the immune system in different ways and suggest that best detection and dissection of agent-induced immunomodulation should include a battery of both *in vivo* and *in vitro* assays of the type described.

MATERIALS AND METHODS

Experimental Animals

Six to eight week old female B6C3F1 (C3H male x C57B1/6 female) mice were used in all studies. Animals were obtained from the Frederick Cancer Research Center and quarantined for 1 to 2 weeks prior to treatment. Mice were housed five per cage in animal rooms having ambient temperatures of 23°C and 12 hr light/dark cycles.

Chemical Treatment

DES: Diethylstilbestrol, lot 29-C-0318 was obtained from Sigma Chemical Company (St. Louis, MO). Mice were injected subcutaneously (sc) daily for 14 days with 0.2 ml of corn oil (Mazola, C.P.E. International) or oil containing the equivalent of 4 mg;kg of DES. Two days following the last sc injection the mice were challenged with infectious agent or with tumor cells or sacrificed for evaluation of immune function.

DMN: N-nitrosodimethylamine, lot no. 22F-0127 was obtained from Sigma. Mice were injected intraperitoneally (ip) daily for 14 days with 0.2 ml of phosphate buffered saline (PBS) alone or PBS containing the equivalent of 5 mg/kg of DMN. Two days following the last ip injection the mice were challenged with infectious agent or with tumor cells or sacrificed for evaluation of immune function.

Assay Systems

Tables 1 and 2 summarize the assays used to measure host resistance and immunity, the endpoints measured, and specific references for the methodology.

TABLE 1
HOST RESISTANCE ASSAYS

Host Resistance Model	Endpoint Measured	Protective Mechanism	Methodology Reference
B16-F10 Melanoma	Measurement of lung tumor burden 21 days post-challenge	CMI[a], macrophage NK[b]	8, 14
Listeria monocytogenes	Cumulative percent mortality 14 days post-challenge, mean survival time	CMI, macrophage	8, 14
Streptococcus zooepidemicus	"	AMI[c], polymorphonuclear leukocytes, nonspecific immunity	14
Influenza A2; Taiwan virus	"	AMI, interferon	14
Herpes simplex types 1 and 2 viruses	Cumulative percent mortality 21 days post-challenge, mean survival time	CMI	14

TABLE 1 (continued)

Host Resistance Model	Endpoint Measured	Protective Mechanism	Methodology Reference
Trichinella spiralis	Worm explusion rates measured 14 days post-infection	CMI, AMI?	8, 14

[a]Cell-mediated immunity
[b]Natural killer cell function
[c]Antibody-mediated immunity

TABLE 2

IMMUNE FUNCTION ASSAYS

Assay System	Endpoint Measured	*In Vivo* Immune Correlate	Methodology Reference
Lymphocyte mitogenesis to PHA		CMI (mature T-cells)	6, 9, 17, 25
Lymphocyte mitogenesis to Con A	Incorporation of radiolabeled nucleic acid precursors into DNA of dividing cells	CMI (immature T-cells)	
Lymphocyte mitogenesis to LPS		AMI	
Mixed lymphocyte culture		CMI	
NK cell function	Percent cytotoxicity of spleen cells vs ^{51}Cr-labeled YAC-1 lymphoma target cells	Natural or innate immunity	21
Plaque forming cell (PFC) response to sheep red blood cells (SRBCs)	Quantitation of IgM antibody producing PCFs/ 10^6 spleen cells 4 days after immunization	AMI, macrophage	7, 9, 11, 23
Delayed hypersensitivity response to keyhold limpet hemocyanin (KLH)	Measurement of influx of ^{125}IUdR labeled, monocyte precursors into the site of elicitation of response to KLH antigen	CMI	12, 17
Macrophage cytostasis	Inhibition of growth of MBL-2 leukemia cells	—	10
Macrophage phagocytosis	Phagocytosis of ^{51}Cr-labeled SRBCs	—	18
ATP/unit protein	Macrophage ATP levels	—	2
Alveolar Macrophage bactericidal activity	Pulmonary Clearance of inhaled ^{35}S-labeled *Klebsiella pneumoniae*	Respiratory defense	3

Statistical Analyses

The mixed model analysis of variance (27) followed by individual post-hoc comparisons using Student's and Dunnett's T-tests were chosen for continuous response data. In addition to the univariate analyses, multivariate test statistics (1,5) also were included. A log linear model was used to evaluate mortality data (4, 15,).

RESULTS

The results for each assay system shown in Figures 1 to 5 represent combined data from two to four replicate experiments. These data were analyzed statistically and are presented in summary form as percent change relative to corresponding vehicle controls. The host resistance data are interpreted as increased resistance or increased susceptibility to infection or tumor challenge. The data from the immune function assays are interpreted as immunosuppression or immunostimulation relative to controls.

Effect Of DES Exposure

Figure 1 summarizes the effects of exposure to 4 mg/kg DES for 14 days on host resistance to microbial or tumor challenge 2 days later. DES treatment significantly enhanced resistance to B16-F10 melanoma tumor cells, as measured by a 37 percent decrease in pulmonary tumor weights 21 days post-challenge compared to controls. In contrast, mortality following challenge with *Listeria monocytogenes* organisms and with *Herpes simplex* type 1 and 2 viruses (HSV-1, HSV-2) was significantly increased by 55, 26 and 18 percent, respectively. DES-treated animals retained 42 percent more *Trichinella spiralis* worms in the gut than controls, showing that the compounds significantly impaired the host's capacity to resist infestation. DES treatment had no effect on resistance to challenge with either Streptococcus or influenza virus. Animals similarly treated with DES exhibited significantly reduced splenic lymphocyte blastogenic responses to the mitogens phytohemagglutinin (PHA), concanavalin A (Con-A), and lipopolysaccharide (LPS) compared to controls (Fig. 2). A significant, 32 percent decrease in blastogenesis of spleen cells was noted in the mixed lymphocyte culture (MLC) responses in DES-treated mice compared to controls. DES exposure also significantly impaired the natural killer (NK) response, anti-sheep red blood cell (SRBC) plaque-forming-cell (PFC) response and delayed hypersensitivity response (DHR) to keyhold limpet hemocyanin (KLH) antigen by 51, 9, and 63 percent, respectively (Fig. 2).

DES treatment significantly increased peritoneal macrophage cytostasis of MBL-2 leukemia cells and phagocytosis of ^{51}Cr-SRBCs by 46 and 72 percent, respectively compared to controls (Fig. 3). However, DES-treated mice were significantly impared in their ability to clear ^{35}S-labeled *Klebsiella pneumoniae* from the lung compared to controls suggesting some impairment of pulmonary host defenses. DES treatment did not alter macrophage ATP levels when compared with controls.

Effects of DMN Exposure

Figure 4 summaries the effects of exposure to 5 mg/kg of DMN on host resistance. As was seen with the DES-treated animals, DMN also significantly increased host resistance to B16-F10 tumor challenge as shown by a 47 percent decrease in tumor weights 21 days post-challenge. DMN-exposed mice exhibited a significant 50 and 29 percent increase in mortality following challenge with Streptococcus and influenza virus, respectively. In contrast to the effects of DES, compared to controls, DMN exposure did not alter host resistance to Listeria, HSV-1, HSV-2 or Trichinella challenge.

ASSAYS FOR CHEMICAL-INDUCED IMMUNOMODULATION   217

Figure 1   EFFECT OF EXPOSURE TO 4 mg/kg DES FOR 14 DAYS ON HOST RESISTANCE

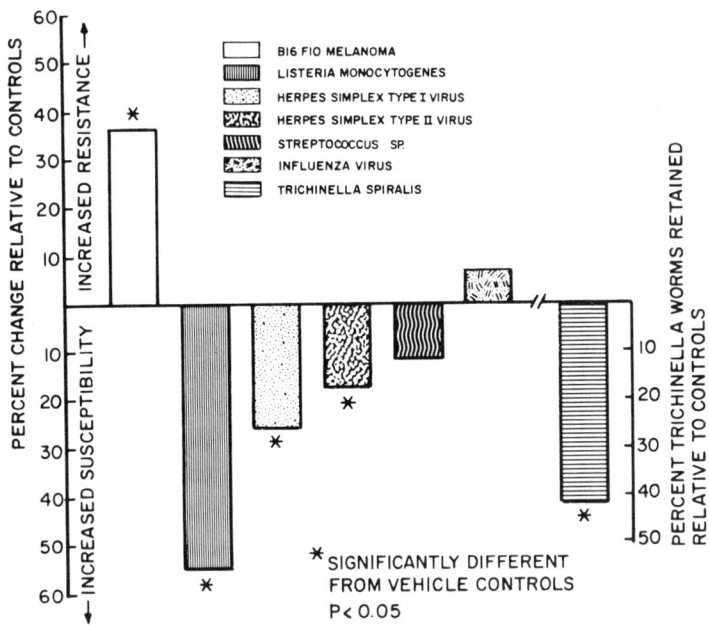

- B16 F10 MELANOMA
- LISTERIA MONOCYTOGENES
- HERPES SIMPLEX TYPE I VIRUS
- HERPES SIMPLEX TYPE II VIRUS
- STREPTOCOCCUS SP.
- INFLUENZA VIRUS
- TRICHINELLA SPIRALIS

* SIGNIFICANTLY DIFFERENT FROM VEHICLE CONTROLS $p < 0.05$

Figure 2   EFFECT OF EXPOSURE TO 4 mg/kg DES FOR 14 DAYS ON IMMUNITY

- BLASTOGENESIS TO PHA
- BLASTOGENESIS TO CON-A
- BLASTOGENESIS TO LPS
- MIXED LYMPHOCYTE CULTURE
- NATURAL KILLER CELL
- α SRBC PFC (DIRECT)
- DELAYED HYPERSENSITIVITY

* SIGNIFICANTLY DIFFERENT FROM VEHICLE CONTROLS $p < 0.05$

Figure 3 EFFECT OF EXPOSURE TO 4mg/kg DES
FOR 14 DAYS ON MACROPHAGE FUNCTION

- CYTOSTASIS
- PHAGOCYTOSIS
- ATP/UNIT PROTEIN
- ALVEOLAR MACROPHAGE BACTERICIDAL ACTIVITY

* SIGNIFICANTLY DIFFERENT FROM VEHICLE CONTROLS $p < 0.05$

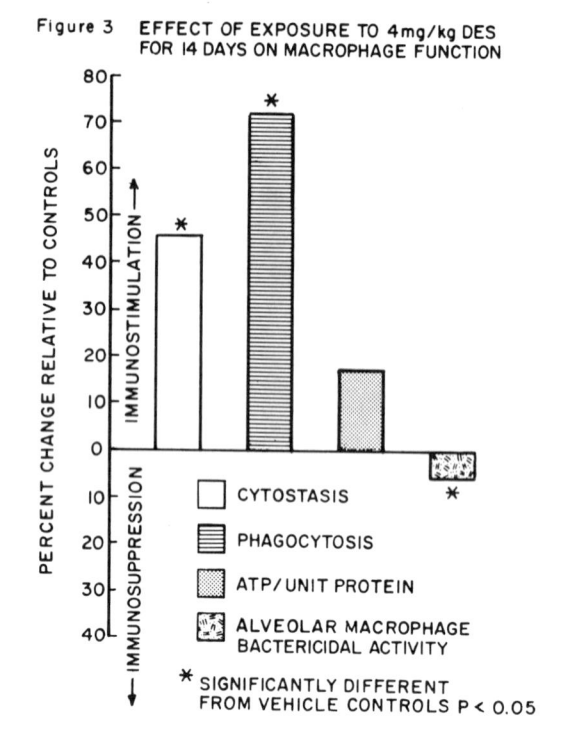

Figure 4 EFFECT OF EXPOSURE TO 5mg/kg DMN FOR
14 DAYS ON HOST RESISTANCE

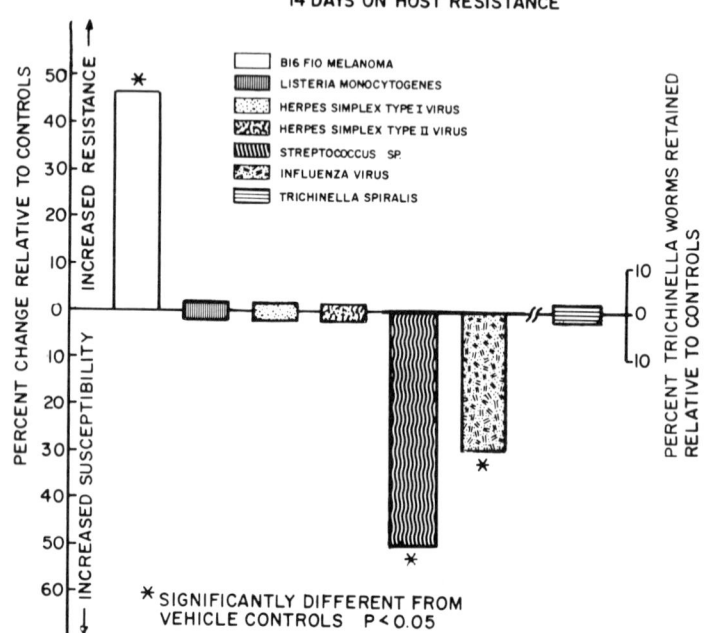

- B16 F10 MELANOMA
- LISTERIA MONOCYTOGENES
- HERPES SIMPLEX TYPE I VIRUS
- HERPES SIMPLEX TYPE II VIRUS
- STREPTOCOCCUS SP.
- INFLUENZA VIRUS
- TRICHINELLA SPIRALIS

* SIGNIFICANTLY DIFFERENT FROM VEHICLE CONTROLS $p < 0.05$

DMN exposure significantly suppressed the blastogenic response to PHA and Con-A by 46 and 19 percent, respectively and reduced the anti-SRBC PFC response by 53 percent compared to controls (Fig. 5). Conversely, lymphocyte blastogenesis to LPS and NK and DHR reactivity of DMN-exposed mice was significantly enhanced. There was no effect of DMN on MLC responses in any experiments performed.

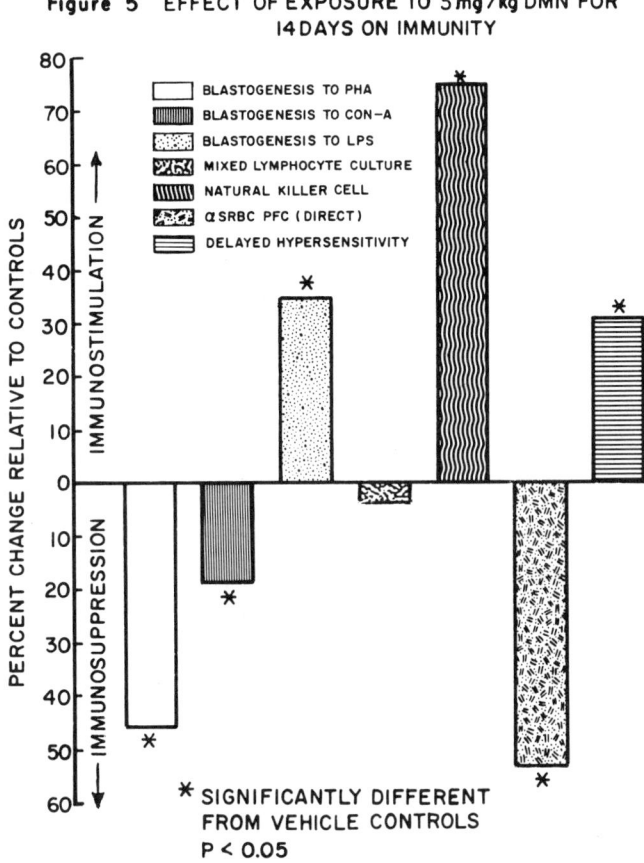

Figure 5 EFFECT OF EXPOSURE TO 5 mg/kg DMN FOR 14 DAYS ON IMMUNITY

* SIGNIFICANTLY DIFFERENT FROM VEHICLE CONTROLS $p < 0.05$

DISCUSSION

The immune system is an extremely complex, highly regulated system where interaction and communication occurs at both the molecular and cellular levels. Manifestations of immunologic disorders range from hypersensitivity and autoimmune disease to alterations in susceptibility to infectious disease and even to the development and course of the malignant process. The complex mechanisms responsible for these variations are only beginning to be understood. Owing to the nature and complexity of the immune system, two levels of investigation are important when assessing immune effects following exposure to a test material.

The first is a holistic assessment of immunologic interactions as measured by host response to challenge with a variety of infectious agents or tumor cells. The second is an investigation of the underlying mechanisms which are responsible for observed alterations in host resistance. As more information is gathered concerning the function of the immune system on a mechanistic level, more sophisticated tests can be devised to dissect the effect of chemicals on the immune response.

The purpose of these studies was to develop and standardize a battery of host resistance and immune function assay capable of detecting both positive and negative alterations in immune function. DES and DMN were selected for these studies because of their known and presumed effects on immunity and the fact that they have different pharmacologic properties.

It is clear from the data that each compound affected the immune system differently. DES is a synthetic estrogenic compound which is thought to exert its immunomodulatory effects in part by altering hormone levels. Its effects on immunity and host resistance are well characterized (8, 14, 17). DMN is a potent hepatic carcinogen and alkylating agent (19). Its effects on immunity are not well understood but available evidence suggests that this compound alters serum antibody and PFC responses (22, 26). To our knowledge, nothing has been reported concerning the effects of DMN on host resistance.

The exposure levels of DES and DMN used in these studies did not produce overt symptoms of toxicity in the B6C3F1 mouse, which is one strain utilized in the National Toxicology Program's bioassay program. The data show that alterations in host resistance following exposure to each of the agents were detected by different assays and by more than one but not all assays. The immunologic mechanisms thought responsible for maintenance of host resistance *in vivo* in general, correlated with those *in vitro* measurements of specific immune responses. For example, DES-induced impairment of cell-mediated immunity was accompanied by increased susceptibility to those host resistance models thought to measure T-cell responses. Resistance to challenge with those infectious models which measure primarily humoral immunity were unaffected.

Chronic, long-term exposure of humans to ambient concentrations of chemicals or environmental toxicants may not result in the extremes of immunologic responsiveness noted here. However, the questions of whether or not these long-term ambient exposures cause immunomodulation, and how much change in either direction is tolerable to maintain homeostasis are fundamental questions which remain unanswered.

The broad spectrum of immunologic responses possible following exposure to an increasingly wide variety of drugs, chemicals and environmental toxicants makes the development of a single, comprehensive test for immunomodulation highly unlikely. Therefore, we believe that the effect of exposure on the overall, holistic host response to bacterial, viral, and tumor challenge followed by selected *in vitro* measurements of immunity designed to dissect the mechanism(s) responsible for any *in vivo* alterations will best serve to detect any immune alteration.

We conclude that the battery of host resistance and immune function assays described here is capable of detecting immunomodulation resulting from exposure to compounds having a variety of pharmacologic properties. We feel that they represent both a comprehensive and cost-effective means of evaluating a wide variety of drugs, chemicals and environmental toxicants for potential modulation of the immune system.

ACKNOWLEDGEMENTS

The authors wish to thank Terri Caprio, Linda Nelson, Jeannie Bradof, and Peter Barbera for expert technical assistance.

These studies were sponsored by the National Institute of Environmental Health Sciences under Contract NO1-ES-1-5000.

REFERENCES

1. *Anderson, T. W.*: An Introduction to Multivariate Statistical Analysis. New York, Wiley, 1958.

2. *Aranyi, C. A.; Gardner, D. E., and Huisingh, J. L.*: Health Effects of Synthetic Silica particulate. In: ASTM STP 732. Dunnom, D., ed., Amer. Soc. for Testing and Materials, 1981.

3. *Aranyi, C. A.; Vana, S. C.; Thomas, P. T.; Bradof, J. N.; Fenters, J. D.; Graham, J. A., and Miller, F. J.*: Effects of subchronic exposure to a mixture of O_3, SO_2, and $(NH_4)_2SO_4$ on host defenses of mice. *J. Toxicol. Env. Health, 12*:55, 1983.

4. *Bishop, T. M. M.; Fienberg, S. E., and Holland, P. W.*: Discrete Multivariate Analysis: Theory and Practice. Cambridge, MIT Press, 1975.

5. *Bock, R. D.*: Multivariate Statistical Methods in Behavoiral Research. New York, McGraw-Hill, 1975.

6. *Bradley, L. M.*: Cell proliferation. In: *Selected Methods in Cellular Immunology,* Chapter 6, Mishell, B., and Shiigi, S., eds., San Francisco, W. H. Freeman and Co., 1980.

7. *Cunningham, A. J., and Szenberg, A.*: Further improvements in the plaque technique for detecting single antibody-forming cells. *Immunol., 14*:599, 1968.

8. *Dean, J. H.; Luster, M. I.; Boorman, G. A.; Leubke, R. W., and Lauer, L. D.*: Effect of adult exposure to diethylstilbestrol in the mouse: Alterations in tumor susceptibility and host resistance parameters. *J. Reticuloendothel. Soc., 28*:571, 1980.

9. *Dean, J. H.; Padarathsingh, M. L., and Jerrells, T. R.*: Application of immunocompetence assays for defining immunosuppression. *Ann. N.Y. Acad. Sci., 320*:579, 1979.

10. *Dean, J. H.; Padarathsingh, M. L., and Keys, L.*: Response of murine leukemia to combined BCNU-maleic anhydride-vinyl ether (MVE) adjuvant therapy and correlation with macrophage activation by MVE in the in vitro growth inhibition assay. *Cancer Treat. Rep., 62*:1807, 1978.

11. *Dresser, D. W.*: Assay for immunoglobulin-screting cells. In: *Handbook of Experimental Immunology,* 3rd Edition, Vol. 2, Chapter 28, Weir, D. M., ed., Oxford, England, 1978.

12. *Eipert, E. F., and Miller, H. C.*: Contact sensitivity in mice measured with thymidine labeled lymphocytes. *Immunol. Commun., 4*:361, 1975.

13. *Faith, R. E.; Luster, M. I., and Vos, J. G.*: Effects of immunocompetence by chemicals of environmental concern. *Rev. Biochem. Toxicol., 2*:173, 1980.

14. *Fugmann, R.; Aranyi, C. A.; Barbera, P. W.; Bradof, J. N.; Gibbons, R. D., and Fenters, J. D.*: The effect of diethylstilbestrol as measured by host resistance and tumor susceptibility assays in mice. *J. Toxicol. Env. Health, 11*:827, 1983.

15. *Haberman, S. J.*: Analysis of Qualitative Data. New York, Academic Press, 1979.

16. *Koller, L. D.*: Effects of environmental contaminants on the immune system. *Adv. Vet. Sci. Comp. Med., 23*:267, 1979.

17. *Luster, M. J.; Boorman, G. A.; Dean, J. H.; Leubke, R. W., and Lawson, L. D.*: The effect of adult exposure to diethylstilbestrol in the mouse: Alteration in immunological function. *J. Reticuloendothel. Soc., 28*:561, 1980.

18. *Meltzer, M. S., and Stevenson, M. M.*: Macrophage function in tumor-bearing mice: Dissociation of phagocytic and chemotactic responsiveness. *Cell. Immunol., 35*:99, 1978.

19. N-nitrosodimethylamine. In: *IARC Monographs on the Evaluation of the Carcinogenic Risk of Chemical to Humans, 17*:125, WHO, Lyon, 1978.

20. *Oppenheim, J. J., and Schecter, B.*: Lymphocyte transformation. In: *Manual of Clincal Immunology.* Rose, N. R., and Friedman, H., eds., Am. Soc. Microbiol., Washington, 1976.

21. *Reynolds, C. W.; Timonen, T., and Herberman, R. B.*: Natural killer cell activity in the rat I. Isolation and characterization of the effector cells. *J. Immunol., 127*:282, 1981.

22. *Scherf, H. R.*: Untersuchungen an Männlichen Sprague-Dawley-Ratteniiber Zusammenhänge Zwischen der Immun-depressiven und der carcinogen Wirkung bei vier N-Nitrosoverbindugen. *Z. Krebsforsch, 77*:189, 1972.

23. *Thomas, P. T., and Hinsdill, R. D.*: The effect of perinatal exposure to tetrachlorodibenzo-p-dioxin on the immune response of young mice. *Drug Chem. Toxicol., 2*:77, 1979.

24. *Vos, J. G.*: Immune suppression as related to toxicology. *CRC Crit. Rev. Toxicol., 5*:67, 1977.

25. *Waithe, W. I., and Hirschhorn, K.*: The lymphocyte response to activation. In: *Handbook of Experimental Immunology,* 3rd Edition, Vol. 2, Chapter 26, Weir, D. M., ed., Oxford, England, 1978.

26. *Waynforth, H. B., and Magee, P. N.*: The effect of N-Nitroso-N-Methylurea and N-dimethylnitrosamine on cell mediated and humoral immune responses in rats and mice. *Brit. J. Cancer, 30*:512, 1974.

27. *Winer, B. J.*: *Statistical Principles in Experimental Design.* New York, McGraw-Hill, 1975.

New Approaches in Toxicity Testing and Their Application in Human Risk Assessment, edited by A. P. Li. Raven Press, New York © 1985.

Discussion

Dennis Flaherty: Dr. Bick you have worked toward developing a battery of assays which can be used to assess immunotoxic potential. Peter Thomas at IIT and Jack Dean at CIIT are working in the same area. How soon can we expect a battery of validated tests that we can use in the laboratory. Peter, you might want to comment on that if you are still here.

Peter Bick: I think as a result of the two contracts that NIEHS has let along with the National Toxicology Program and the success we have had in validating between laboratories that we should have a panel of useable tests, at least some basic guidelines within certainly the next two years. I think we are making rapid progress in that area. There are a few areas we really haven't delved into yet. Of course, any panel can be added to later, but a basic panel will be useable fairly shortly. Many of the assays I had in the tier system here plus the infectious models may be in a panel. I didn't want to deal with those today, but I think many of those will be available as well. Some of them are shown in Peter's poster as well.

Peter Thomas: Listening to Dr. Beaudoin's talk on the *in vitro* immunoassay for immunoteratogenesis, I think immunotoxicology and methodologies used are probably a couple years, maybe three or four years, ahead of Dr. Beaudoin's comment on the need for intervalidation studies. Within, as Peter mentioned, the next couple of years we should have a pretty good idea which tests are most sensitive, which ones are validated between laboratories, and ones which are cost effective to do and which are predictive of what goes on in the whole animal system.

Dennis Flaherty: Let me just throw open a theoretical question. If, one were asked to develop assays to measure transplacental carcinogenesis or teratogenic effects, how would you go about it? What assays would you use? What do you think would give you the best results, and the most reproducible data?

Art Beaudoin: I guess if you wanted a test, you have to pick one that will cover as many developmental features of a human embryo that could possibly be found. Therefore, you would probably immediately think of the chick embryo or an amphibian embryo or some other embryo that would have cell divisions, cell recognition, cell differentiation, cell movement and so forth - all these phenomena associated with the period of organogenesis. I still am stuck on this problem that it seems to me that everyone wants to be the one to come up with the Ames test for teratology and we are passing over alot of tests. If enough people would start to work on some of these systems to know whether it can be repeatable from one laboratory to the next. There is an interesting system in Hydra right where you dissociate the adult Hydra and make an artificial embryo and then subject the growth of the artificial embryo to a variety of agents and it seems to have a fairly predictive value for toxic chemicals. As far as I know, only one laboratory has done this. No one else has picked it up. Drosophila embryos - there is a new test in drosophila embryos that covers ectoderm, the maturation of neurocells, mesoderm, the formation of myotubes. These are both things that would occur in a mammalian embryo and there seems to be some correlation here. Again, as far as I know only one lab has done it and only a few teratogens have been tested. I guess what I still would like to see is perhaps somebody sit down, maybe in the teratology society, and say, look why don't we pick these tests because they do contain most of the developmental or the largest number of developmental phenomena and see how many people would work it and see what we can come up with.

Lucy Anderson: I think that my responses would be a little controversial to people that like the rat as a model. The first thing that would need to be done, obviously, would be to expand these models and validate them and test them with a lot of additional carcinogens and noncarcinogens. If the need is for screening, I personally would start with this *in vivo/in vitro* mutagenesis assay, and after having validated it for a lot more chemicals than had been tested so far. I would pick out from that test those that appear to be particularly potent and then take them to the Swiss mouse model with chronic exposure from preconception throughout the gestation and lactation and take as the endpoint lung tumor at about say 6 or 7 months of age. Again, this is something that needs to be validated by applying the model with that specific goal in mind which has not been done as far as I know. It seems to me considering all approaches in transplacental carcinogenesis as well as the cost factors, sensitivity factors and so forth that this would be the most rationale approach in responding to the needs you stated.

Unidentified Speaker: I think prenatal exposure of the toxicant can very well express itself postnatal. Humanate can be born normally to look at what's been made for example retardation or maturation can be affected such that later on in the growth of the animal you can see signs of delayed development. Also, I think we want to touch on behavior. It is very important. I do not think any of these *in vitro tests* will cut behavioral tests. Even when the use of classical strategies, there is a level at which we're not going to bring about a typical type of teratogenic effect. In other words, we are not going to see a full effect, but there is a level of so-called non-teratogenic level will express itself for taking in the form of behavior (effects). I think we are very far from being able to detect subtle toxicity.

Dose-Response Models, Environment, and Epidemiology

Section Editor: W. E. Ribelin

New Approaches in Toxicity Testing and Their Application in Human Risk Assessment, edited by A. P. Li. Raven Press, New York © 1985.

Assessment of Various Dose-Response Models in the Determination of Risk

Tom Downs

The University of Texas School of Public Health, Houston, Texas 77025

Carcinogenicity of a test substance is frequently established only at high doses. The question then arises as to the effects of the substance at the relatively low doses to which humans may be exposed. This question is not easily answered since risks on the order of a few percent or less are generally not demonstrable experimentally or epidemiologically, even in very large studies. Yet the question is an important one since an excess risk of one in a thousand could result in nearly a quarter of a million excess cases nationwide.

To protect against such eventualities it has been considered prudent to extrapolate effects observed at relatively high doses to the low doses commonly encountered by man, with a view to adjusting human exposures to extrapolated "safe" levels. Such extrapolations must necessarily be done via mathematical models. However, current knowledge of carcinogenic processes is inadequate to determine in a given situation which mathematical model, from a multitude of potential models, is most appropriate. In this paper we describe and compare some of the methods and techniques used in this important area.

DOSE UNITS

Administered Dose

We denote the administered dose by x, and the corresponding response by P_x : P_x is the probability of contracting cancer (at some specific site) when exposed to a dose x of the test substance.

The choice of units for x can have a profound effect on the graph of P_x versus x, as well as on the estimated risk when extrapolating from one species to another. To illustrate this latter point, suppose test animals weighing 1 pound and having body surface areas of 1 square foot have been continuously dosed with 1 mg/day of a test substance. The administered dose x could be expressed as either x = 1 mg/lb/day or as x = 1 mg/ft^2/day. But for a 100 pound human whose body surface area is 10 square feet, a dose of 1 mg/day is either 0.01 mg/lb/day or 0.1 mg/ft^2/day. For simplicity, suppose the test animals have a risk proportional to x, say P_x = bx. If human risk is calculated by direct extrapolation, then the human risk for daily intake of 1 mg off the test substance will be b/100 when the dose units are mg/lb/day, and will be b/10 when the units are mg/ft^2/day. These differ by an order of magnitude, due solely to the choice of units.

The ideal dose units should be tailored to the biological action of the test substance. Unfortunately this action is seldom known in sufficient detail. There are situations, though, where certain units are contraindicated. For example, a dose scale in common use is the amount of the total intake of a substance. This choice of units is especially appealing in occupational studies of cancer because lower and upper bounds for the total intake may sometimes be estimated from historical data, whereas more precise estimates of dose are as a rule unobtainable. But this scale may be biologically unsound since, for instance, a man taking 2 aspirin tablets a day for 300 days has the same total intake as another man taking 600 aspirin tables in one day, yet their risks of toxic effects are different. More generally, total intake dose units are inappropriate when small amounts of the test substance are safely excreted or detoxified, but where large amounts overwhelm these defense mechanisms.

Effective Dose

Any dose-response model can be put in the form:

$$P_x = F(y) \qquad (1)$$

where F (•) is a strictly increasing cumulative probability distribution function. The argument y is called the *effective dose* and is conceptually defined as that function of the administered dose x which has reached the target site and is capable of producing damage. Hoel *et al.,* (1983) give a number of arguments and references in support of taking y to be the concentration of DNA adducts in the target organ for test substances whose metabolites interact with DNA. The pioneering work by Gehring *et al.,* (1977, 1978) helped lay the groundwork for this approach. However, since carcinogenic processes are poorly understood the effective dose y is considered herein as a metaphor for a variety of possible measures of direct potential damage.

Historically the forms of y as a function of the administered dose x have been simple polynomials; y = bx, y = bx + cx^2 + ..., y = bx^k, or logarithmic transformations: y = klogx. The parameters b,c, ..., k are non-negative by convention. Recent work by Gehring and Blau (1977), Downs and Frankowski (1982), and Hoel *et al.,* (1983) on nonlinear pharmacokinetics leads to expressions for y involving linear ratios in x.

COMMON DOSE-RESPONSE MODELS

In the general dose-response expression $P_x = F(y)$, the function F(•) is usually taken as the exponential, logistic, gamma or normal probability distribution.

The exponential distribution F(y) is given by:

$$F(y) = 1-\exp(-y). \qquad (2)$$

Three common dose-response models are special cases of (2). When the effective dose y is proportional to the administered dose x, (2) becomes the *one-hit* model:

$$P_x = 1-\exp(-bx), \qquad (3)$$

where b is a non-negative proportionality constant. The greater b the greater the risk P_X for any given x, so b is called the potency. The one-hit model is called such because of the following: suppose particles of the test substance or its metabolites "hit" the target tissue in accord with a Poisson process whose mean is y = bx. If cancer occurs whenever there are one or more "hits" then

$$\Pr(\text{cancer}) = 1\text{-}\Pr(\text{no hits}) = 1\text{-}\exp(\text{-}bx)$$

When bx is less than 1/20, then an excellent approximation to (3) is the linear model:

$$P_X = bx. \tag{4}$$

The one-hit model is the simplest of all the common dose-reponse models, both conceptually and mathematically. However, the shape of the dose-reponse curve for the one-hit model is inflexible, being always convex upward for all values of x.

The *multistage* model can be obtained from the exponential distribution (2) by taking the effective dose y to be a polynomial in x: $y = bx + cx^2 + \ldots$ Then

$$P_X = 1\text{-}\exp(\text{-}bx\text{-}cx^2\text{-}\ldots). \tag{5}$$

The linear approximation (4) is also valid for the multistage model when x is small. The multistage model is more flexible in shape than the one-hit; however, it is limited in its ability to be applied to data sets with threshold-like behavior. A rationale for the multistage model has been put forth by Armitage and Doll (1954), and again by Crump et al., (1976). The multistage model can also be construed as a one-hit model, as above, by taking the mean of the Poisson process to be the polynomial $y = bx + cx^2 + \ldots$ To avoid such ambiguities the one-hit model (3) is often called the linear one-hit. Thus the multistage model would be a polynomial one-hit model.

The *Weibull* dose-response model is the third special case of the exponential distribution and can be derived as a "hit" model by taking the mean of the Poisson process to be $y = bx^k$. The resulting Weibull model is given by

$$P_X = 1\text{-}\exp(\text{-}bx^k). \tag{6}$$

This model, unlike the previous two, is adaptive in shape. The graph of the dose-response curve at low doses is convex upward, linear, or convex downward according as the shape parameter, k, is less than, equal to, or greater than unity. By convention k is non-negative.

The *multi-hit* or *k-hit* model can be derived by supposing that "hits" occur as a Poisson process with mean bx, and requiring that cancer occurs when there are k or more hits. Then:

$$P_X = 1 - \sum_{j=0}^{k-1}(bx)^j \exp(\text{-}bx)/j!, \tag{7}$$

where k is any positive integer. The k-hit model can be generalized to any positive number k by means of the gamma distribution. This general model has been extensively studied by Cornfield et al (1978). The k-hit model is an improvement over the one-hit because it is adaptive in shape, with its low-dose shape determined by k in the same manner as the Weibull model. Fitting the k-hit model to a data set is computationally involved, though computer programs for this have been developed (Rai and Van Ryzin, 1980). The Weibull model is mathematically much more tractable than the k-hit.

The *logistic* model is derivable from kinetic theory and has the form

$$P_X = bx^k/(1+bx^k). \qquad (8)$$

This model was proposed for bioassay use by Berkson (1944). The graph of the logistic model is similar to those of the k-hit and Weibull, and the shape parameter k plays the same role here as for those models.

The *probit* or *log-normal* distribution was proposed by Mantel and Bryan (1961) for risk assessment, and later improved by Mantel *et al.*, (1975) to better account for spontaneous tumors and multiple-dose data. This model has a long history of success in bioassays, and there is a wealth of experimental data supporting it. However, its low-dose behavior is non-analytic, and the low-dose extrapolated risk for this model tends to zero faster than any power of x. For this reason the probit model has been criticized for possibly underestimating low-dose risks.

Krewski and Van Ryzin (1981) have compared the six models above with respect to (essentially) the relative risks that they predict for very low doses. Twenty data sets were used, and nineteen of these were convex downward in the observed range of low to moderate doses. The typical ordering of risks resulted in the one-hit model predicting the highest risk, the multistage the next highest, followed by the Weibull, logistic and multihit each predicting roughly the same risk. The probit model predicted the lowest risk. For the single data set (vinyl chloride) which had upward convexity, this order was completely reversed.

The extremes of the risk estimates often differed by several orders of magnitude. In general, the models which were the most flexible and adaptive in shape (logistic, Weibull, and multihit) gave better fits. However, a common problem with many data sets is that any one of many models will fit the data equally well over the observed dose range. It is in the low-dose extrapolation that they differ so markedly. The problem is further compounded by the practice of dosing bioassay test animals only at the MTD (maximum tolerated dose), and at one-half or one-fourth the MTD. This provides maximal information on carcinogenic potential, but gives no information about the shape of the dose-response curve at low doses.

KINETIC MODELS

The Gehring-Blau Model

A significant breakthrough in quantitative risk assessment was achieved by Gehring and Blaus (1977), who developed a simple yet plausible pharmacokinetic model for carcinogenic action. A modified version of this appears in Figure 1. The test substance X therein leads ultimately to the retained genetic program Y. If one denotes concentrations of substances by lower-case letters, x corresponds to the administered dose and y to the effective dose. Estimation of the rate constants for the reactions in Figure 1 permits numerical determination of the effective dose y as a function of x. While the pharmacokinetic model sheds no light on which dose-response model is appropriate, it does aid in deciding whether y is a convex upward, linear, or convex downward function of x at low doses.

FIGURE 1

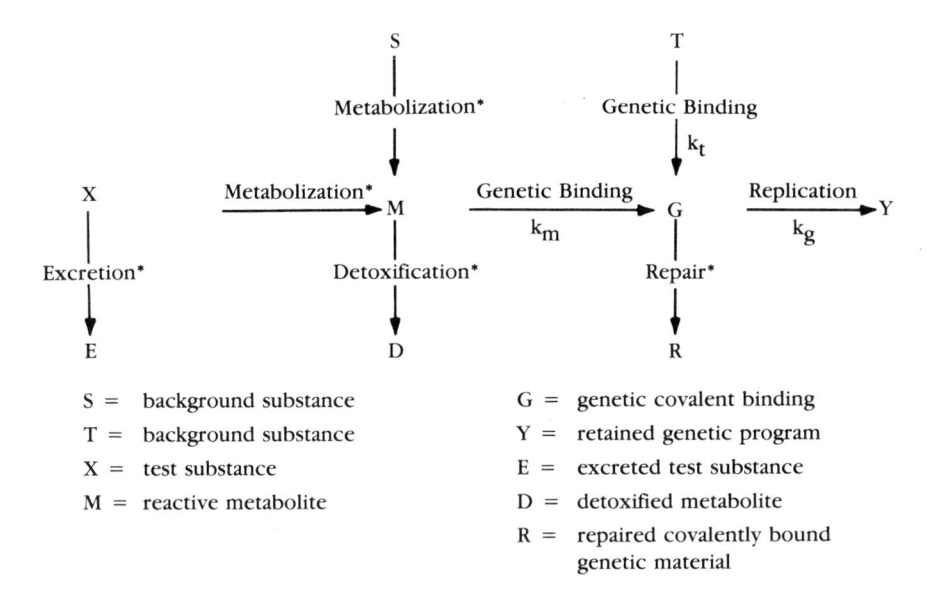

MODIFIED GEHRING-BLAU PHARMACOKINETIC MODEL

```
                    S                         T
                    |                         |
             Metabolization*            Genetic Binding
                    |                         | k_t
                    ▼                         ▼
   X    Metabolization*    Genetic Binding        Replication
   |   ───────────────► M ─────────────────► G ──────────────► Y
   |                          k_m                    k_g
Excretion*       Detoxification*              Repair*
   |                    |                         |
   ▼                    ▼                         ▼
   E                    D                         R
```

S = background substance   G = genetic covalent binding
T = background substance   Y = retained genetic program
X = test substance   E = excreted test substance
M = reactive metabolite   D = detoxified metabolite
    R = repaired covalently bound genetic material

Hypothetical model of the fate of three chemical carcinogens (S.T.X.) with similar actions. Dose-dependent reversible reactions in accord with Michaelis-Menten Kinetics are starred (*). First-order linear reactions are listed with rate constants. Modified from Gehring and Blau (1977).

All dose-reponse models must somehow account for spontaneous tumor rates due to background substances. There are two customary means of doing this: by assuming that the background and test substances operate independently, or by assuming that they operate in an additive fashion. Mixtures of these two have also been proposed. At any rate the method of dealing with spontaneous tumors can have an enormous effect on risk estimates (Hoel, 1980). The background substances S (with a mechanism similar to X) and T (with a different mechanism, but the same endpoint Y) appear, however, to operate neither additively nor independently. The kinetics provide here a third means of dealing with spontaneous tumors.

Vinyl Chloride Example

When Krewski and Van Ryzin fitted the six models described previously to 20 different data sets, the only case where the adaptive models indicated high potency, via upward convexity at low doses, was with vinyl chloride. Hoel *et al.*, (1983) used the kinetic model and numerical results on vinyl chloride of Gehring and Blau and noted that the vinyl chloride dose-response curve may well be convex downward at low doses, and that in none of an array of possibilities was the estimated dose-response curve actually convex upward. These conclusions were reached even though the one-hit model $P_x = 1-\exp(-by)$ was used, with y determined from the kinetic model. Hoel *et al.*, concluded that simple dose-response models tend to overestimate low-dose effects because of possible downward convexity.

This example illustrates the pitfalls that can be encountered in fitting mathematical models to data sets without some awareness of the pharmacokinetics involved. Unfortunately, there are at this time very few substances wherein the pertinent data is as available as that for vinyl chloride.

Adapative Repair

Downs and Frankowski (1982) used a simple kinetic model with a stochastic adaptive repair system to derive a very flexible class of dose-response models. It is possible, for instance, to have one of their models portray a dose-response curve wherein the response at low doses is actually smaller than the spontaneous response.

CONCLUSION

Some dose-response models are less useful than others for unbiased low-dose risk estimation because their shapes are relatively inflexible and unable to accommodate diverse sets of data. Among these are the linear one-hit, multistage and lognormal models. Of the flexible models remaining, my personal choice is the Weibull because of its relatively simple form and its ready extension to include time-to-tumor data and to account for competing risks.

Pharmacokinetic models hold much promise for greater understanding of carcinogenic processes, and for development of more biologically meaningful dose-response curves. It is surprising that none of the dose-response models in common use allow for Michaelis-Menten processes. I anticipate this situation will change as work progresses in this important area.

REFERENCES

Armitage, P. and Doll, R.: (1954). The age distribution of cancer and a multistage theory of carcinogenesis, *British J. Cancer,* 8:1-12.

Berkson, J.: (1944). Application of the logistic function to bioassay. *J. Amer. Statist. Assoc.,* 39:134-167.

Brown, C. C. and Koziol, J. A.: (1983). Statistical aspects of the estimation of human risk from suspected environmental carcinogens. *SIAM Review,* 25:151-181.

Cornfield, J.: (1977). Carcinogenic risk assessment. *Science, 198*:693-699.

Cornfield, J., Carlborg, F. W., and Van Ryzin, J.: (1978). Setting tolerances on the basis of mathematical treatment of dose-reponse data extrapolated to low doses. In: *Proceedings of the First International Congress on Toxicology,* Plaa, G. and Duncan, W. (eds), Academic Press, New York, 143-164.

Crump, K. S., Hoel, D., Langley, C., and Peto, R.: (1976). Fundamental carcinogenic processes and their implications for low-dose risk assessment. *Cancer Research 36* :2973-2979.

Downs, T.D. and Frankowski, R. F.: (1982). Influence of repair processes on dose-response models. *Drug Metab. Reviews, 13*:839-852.

Druckrey, H.: (1967). Quanticative aspects of chemical carcinogenesis. In: *Potential Carcinogenic Hazards from Drugs. Evaluation of Risks.* UICC Monograph Series, Vol. 7, Springer-Verlag, New York: 60-78.

Gehring, P. J. and Blau, G. E.: (1977). Mechanisms of carcinogenesis: dose-response. *J. Environ. Pathol. Toxicol., 1*:163-179.

Gehring, P. J., Watanabe, P. G., and Park, C. N.: (1978). Resolution of dose-response toxicity data for chemicals requiring metabolic activation: example-vinyl chloride. *Toxicol. Appl. Pharmacol., 44*:581-591.

Hartley, H. O. and Sielkin, R. L. Jr.: (1977). Estimation of "safe doses" in carcinogenic experiments. *Biometrics, 33*:1-30.

Hoel, D. G.: (1980). Incorporation of background responses in dose-response models. *Federation Proceedings, 39*:67-69.

Hoel, D. G., Kaplan, N. L., and Anderson, M. W.: (1983). Implications of nonlinear kinetics on risk estimation in carcinogenesis. *Science, 219*:1032-1037.

Krewski, D. and Van Ryzin, J.: (1981). Dose response models for quantal response toxicity data. In: *Statistics and Related Topics,* M. Csorgo D. Dawson, J. N. K. Rao and E. Saleh (eds.), North Holland, New York, 201-231.

Mantel, N., and Bryan, W. R.: (1961). "Safety" testing of carcinogenic agents. *J. Nat. Cancer Inst., 27*:455-470.

Mantel, N., Bohidar, N. R., Brown, D. C., Chiminera, J. L., and Tukey, J. W.: (1975). An improved "Mantel-Bryan" procedure for "safety testing" of carcinogens. *Cancer Res., 35*:865-872.

Rai, K. and Van Ryzin, J.: (1980). MULTI 80: A computer program for risk assessment of toxic substances. Rand Publications N-1512, Santo Monica, California: The Rand Corporation.

Raiffa, H.: (1982). Science and policy: their separating and integration in risk analysis. *The Amer. Statist., 36*:225-231.

Environmental Distribution and Fate: Its Role in Risk Assessment

W. Brock Neely

Environmental Sciences Research, The Dow Chemical Company, Midland, Michigan 48640

Before discussing the role of environmental distribution and fate it will be well to define risk assessment. This is a phrase that has been used and abused for many years. The controversy and conflict surrounding its use caused the government to enlist the services of the National Academy of Sciences to address the issue (1). One of their conclusions was that risk assessment is a prelude or input to the overall risk management operation and the distinction between the two processes (i.e. of assessment and management) should be sharply defined. The former is the use of a factual scientific base to define and interpret the health effects of exposure of individuals and populations to hazardous materials and situations. The management side of the process involves choices between the broader social and economic values. This paper will not discuss the mangement issue but will concentrate on the assessment question. In this regard the Academy outlined the following items that need to be considered in performing a risk assessment (1).

Hazard Identification is a process of determining whether exposure to an agent can cause an increase in the incidence of a health condition (cancer, birth defect, etc). It involves characterizing the nature and strength of the evidence of causation.

Dose-response assessment is a process of characterizing the relation between the dose of an agent and the incidence of an adverse effect.

Exposure assessment is a process of measuring or estimating the intensity, frequency and duration of human exposure to an agent currently present in the environment or of estimating hypothetical exposures that might arise from the release of new chemicals into the environment.

Risk characterization is a process of estimating the incidence of health effects under the various conditions of exposure described in exposure assessment.

EXPOSURE ASSESSMENT

The role of environmental fate and distribution analysis thus is to help estimate the extent of the exposure. In all of these assessment schemes the customary practice is to begin with the minimum amount of data and then to generate new data until the uncertainty in the risk estimate is acceptable from a management point of view. This relation between exposure and effect has recieved a great deal of attention in the aquatic toxicological area (2). One of the important concepts that emerged from these studies is that testing of a chemical should proceed through a sequence of tests where each succeeding level is closer to real world conditions and has a greater degree of confidence associated with the result. This is illustrated in Figure 1. Along the ordinate is listed the concentration of the chemical showing both the highest expected environmental concentration and the highest test concentration producing no observable biological effects. The abscissa indicates the increasing sophistication of testing that is required to reduce the uncertainty of the experimental result. The dashed lines represent the confidence interval that can be placed around the final numbers. The logic indicates that testing proceeds until there is no overlap in the confidence regions of the test. Once this level is accomplished the risk is said to be minimal and no further testing is required.

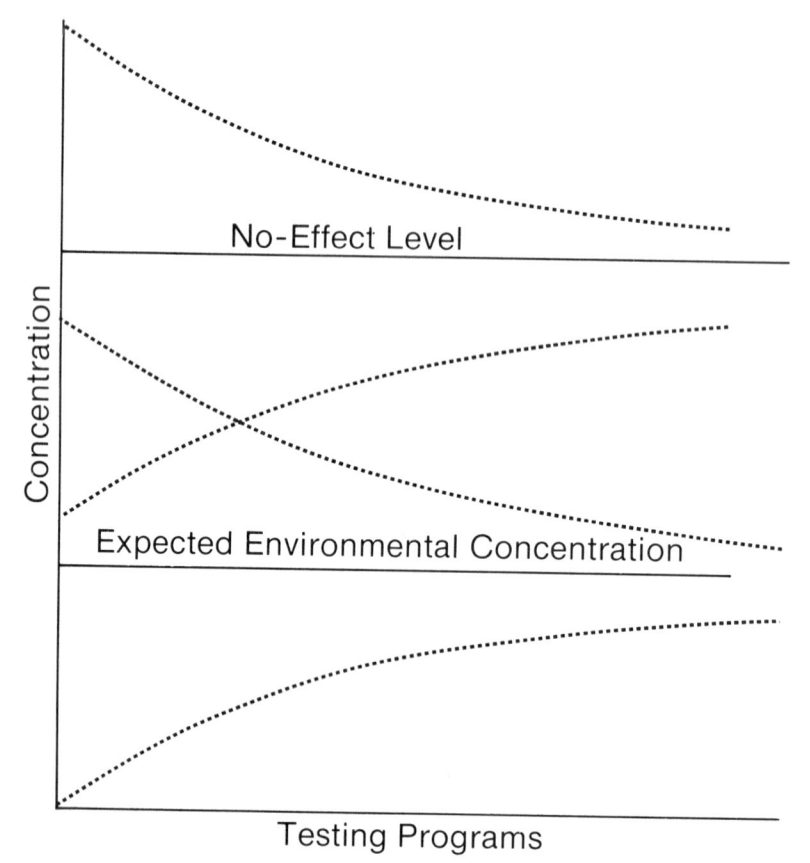

FIGURE 1. Schematic representation demonstrating how more sophisticated testing narrows the confidence region to the point where a risk assessment can be made.

At a recent workshop sponsored by the Office of Toxic Substances of EPA(3a) several recommendations were made regarding the tiered or sequential approach to estimating the environmental exposure from chemicals. In addition to the recommendations there was a discussion of the uncertainty factors associated with increasing sophistication of analysis. The models and associated uncertainties are reproduced in Table I. It should be noted that the uncertainty factors are not consensus numbers but were presented at the Workshop for discussion purposes only(3a). The next section will discuss the models and illustrate their use with examples.

TABLE I.

Uncertainty Associated with Estimating Procedures for Environmental Concentrations[a]

Model	Uncertainty Factor
Unit World	100
Site Specific	10
Field Data	1

[a]Taken in part from Reference 3.

MODELS FOR ESTIMATING ENVIRONMENTAL DISTRIBUTION AND FATE

UNIT WORLD

At the first level of modeling the technique is to use a screening approach where the objective is to gain a preliminary idea of what can happen to a chemical once it enters the environment. The Unit World has been designed for this purpose (4-6). It is particularly applicable to chemicals released or expected to be released into the environment in large quantities on a regional or global basis. The basic model is illustrated in Figure 2 where the major compartments are illustrated. The scaling is such that 510 million units are equivalent to the world. The volumes and physical properties have been described previously (5) and will not be discussed further in this report. The processes that are operating in the Unit World are given in Table II. Integrating the partition coefficients between the various phases with the input data yields three main results:

1. An indication of how much of the chemical is located in each of the four main compartments; air, water, bottom sediments and ground.
2. The water concentration at steady state.
3. The residence time, or the length of time required for the chemical to be cleared. This number becomes an index of persistence.

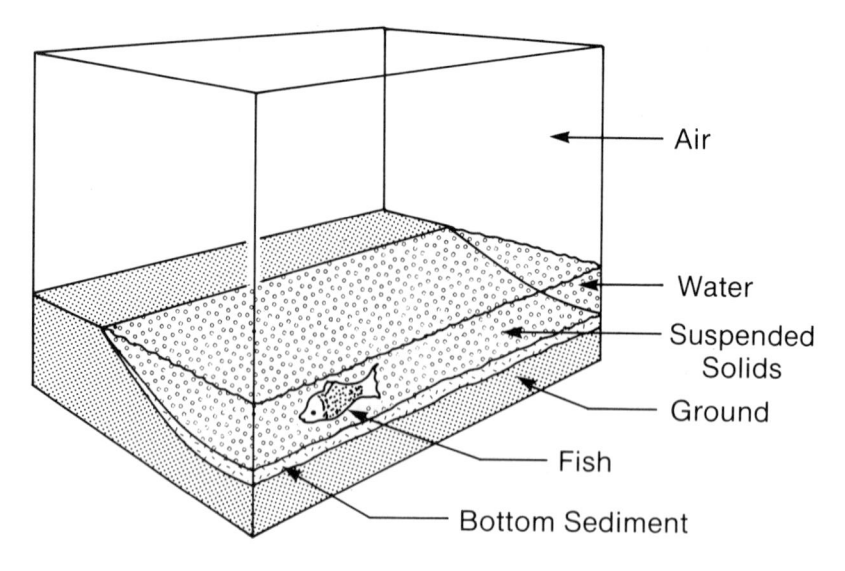

FIGURE 2. Schematic representation of the unit world showing the major compartments.

TABLE II.

Processes Operating in the Unit World

Transport

1. Exit to the stratosphere   41. x 10^{-5}/day
2. Burial in the bottom sediments   2 x 10^{-4}/day

Both of these processes remove chemical from the Unit World and are assumed to be operating all of the time.

Transformation

1. Hydrolysis occurs at pH 7 and 25°C
2. Atmospheric oxidation occurs as second order reaction with hydroxyl radicals. These radicals are present at a concentration of 5 x 10^5 molecules/cm^3.
3. Microbial degradation is a second order reaction in which the concentration of cells is 1 x 10^5 cells/mL and 1 x 10^6 cells/mL of sediment.
4. Aqueous photolysis is estimated by the method of Zepp and Cline (10). For this purpose the Unit World is located at 40°N latitude with no cloud cover.

Data requirements - It is important to have an estimate of the amount released to the environment. For most common solvents and pesticides the amount is nearly equivalent to the production figure. At the other end of the spectrum there are intermediates produced and used in a chemical reaction which are essentially never released. In this situation the input to the environment will be assigned a value equal to 0.01 of the production. A range of values for some well known chemicals between these two extremes is given by Stephanson (7).

In addition to the input data it is necessary to have some knowledge of the chemical and physical properties. the minimum set of data for an analysis include the molecular weight, vapor pressure and water solubility. These latter two items need to be determined for the temperature of interest usually in the range of 20-25°C. The data are then integrated by the model and concentrations in each compartment are estimated. To refelct the uncertainty in comparing with anticipated real world situations the results are increased by a factor of 100 (see Table 1). For example, the water concentrations that result under actual use conditions might be 100 times as large as the numbers generated by the model. This maximum number is then matched with toxicity data or preferably with an accepted water quality criteria number. If the predicted water concentration number is greater than the toxicity data would suggest, an investigation should be initiated for degradation reactions. The partitioning pattern will give an indication of where to look. For example, if the pattern indicates that the bulk of the chemical is located in the air then it would be a waste of time to examine the water compartment for degradation reactions. Several examples will illustrate the details.

a) *DDT* — For this example the input will be equated to the world production which reached a level of 350×10^6 pounds/year in the early 1970's. Equation 1 converts pounds/year in the early 1970's. Equation 1 converts pounds/year to an input of nmoles/day for the Unit World.

$$\text{Input (nmoles/day)} = \frac{\text{Production} \times 453 \times 10^3}{365 \times \text{mol wt} \times 510 \times 10^6} \times \text{Release} \quad (1)$$

Release = fraction of production released to the environment

510×10^6 = number of units in the world

Since DDT is a pesticide the release factor is 1. The properties for DDT are assembled in Table III and the results are given in Table IV. The partitioning pattern indicates the strong sorption of the pesticide to soil while the residence time suggests a very persistent chemical. By comparing the predicted water concentration of 5.6 ppt with the conservative guideline estimate of 1 ppt as suggested by the water quality criteria documents (8) it is readily apparent that even without including the uncertainty factor the predicted exposure from DDT is too close to the guideline number. Such an analysis would immediately suggest further studies to see if either the exposure could be decreased of if the action number as proposed by the criteria could be increased. Thus by focusing on both aspects of the hazard equation society might have eliminated the need to ban this useful pesticide.

b) *2,4-D* — The world production of 2, 4-D when reduced to an input for the Unit World has a value of 0.66 mmoles/day. This and the other key data are shown in Table III. The results of the analysis in Table IV indicate that the water compartment is favored. Assuming that no dissipating reactions are operating, the water concentration has a value of 960 ppt which should be increased to 96 ppb by application of the uncertainty factor (Table I). The chronic no-effect concentration for a full life cycle test on fathead minnows has been reported as 300 ppb (9). Reducing this value by the proposed uncertainty (3b) factor of 10 yields 30 ppb for the toxicity. Thus, the exposure is greater than the no effect level, which necessitates a further investigation into possible degradation reactions. When the photolytic rate constant of 0.0345/day (10) is incorporated into the analysis the water concentration is estimated at 0.6 ppt (for a maximum of 60 ppt) and the residence time becomes 35 days. This revised prediction of exposure is well below the action level of 30 ppb. If soil degradation is also incorporated, the water concentration would be reduced even further. The risk assessment from this study implies that no further work is necessary from an environmental perspective. In view of the widespread use of these herbicides over the years with little or no impact being reported such a conclusion is justifiable.

TABLE III

Properties Required for Operating the Unit World

Property	DDT	2,4-D	Benzene
World Production ($\bar{M}$ lbs/year)	350	60	20,000
Release Rate	1	1	0.1
Input to Unit World (nmoles/day)	2.4	0.66	62
Molecular Weight	354	221	78
Vapor Pressure (mm Hg)	2×10^{-7}	6×10^{-7}	95
Water Solubility (ppm)	0.005	900	1780
Rate Constant (1/day)	0	0.0345[a]	0.06[a]

[a] The rate constant for 2,4-D is the photolysis rate in water while the value for benzene is the oxidation in air.

TABLE IV

Results from Using the Unit World Model on the Data in Table III.

Results		DDT	2,4-D	Benzene
Partitioning Pattern	Air	0.003	0	0.990
	Water	0.004	0.820	0.005
	Bottom Sediment	0.479	0.090	0
	Ground	0.51	0.094	0
Residence Time (days)		10,000	5700[a]	25000[a]
			35[b]	16[b]
Water Concentration (ppt)		5.6	960[a]	90[a]
			0.6[b]	0.06[b]

[a] These figures are the residence time and the water concentration assuming that no degradation reactions are operating.

[b] These figures are the residence time and the water concentration as a result of using the degradation rate constants given in Table III.

c) Benzene — The production figure for benzene (11) is 20,000 million pounds/year. Stephanson (7) estimated that only a tenth of the production actually entered the environment. Combining this with the other properties from Table III gives the results in Table IV. Once again the impact that the dissipating reaction (12) has on both the residence time and the predicted water concentraton is quite apparent. Thus, without degradation the predicted water concentration from the Unit World is 9 ppb (0.09 x 100). By incorporating the photodegradation rate constant the water level is estimated to be 0.06 ppt for a maximum of 6 ppt. This is three orders of magnitude smaller than the first estimate.

SITE SPECIFIC

At this second level of evaluation more extensive data is needed since the analyst is now attempting to make more accurate exposure predictions of what might be expected at a particular site. For example, if a manufacturing plant is located on a river it may be necesssary to make an estimation of the concentration of the material that is added to a stream as a result of the manufacturing process. The type of site specific parameters that must be developed for this ecosystem are shown in Table V.

TABLE V.

Site Specific Parameters Associated with a River

1. Volumetric flow
2. Dispersion coefficient
3. Width
4. Depth
5. Velocity
6. Suspended sediments
7. Attenuation coefficient
8. Trophic status

While many of the parameters are self-explanatory a few need interpretation. The dispersion coefficient helps define the turbulent properties which in turn help characterize the mixing zone (13). The suspended sediment concentration will determine what sorption is taking place and what the expected water concentration will be. The attenuation coefficient is necessary only if the chemical is subjected to photodegradation. The trophic status will provide information as to what species may be the most sensitive and thus what species should be examined for adverse effects.

Three examples will be described where site specific modeling has been used. The examples chosen are for illustrative purposes and do not imply that an exhaustive literature search has been performed on the subject.

a. Chlorpyrifos applied to a fish pond — Macek (14) performed a field study where chlorpyrifos was applied to several fish ponds in Missouri at the rate of 0.05 pounds/acre of water. Water and fish samples were collected on days 1, 3, 7, 14 and 28. Neely and Blau (15) built a model to stimulate this field study. By performing a mass balance on the pond the following model was formulated.

$$\frac{V_d C_w}{dt} = -k_1 A C_w - k_2 V C_w - k_3 F C_2 + k_4 F C_f - k_5 S C_w + k_6 S C_s$$

$$F \frac{dC_f}{dt} = k_3 F C_w - k_1 C_f$$

where:

V	=	Volume
A	=	Area
F	=	Mass of fish
S	=	Weight of active sediment layer
k_1	=	Rate constant for evaporation
k_2	=	Rate constant for hydrolysis
k_3	=	Rate constant for uptake by fish
k_4	=	Rate constant for clearance by fish
k_5	=	Rate constant for uptake by soil
k_6	=	Rate constant for desorption from soil
C_f, C_w, C_s	=	concentration in fish, water and soil

Using laboratory derived values for the rate constants and field data for the site-specific parameters the differential equations were readily solved on the computer and the results in Figure 3 were obtained (15). It is apparent that the match of the observed data with the predicted is reasonably close. Such a comparison lends credibility to using this type of model for similar situations where field data might be absent.

b. Alachlor and Atrazine in Rathbun Reservoir — Schnoor et al., (16) applied a mass balance model to predict concentrations of the pesticides in a reservoir in Iowa. The study was conducted in the south central part of the state where the watershed for the reservoir was 535 square miles of agricultural land. Using flow data from the United States gauging stations and field measurements of the concentrations of the two pesticides entering the reservoir the authors were able to generate an actual concentration profile. This was then matched with the predicted concentration from the mass balance model. For the more water soluble herbicide (Alachlor) the match was close. The results on Atrazine were not quite as good. However, even in this case the predicted values were well within the order of magnitude that was suggested by the workshop (3a) for site specific models (Table I).

c. Chlorinated Solvents — Chlorinated solvents (and PCB's section d) illustrate the importance of having a good input parameter. In all models, whether they are like the Unit World or more sophisticated as in the case of site specific models, an input function is required. In the case of the chlorinated solvents the emission becomes the production since it may be assumed that if the solvent is produced most of it will eventually end up in

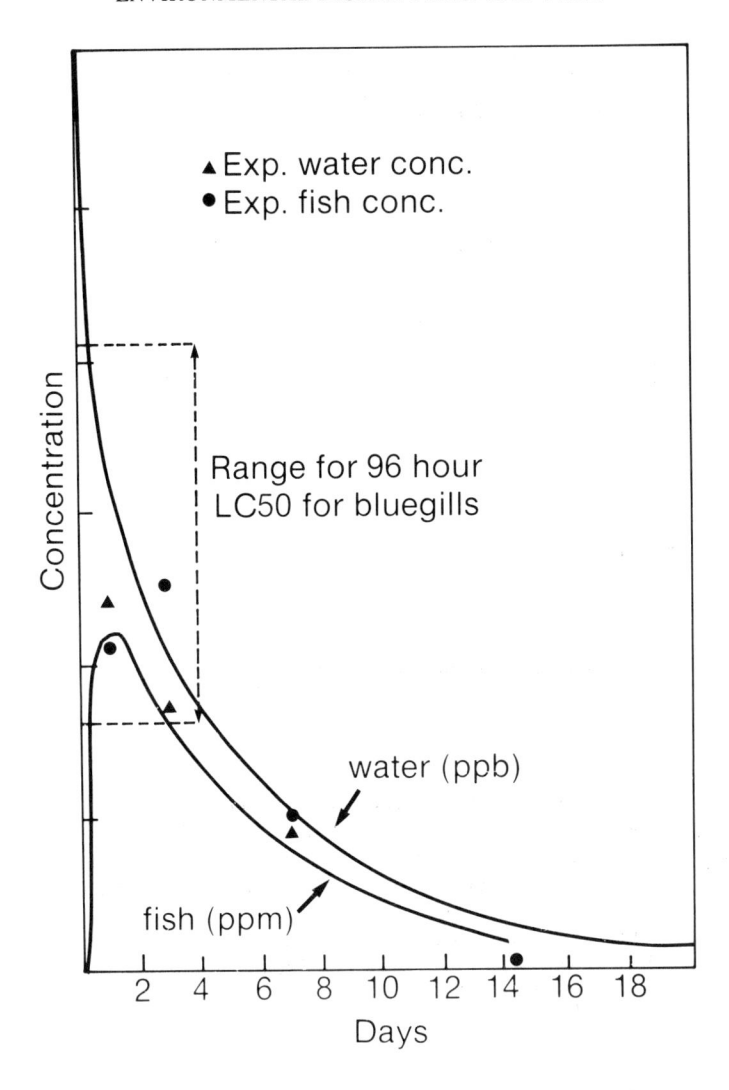

FIGURE 3. Computer simulation of the concentrations of Chlorpyrifos in both fish and water.

the atmosphere. Thus, the main problem is in estimating the worldwide production. Once this is accomplished there are many models that have been developed which are capable of predicting average global concentrations in the troposphere. The models range from simple box models (17) to complicated two-dimensional models of the atmosphere (18-20). Figure 4 matches the actual tropospheric concentrations of methylchloroform with those that are predicted from a simple box model (17). The close match indicates that if knowledge of the production and dissipating reactions are known then the simple model is adequate to predict atmospheric concentrations.

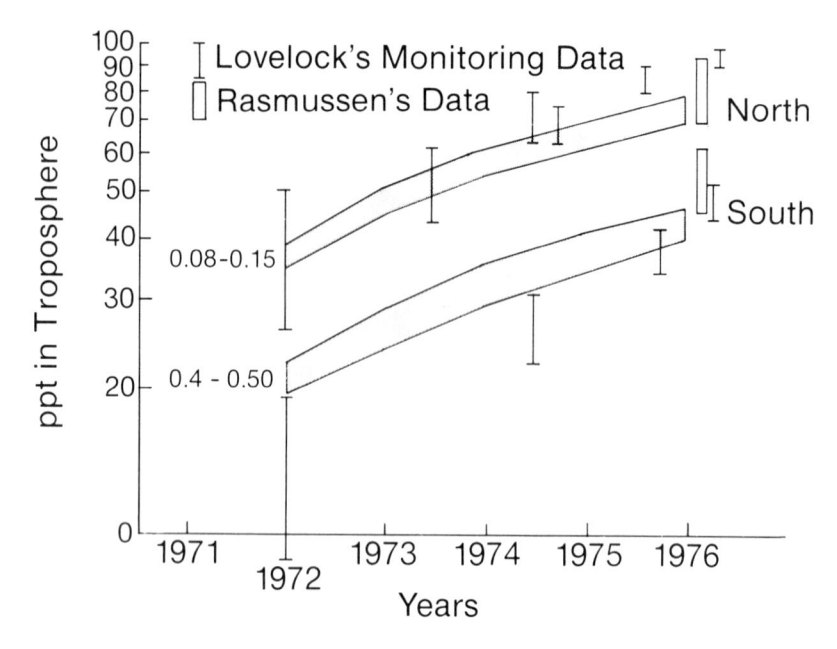

FIGURE 4. Computer simulation of the tropospheric concentrations of methylchloroform matched to the actual monitoring data. The shaded region represents a variation in the photodegradation rate constant for the solvent.

d. Polychlorinated Biphenyls (PCB) — The polychlorinated biphenyls illustrate a more complicated problem associated with estimating input. Given the diversity of uses that occurred for these versatile chemicals prior to 1970 it becomes impossible to estimate with a reasonable degree of accuracy how much of the production entered the environment. The reader is referred to the chapter by Conway et al., (21) for a better understanding of the problems connected with determining environmental release. Suffice to say that in modeling the environmental fate and distribution of PCB, the main problem is not in the fate and distribution analysis but in estimating the input that should be used in the model of choice.

CONCLUSION

A tiered approach to exposure assessment is possible as these various case studies have shown. By starting with a minimum set of data, tentative conclusions may be reached regarding the expected concentrations that might be observed. If, after applying the uncertainty factors, the exposure is still higher than the effect, then more detailed site specific modeling is required to generate a more reliable measure of exposure. By proceeding in a logical stepwise fashion, intelligent decisions can be made regarding the life of a product. Such planning will help minimize future environmental crises. In addition, if there is an identified hazard where the benefit to society is great it becomes possible to manage the associated risk with a greater degree of confidence.

REFERENCES

1. National Academy of Sciences: *"Risk Assessment in the Federal Government: Managing the Process"*, NAS, Washington, D.C., 1983.
2. *Cairns, J.; Dickson, K. L.; and Maki, A. W.: "Estimating the Hazard of Chemical Substances to Aquatic Life"* Amer. Soc. Test. Materials, Philadelphia, PA, 1978.
3. *a) Glennon, J. R.*: "Testing Triggers Workshop". Environ. Prot. Agency. Contract No. 69-01-6554, May 19, 1983. b) This same workshop suggested that an uncertainty factor of 10 should be applied to chronic data. Thus, a chronic number would be reduced by 10.
4. *Mackay, D.: Env. Sci. & Technol., 13*:1220, 1979.
5. *Neely, W. B.; and Mackay, D.: Modeling the Fate of Chemical in the Aquatic Environment.* Ann Arbor Press. Ann Arbor, Mich., 1982.
6. *Neely, W. B.: Env. Toxicol. & Chem., 1*:259, 1982.
7. *Stephanson, M.: Ecotoxicol. Environ. Safety, 1*:39, 1977.
8. *Costle, D.: Fed. Register, 45*, p. 79318, Nov. 28, 1980.
9. *Mount, D. L.; and Stephan, C. E.: Trans. Am. Fish. Soc., 96*:185, 1967.
10. *Zepp, R.; and Cline, D. M.: Environ. Sci. & Technol., 11*:359, 1977.
11. *Anonymous. Chem. and Eng. News, May 4*, p. 35, 1981.
12. *Neely, W. B.: Chemicals in the Environment.* Marcel Dekker, New York, 1980.
13. *Neely, W. B.: Env. Sci. & Technol., 16:518, 1982.*
14. *Macek, K. J.; Walsh, D. F.; Hogan, J. W.; and Holz, D. D.: Trans. Am. Soc., 191*:420, 1972.
15. *Neely, W. B.; and Blau, G. E.: Pesticides in the Aquatic Environment.* Plenum Press, New York, 1977.
16. *Schnoor, J. L.; Rao, N. B.; Cartwright, K. J.; and Noll, R. M.: Modeling the Fate of Chemical in the Aquatic Environment.* Ann Arbor Press, Ann Arbor, Mich. 1982.
17. *Neely, W. B.; and Plonka, J. H.: Envion. Sci. & Technol., 12*:317, 1978.
18. *Crutzen, P. J.; and Fishman, J.: Geophys. Res. Let., 4*:101, 1977.
19. *Rasmussen, R. A.; and Khalil, M. A. K*: Geophys. Res. Let., 8:1005, 1981.
20. *Derewent, R. J.; and Eggleton, A. E. J.: Atmos. Environ., 1*:1261, 1978.
21. *Conway, R. A.; Whitmore, F. C.; and Hansen, W. J.: Environmental Risk Analysis for Chemicals,* Van Nostrand, Reinhold Co., New York, 1982.

… continued

Use of Epidemiology in Risk Assessment

William R. Gaffey

Department of Epidemiology, Monsanto Company, St. Louis, Missouri 63167

As one of the two token epidemiologist on this program, I would like to examine the usefulness of epidemiology as a tool for risk assessment, and to say something about the complementary roles of epidemiology and toxicology. From the titles of the other presentations it is clear that to most of us risk assessment means the assessment of carcinogenic risk. Perhaps that is not a proper preoccupation, but it is one which I share, and it will be reflected in this talk. Also, I will tend to talk about occupational epidemiology and industrial toxicology, although most of what I will say has a wider applicability. Let us look first at some of the inherent differences between the two, from Table 1.

TABLE 1

Toxicology	Epidemiology
Before the fact	After the fact
Experimental	Observational
Dose-response study usually feasible	Dose-response study usually not feasible
Not easily generalizable	Can be generalized

Before the Fact Versus After the Fact

Epidemiology and toxicology differ radically in their research designs and the relevance of their findings, sometimes to the detriment of one or the other of the two disciplines. The greatest difference between them is that toxicology tends to concern itself with substances to which human beings are not yet exposed, while epidemiology of necessity is carried out after the fact, that is, after an exposure is present in a human population. Of course, the first half of the preceding sentence is not entirely true, because as new insights arise toxicologists may often reexamine substances that either were ignored in the past or given a clean bill of health based on outdated methodology.

Nevertheless the crucial difference between epidemiologists and toxicologists is that the latter have the opportunity to intervene before there is any human exposure.

This leads to some interesting differences in how one defines the successes and failures of the two disciplines. Of the known human carcinogens, practically all have been discovered by epidemiologic studies (1). I suppose that could be called "success." The successes of toxicology, on the other hand, are in terms of things that do not happen. Many substances are not present in our environment because toxicological investigation has raised suspicions about their effects on humans. Were it not for such investigations there might now be many more carcinogens for epidemiologists to find. The other side of the coin, of course, is that in the absence of human exposure no one can be sure of what is toxic to humans. This means that those substances that have passed muster, toxicologically speaking, must be constantly monitored for their possible effects on human beings.

One role of epidemiology is therefore to look at real exposures of human beings, under real life conditions, to those substances that have been given a clean bill of health by the toxicologist (as well as to those substances that have not yet been investigated by the toxicologist). Another way to put it is that epidemiologists count bodies and report the result. Unfortunately, there is a tendency to think that because the epidemiologist presents a body count he is somehow responsible for the deaths which he documents. Many of you have heard or seen the expression "We can't wait to count the bodies." This is a disreputable cliché intended to confuse finding the bodies with creating them. It suggests that epidemiologists would prefer to bypass toxicology and experiment on human beings. I hope I have made it clear that such is not the case.

Experimental Versus Observational Studies

Toxicology studes are true experiments, in the sense that experimental animals can be randomly assigned to different treatment groups. Epidemiology studies in practially all cases are observational. This has several implications. First, if a substantial effect is found in an animal study it is almost always due either to chance or to the treatment, and standard statistical techniques are designed to deal with precisely these alternatives. It can happen, of course, that some event such as an epidemic in a control group can introduce a confounding factor, but it is always physically possible to do the study over.

By contrast, a substantial effect in an epidemiology study is due either to chance *or* to the effect of exposure *or* to the presence of some systematic difference between the exposed and control groups that the investigator was not clever enough to recognize. The latter is always a possibility because the epidemiologist cannot randomly assign people to an exposed or control group. One result is that epidemiology studies tend to generate polemics over interpretation, and epidemiologists have a long standing fascination with an assortment of statistical techniques for dealing with, or at least making the epidemiologist more comfortable about, confounding factors (2).

Another result is that what the epidemiologist can measure is usually determined for him. This is particularly true of chronic diseases such as cancer, where the exposure that might have caused the cancer will have occurred several decades ago. In addition, many covariables of interest were probably never recorded. This is generally true, for example, of smoking. When the time comes to do a study of persons exposed to Substance X 20 years ago, a large number of them will have left employment and some will have died. There is no practical way to determine their smoking practices retrospectively. The same thing is true, to an extent, of the outcome measurements that are available to the epidemiologist. Even if we could reach former employees, we would doubt the accuracy of their reports as to their health in the past two decades. Circumstances therefore virtually compel the epidemiologist to concentrate on mortality, although many will feel that this is an overly stringent measure of ill health.

In reaction to these limiations, we are trying to anticipate the future by measuring, on a current basis, all those covariables that we think might be important in future studies. My successor will have no trouble with smoking, as far as being able to adjust for it as a covariable. He will have no trouble dealing with weight, hypertension or a host of other such variables.

He may well have trouble with some other confounding variables that are not being currently measured, since surveillance schemes can never perfectly anticipate the future.

Dose Versus Response

Epidemiology studies, especially of chronic diseases, can often measure effects better than causes. I can tell with a fair degree of certainty whether or not someone is dead, for example. However, I have the greatest of difficulty determining what his exposure was to vinyl chloride 30 years ago, partly because nobody tried to measure it, and partly because if they had tried, the existing technology would have made those measurements both expensive and unreliable. Toxicology studies, on the other hand, generally can measure both causes and effects reasonably adequately. One result is that various surrogates for exposure are used in epidemiology studies, such as duration of employment at sites where there is a potential exposure (but one which has not been reliably measured in the past). If there is no relationship between an outcome measure and the surrogate for exposure, this may, subject to some uneasiness on the part of the investigator, be taken as evidence that there is no exposure effect. If the converse occurs we may believe that we have a dose response relationship, but it is not possible to quantify it. In addition, exposures in human populations are seldom pure, as they are in toxicology studies, so that some way of adjusting for this complication are often required. For example, I am familiar with a lead smelter in which, several years ago, a considerable number of employees had unacceptably high blood lead levels, in spite of an industrial hygiene pogram of which the smelter was justifiably proud. The convariable here was that the workers were of Italian ancestry. They made their own wine at home, in lead lined vessels, and therefore were subject to exposure completely independent of their employment. In this case the confounding exposure was uncovered by chance, but in other cases it may exist undetected.

Generalizability

The least worrisome problem that the epidemiologist faces in contrast to the toxicologist is that of generalizing beyond the population under study. It is often true that the epidemiologist studies relatively heavily occupationally exposed populations, even though his real interest may be in low level exposures in the general environment, but if he finds no untoward results it is reasonable to conclude that people exposed to those lower levels in the general environment are not in any trouble. If the occupationally exposed group is experiencing some health effect the problem of extrapolating to low level exposure exists, but at least the epidemiologist has no species differences to content with.

What Can Epidemiology Uncover?

Table 2 shows the more important things that we can find out from epidemiology studies. First, a reasonably well done study can find substantial excesses in various causes of death such as cancer, the classical example being that of lung cancer among cigarette smokers (3). Second, an epidemiology study can find effects unique to human beings. Lung cancer in cigarette smokers is one such example. Another is finding that men who are substantially underweight for their height have an excess mortality from stomach cancer (4). A third is the finding that women whose first pregnancies occur at younger ages have less breast cancer (4).

TABLE 2

What can epidemiology uncover?

1. Substantial excesses
2. Effects unique to human beings
3. Verification of toxicological findings
4. Absence of a substantial effect

A third and very important function of epidemiology is to verify the predictions of toxicology. In the case of vinyl chloride toxicological findings from animal studies were indeed confirmed in human studies (5). In the case of formaldehyde the animal findings do not appear to be confirmed by human data (6).

This brings us to the fourth thing that epidemiology can do, which is to establish the absence of an effect in human beings. This situation is particularly difficult to deal with when animal studies come to the opposite conclusion, as has been the case with formaldehyde. For statistical reasons it is always possible that a study which finds no health effect could have missed a real effect which would have appeared had the sample size been larger. Negative studies therefore tend to be given less weight than positive ones. However, in the case of formaldehyde there are now twelve human studies with sample sizes ranging from a few hundred to more than 17,000, none of which confirm the animal data. It is my judgement that the human data in this case carry more weight, but the ground rules for resolving this kind of contradiction have not yet been agreed upon. A further complication, of course, is the refusal of some journals to publish studies unless they show adverse effects.

In summary, although epidemiology is a "softer" discipline than toxicology, it can detect large excesses in mortality in human populations, it can detect effects that are unique to human beings, it can verify the predictions of toxicology concerning effects on humans, and in some circumstances it can convince us that, in spite of the findings of animal studies, the practical consequences of human exposure are minimal.

One final comment is appropriate with respect to the use of epidemiology studies in the area of risk assessment. When we consider chronic effects such as cancer, the data to evaluate human effects is generally available. In a sense, the study has been done, and the data are waiting to be analyzed. The existence of the data requires us to analyze it in order to fulfill our responsibility for health surveillance.

REFERENCES

1. *Higginson, J.*: Chronic Toxicology - An Epidemiologist's Approach To The Problem of Carcinogens. *Essays in Toxicology* 7:29-72, 1976.

2. *Fletcher C.M., Peto R, Tinker C.M.: et al. The Natural History Of Chronic Bronchitis and Emphysema.* Oxford: Oxford University Press, 1976.

3. *Doll R., Hill A.B.:* A Study of The Aetiology of Carcinoma of The Lung. *Br. Med.* 2:1271-1286, 1952.

4. *Lew E.A., Garfindel L.:* Variations in Mortality By Weight Among 750,000 Men and Women. *J. Chronic Dis.* 32:563-576, 1979.

5. *Tabershaw I.R., Gaffey W.R.:* Mortality Study of Workers in The Manufacture of Vinyl Chloride and Its Polymers. *J. Occup. Med.* 16:509-518, 1976.

6. *Formaldehyde Newsletter,* September 1983.

Human Biologic Parameters as Epidemiologic Tools in Environmental Risk Assessment

Clark W. Heath, Jr.

Masters of Public Health Program, Department of Community Health, Emory University School of Medicine, Atlanta, Georgia 30322

Assessment of human health risks should ideally be based on direct observations of the frequencies of illness in exposed and non-exposed human populations. In places where public health attention is preoccupied with acute disease, such methods of risk assessment are relatively easy to apply. This is so in most developing countries where preventable infectious diseases are principal causes of morbidity and mortality.

TABLE 1

FACTORS WHICH COMPLICATE DIRECT ASSESSMENT OF HUMAN HEALTH RISK FROM EXPOSURE TO ENVIRONMENTAL TOXINS

1. Long and variable latency between exposure to toxin and appearance of illness.

2. Low frequency of disease requiring large population sizes for estimating statistically stable rates.

3. Clinical non-specificity whereby individual cases of illness caused by toxic exposure cannot be distinguished from cases arising from other causes.

Where chronic illness is a main concern, however, simple risk assessment by direct measurement of illness frequencies has limited application and must be supplemented by other approaches. The reasons for this are three-fold (Table 1). First, chronic diseases such as cancer or neurologic disability are likely to require the passage of many years after exposure to disease-producing agents before clinical symptoms appear. Such long latency makes it difficult, if not impossible, to associate illness with preceding causation.

Second, the problem of long latency is intensified by the fact that very few chronic diseases can be attributed to single causes. Only rarely can a physician identify the particular cause of a particular case of cancer (the association of mesotheliomas with asbestos exposure being a conspicuous exception). For most chronic, non-infectious diseases many different causes, working separately or in synergy, may be equally likely. Expressed differently, chronic illnesses, unlike many acute infectious diseases, are clinically nonspecific when considered in relation to particular etiologic factors.

Third, the frequency of most chronic diseases such as cancer is usually so low that, even if a particular exposure were to increase their incidence as much as 10 to 20 fold, that increase might still be statistically indistinguishable from the expected incidence in non-exposed populations. This problem is particularly apparent when risk assessment is undertaken in populations of small or limited size.

In the face of these difficulties which accompany direct measurements of the frequency of human chronic illness, several indirect approaches have been developed to assist in making useful risk assessments. These approaches can be classified in three groups. 1) observations made in humans, 2) observations made in non-human species (laboratory test animals), and 3) observations made in cell systems *in vitro*. Risk assessment can obviously be made more systematically, with greater control, and with larger numbers of observations in non-human biologic systems. For these reasons, most risk assessment at present is based on extrapolations made from observations in non-human species and in *in vitro* test systems. Ultimately, it will be desirable if cross-species and *in vitro/in vivo* extrapolations can be avoided through use of biologic measurements in humans. This paper reviews the current status of certain kinds of human observations, the results of efforts to apply such approaches in specific human exposure situations, and the limitations involved in their interpretation. Two forms of human biologic observation are considered: first, measurements of abnormal pregnancy outcomes (spontaneous abortion, birth defects, low birth weight) as possible short-latency reflections of environmental risk and, second, measurements of purely subclinical abnormalities, exemplified here by liver function testing and cytogenetic observations.

ABNORMAL PREGNANCY OUTCOMES

Use of pregnancy outcomes to assess environmental risk arises from observations which show that *in utero* chemical and radiation exposure can produce birth anomalies and pregnancy loss both in experimental animals and in humans. This teratogenic effect offers two distinct advantages as a tool for monitoring environmental risk. First, since the developing fetus appears to be particularly sensitive to environmental exposure, measuring abnormal pregnancy outcomes may identify risks at dose levels lower than might be possible through monitoring adult disease. Second, since *in utero* exposure involves latency of less than nine months, relatively rapid assessment of risk may be possible in situations where alternative approaches require observation of long-latency diseases (i.e., cancer). Uncertainty exists regarding the extent to which one can extrapolate from pregnancy effects to cancer risk. On theoretical and experimental grounds, however, it is likely that considerable overlap exists between oncogenesis and teratogenesis.

Systematic monitoring of pregnancy outcomes in relation to specific environmental exposures in human populations has yet to be widely applied. However, programs to this effect are now being developed in occupational settings. An early effort to measure pregnancy outcomes in a general population was undertaken in connection with the Love Canal toxic chemical dump site in Niagara Falls, New York (1). Review of this study illustrates both the uses and the limitations of this kind of risk assessment approach.

The Love Canal was used in the 1940's and 1950's as a dump site for multiple organic chemical waste products from the manufacture of pesticides. The area immediately surrounding the site was developed in later years as a suburban residential neighborhood. In the process of community development, chemicals leached from the dump into the surrounding neighborhood. In 1978, homes immediately adjoining the dump were evacuated, and corrective drainage and sealing of the site was begun. At that time, about 4,000 persons lived in the general Love Canal area, about 300 of whom lived on the two streets bordering the canal itself.

In the spring of 1978, the New York State Department of Health began a survey focused on these families (2). Since public concern encompassed a wide range of illnesses and since chemical exposures from the canal could not be sharply defined, the survey collected data on a wide range of possible medical problems. For the reasons cited above, central attention was given to pregnancy outcomes. Specifically, information was obtained on interview, and checked by review of medical records, regarding outcomes of all pregnancies experienced by women living on the two streets bordering the canal as of June 1978, from the time of their first residence in the area. Over the following year because of growing local concern, the survey was extended to include women living in the larger residential area east of the canal. Within that larger area, homes were identified by location in relation to natural, prexisting drainage channels or swales in the terrain, since it seemed possible that canal chemicals might migrate preferentially along those swales.

Although the final analysis of the full set of data is not yet complete, interim results are summarized in Table 2. Three kinds of abnormal pregnancy outcome were studied: spontaneous abortion, neonatal birth defects, and low birth weight (under 2,500 grams). Frequencies in each category were measured for women whose home adjoined the canal, women who lived east of the canal, either in proximity to drainage swales or not, and women who lived north of the canal. In the course of analysis, adjustments were made for major maternal risk factors which might influence pregnancy outcome (maternal age and history of smoking, in particular).

Although no consistent patterns were seen, the data were clearly limited by the relatively small numbers of pregnancies involved. While increased rates of spontaneous abortions were recorded for homes near swales and near the canal, the differences, when compared either to homes north of the canal or to abortion rates calculated in the medical literature (3), were of questionable statistical significance. They also did not correspond to environmental chemical test results which showed no significant differences in soil chemical levels east of the canal, regardless of location in relation to swales (4). Although low birth weight frequency was higher for homes near swales, no increase was seen for homes near the canal. No significant differences were seen for birth defects.

For both birth defects and spontaneous abortions, the data were compromised by probable observer bias. Despite efforts to confirm questionnaire responses by checking medical sources, there remains the likelihood that persons living near the canal, or in areas where contamination was believed to be especially likely (i.e., near swales), would report pregnancies, especially abnormal ones, more fully than persons living elsewhere. The only solution to this problem would seem to be either to collect interview data prospectively (an obvious impossiblity when assessment must be done after the fact) or to use existing data somehow collected independently of observer bias or prior to exposure awareness. The data regarding low birth weight meet this requirement, since they were obtained from official birth records, and hence they are the most acceptable from a scientific point of view. Of course, the relatively small number of observations, particularly for persons presumed at highest risk, limits the extent to which they can be interpreted statistically.

TABLE 2

REPRODUCTIVE OUTCOMES IN THE LOVE CANAL AREA FOR WOMEN LIVING THERE AS OF JUNE 1978

	Homes Adjoining the Canal	Neighborhood East of Love Canal — Near Swales	Neighborhood East of Love Canal — Not Near Swales	Neighborhood North of Love Canal
Total Number of Pregnancies	79	108	164	125
Total Number of Live Births	65	83	144	110
Spontaneous Abortions				
Number	15	25	21	11
Percent of Pregnancies	19.0	23.1	12.8	8.8
Birth Defects				
Number	4	10	7	8
Percent of Live Births	6.2	12.0	4.9	7.3
Low Birth Weight Births				
Number	1	13	10	3
Percent of Live Births	1.5	15.7	6.9	2.7

Unfortunately no objective measurements were available by which the cumulative exposure of individual persons to canal chemicals could be objectively assessed. Lacking such measurements, all health studies at Love Canal have depended on indirect exposure judgments such as duration of residence in the area or closeness of homes to the canal or to presumed drainage tracks. Precise health risk assessment under such conditions are obviously very difficult to achieve, particularly when it seems likely that most exposures involved relatively low dose levels.

LIVER FUNCTION TESTS

Frequently, toxic chemical exposures involve materials known to have potential for causing hepatic dysfunction or outright liver disease (including malignancy). It is not uncommon, therefore, for risk assessment efforts to focus on subclinical tests of liver function. Although such tests avoid the problems of observer bias which cloud data derived from questionnaires, they must not be interpreted without strict monitoring of potential hepatotoxic exposures other than the chemical toxin of interest (for instance, history of alcohol ingestion or of recent viral hepatitis) and without examining the adequacy of laboratory methodology. Their application can be illustrated by considering data from two recent environmental health field investigations.

In 1977, a community study was performed in the central Indiana city of Bloomington to assess potential health risks associated with exposure to polychlorinated biphenyls

(PCB), both at an industrial plant which manufactured electrical capacitors and among local residents who had used PCB-containing sewage sludge residues for fertilizing home gardens (5). PCB wastes from the plant had been discharged into city sewage lines resulting in sludge contamination. Measurement of serum PCB levels showed increased values both in plant workers and in members of their immediate families. Values were not increased in persons not employed in the plant, whether or not they used PCB-containing sludge. A battery of serum liver function tests was used to assess the possibility of subclinical liver impairment related to PCB exposure. Among six separate tests employed, positive correlation with serum PCB level was observed only for gamma glutamyl transpeptidase (GGTP). The correlation, however, was shown to be the result of alcohol use since it was not present after excluding subjects with a positive history of alcohol consumption (consumption within 24 hours of serum collection or regular use two or more times a week).

Similar liver function tests were incorporated in a study of residents of the small rural community of Triana in northern Alabama (6). Residents of Triana had for years obtained a substantial proportion of their diet from fish caught in a nearby stream which had also served as a dumping site for waste chemical residues from an industrial plant which had produced DDT pesticides from 1947 through 1971. Both stream sediments and fish living in the stream, sampled in 1979, contained high levels of DDT and its congeners DDE and DDD. Serum obtained at the same time from two residents showed marked elevations in total DDT residues, predominently DDE. These serum elevations correlated significantly with age and with history of local fish consumption.

An extensive survey was conducted to assess potential health effects linked to DDT exposure in this population. The survey included performance of three different serum liver function tests. Although no clinical evidence of DDT-related illness was found, a positive correlation was present between total DDT serum levels and GGTP (correlation coefficient = 0.43). Unlike the Bloomington study, when account was taken of alcohol consumption, GGTP levels were found to correlate independently with DDT levels and with history of alcohol use.

It is not yet possible in the Triana situation to know the clinical significance of the observed correlation with GGTP levels. One must recognize the possibility that the finding may foreshadow later toxin-related hepatic illness, since animal experiments clearly associate both PCB and DDT exposures with liver lesions. However, unlike risk assessments in the Love Canal situation, where individual exposures can only be inferred indirectly, the lipophilic persistence of DDT and PCB in tissue has enabled direct individual comparisons between subclinical observations and serum chemical levels in both Bloomington and Triana.

CYTOGENETIC OBSERVATIONS

Another subclinical approach to risk assessment which has received increasing attention is the use of cytogenetic analysis. It is widely recognized that chromosome changes can be induced through exposure to environmental toxins, both chemicals and ionizing radiation. Experience with this potential measure of biologic damage has been extensive for radiation exposures where frequency of chromosome aberrations in short-term, *in vitro* cultures of peripheral blood lymphocytes is recognized as an accurate reflection of cumulative radiation dose. Data regarding chemical exposures, however, especially in humans, are much more limited and may in fact reflect different mechanisms of cell damage and response than those for radiation exposure. Nonetheless, in both settings, the proposition has been advanced that cytogenetic observations may ultimately be useful as a tool for predicting the health risks of environmental exposure. At present, the major difficulty with this idea is the fact that no direct evidence has yet been developed to show that disease frequencies are in fact generally greater in persons with increased frequencies of chromosomal aberrations than in persons with normal chromosome patterns. Although the idea is supported indirectly by clinical associations between certain disease conditions and chromosome changes, direct evidence is lacking.

Again, the example of Love Canal can be used, since it illustrates the recent application of cytogenetic techniques in an effort to assess biologic risk from environmental exposure. Over the winter of 1981-1982, peripheral blood lymphocytes were obtained for short-term, *in vitro* culture and cytogenetic analysis from 46 residents or former residents of the Love Canal area (8). Part of the study group comprised 29 persons who had been living in 1978 in homes directly adjoining the canal itself and in whose homes, at that time, elevated levels of canal-related chemicals had been detected in basement air. Although all of these 29 persons had moved away from the area when their homes were evacuated in 1978, they were considered to represent a group of canal-area residents most likely to have received maximal home-exposure to canal chemicals as confirmed both by the proximity of their homes to the canal and by objective chemical measurement.

The remaining 17 persons were current or former residents of the area east of the canal. Each had undergone cytogenetic analysis on a volunteer basis in 1979. Those analysis were part of a pilot study which was interpreted by some as suggesting increased chromosome damage, largely on the basis of finding large acentric chromosome forms in certain specimens. The 1981 study was partly undertaken to re-examine that earlier cytogenetic suggestion. Peripheral blood specimens from Love Canal participants were interspersed with specimens from 44 matched control participants living about a mile west of Love Canal in a census tract with demographic features similar to those of the census tract containing Love Canal.

Cytogenetic analyses were performed jointly by the Brookhaven National Laboratory in New York and the Oak Ridge National Laboratory in Tennessee. Duplicate specimens were included so that reproducibility of laboratory results could be assessed both between the two laboratories and among individual technologists within each laboratory. Two hundred cells per specimen were scored for frequency of chromosome abberrations and 50 for frequency of sister chromatid exchange (SCE). Work on the study required major effort in both laboratories for more than six months.

Results of analyses (Table 3) showed no statistically significant differences between the Love Canal and control groups, either for various categories of chromosome aberration or for SCE. Measurements of SCE were sufficiently powerful in the study to detect a previously-reported assocation between current cigarette smoking and increased SCE frequency. Inter- and intra- laboratory differences in analytic results seemed no greater than are generally expected in such complex microscopic work.

In addition to technologic laboratory difficulties, time requirements, and cost, this particular study illustrates several important limitations which can be expected in assessments of this sort. First, because of limits in cost, time, and laboratory facilities, the study was necessarily restricted to a relatively small number of specimens. Were it possible to do such work more quickly and cheaply, a greater array of analytic comparisons might have been possible.

TABLE 3

CYTOGENETIC FINDINGS IN PERIPHERAL BLOOD LYMPHOCYTES FROM CURRENT OR FORMER RESIDENTS OF THE LOVE CANAL NEIGHBORHOOD AND FROM RESIDENTS OF A CONTROL NEIGHBORHOOD IN NIAGARA FALLS, NEW YORK, 1981-1982

Cytogenetic Findings*	Love Canal Neighborhood No.	Mean ± 1 SD**	Control Neighborhood No.	Mean ± 1 SD	P Value
Achromatic lesions	45	7.84 ± 3.22	44	7.77 ± 3.69	0.67
Chromatid deletions	45	0.98 ± 0.61	44	1.28 ± 0.72	0.06
Isochromatid deletions	45	0.92 ± 0.74	44	0.97 ± 1.00	0.86
Chromatid exchanges	45	0.08 ± 0.18	44	0.07 ± 0.17	1.00
Rings	45	0.04 ± 0.13	44	0.03 ± 0.16	0.48
Dicentrics	45	0.39 ± 0.59	44	0.28 ± 0.43	0.32
Supernumerary acentrics	45	0.15 ± 0.36	44	0.27 ± 0.50	0.18
Sister chromatid exchanges (SCE)***	46	8.48 ± 1.24	42	8.75 ± 1.02	0.23

*Number of aberrations per 100 cells (except SCE).
**Standard deviation.
***Number of SCEs per cell.

Second, as stated earlier, since the toxic chemicals of prime concern (chlorobenzene, etc.) are largely non-persistent in tissue or blood, no objective measures of individual exposure were available in the Love Canal situation. To make matters more difficult, observations in the Love Canal cytogenetic study were severely retrospective, being made more than three years after remedial drainage and containment of the canal site was begun. This means that in order to interpret the study's results one must either accept the idea that active exposure was not recent enough to produce discernible chromosome effects (in which case the study results would be falsely negative) or one must postulate that chemically-induced chromosome changes, like those caused by ionizing radiation, persist for at least several years and were not detected in the Love Canal setting because increased chemical exposure was small or negligible.

SUMMARY

The use of human biologic observations in assessing risk of illness after exposure to environmental chemical toxins is still largely limited to high-dose, short-latency acute illness problems. For the more common issue of chronic, long-latency diseases such as cancer, risk assessment continues to depend upon indirect extrapolation from experimental observations *in vitro* or in non-human species. Although it is appropriate to study frequencies of biologic events such as abnormal pregnancy outcomes, chromosomal changes, and abnormal liver function in populations with increased exposure to environmental toxins, no direct evidence yet exists regarding how such "biologic markers" may relate to later risk of human illness. Studies using such approaches must pay close attention to population size, data collection biases, and competing risk variables. They also should be used with particular caution where direct measurements of individual toxic dose are lacking and where work must therefore rely on less satisfactory definitions of population exposure.

REFERENCES

1. *Heath, C. W., Jr.*: Field epidemiologic studies of populations exposed to waste dumps. *Envir. Health Perspect., 48*:3, 1983.

2. *Vianna, N. J.*: Adverse pregnancy outcome - potential end points of human toxicity in the Love Canal. Preliminary results. In Porter, I. H., and Hook, E. B. (Eds.): *Human Embryonic and Fetal Death.* New York, Academic Press, 1980, p. 165.

3. *Warburton, D., and Fraser, F. C.*: Spontaneous abortion risks in man: Data from reproductive histories collected in a medical genetics unit. *Amer. J. Hum. Genet., 16*:1, 1963.

4. *Kim, C. S., Narang, R., Richards, A., et al.*: Love Canal: chemical contamination and migration. In: *Proceedings of the National Conference on Management of Uncontrolled Hazardous Waste Sites.* Environmental Protection Agency, 1980, p. 212.

5. *Baker, E. L., Jr., Landrigan, P. L., Glueck, C. J., et al.*: Metabolic consequences of exposure to polychlorinated biphenyls (PCB) in sewage sludge. *Amer. J. Epidemiol., 112*:553, 1980.

6. *Kreiss, K., Zack, M. M., Kimbrough, R. D., et al.*: Cross-sectional study of a community with exceptional exposure to DDT. *J. Amer. Med. Assoc. 245*:1926, 1981.

7. *Bloom, A. D.(Ed.)*: *Guidelines for Studies of Human Populations Exposed to Mutagenic and Reproductive Hazards.* New York, March of Dimes Birth Defects Foundation, 1981.

8. *Heath, C. W. Jr., Nadel, M. R., Zack, M. M. Jr., et al.*: Cytogenetic findings in persons living near the Love Canal, *J. Amer. Med. Assoc. 251*:1437, 1984.

9. *Picciano, D.*: Pilot cytogenetic study of the residents living near Love Canal, a hazardous waste site. *Mammalian Chromosome Newsletter, 21*:86, 1980.

Panel Discussion

Section Editor: T. L. Blank

New Approaches in Toxicity Testing and Their Application in Human Risk Assessment, edited by A. P. Li. Raven Press, New York © 1985.

Panel Discussion: New Approaches in Toxicity Testing and Their Application in Human Risk Assessment

Leon Golberg: The first question that I've received relates to the issue of thresholds, and I think it might be probably directed to Dr. Downs. It is as follows: Is threshold important in risk assessment? Is the determination of the existence of threshold the province of biologists, chemists or statisticians? Associated with that is the question, what dose a zero threshold mean in terms of common thermodynamic measures, for example free energy and entropy? The question points out that there are at least four threshold models in the literature such as those of Cornfield, that he published in Science, Potter and Finnemore, Schaeffer and some name that I can't read and Potter and Wienberg in an Oak Ridge National Lab publication discussing the distribution of individual thresholds. May we start with the threshold question.

Tom Downs: Is the question of thresholds important? Yes, I think it is. Is it practicable to determine, numerically, the value of a threshold for a particular substance? No, it isn't. No amount of experimentation will ever determine whether or not you may have missed somebody that had a lower threshold. Whose province is it? Well, it's certainly not a statistician's, but I would say that is a population of individuals each have their own individual thresholds and they're below which the probability of getting cancer increases with dose, then the average of all those such curves over a population will be a convex downward curve. You can prove this. As to the last question, that definitely is not a statistican's province.

Leon Golberg: Just speaking from my own experience, I was a member of the Scientific Committee of the Food Safety Council and on that Committee we were very privileged to have Dr. Cornfield, and Dr. Van Ryzin. We spent years trying to avoid having to talk in terms of thresholds. The Board of the Food Safety Council took all our labors and immediately scrapped the idea, introduced the threshold concept, the safety factor concept and published it in that form. So it seems that perhaps from a practical point of view there is still a tendency to adhere to the old approaches. We were hoping that with the use of mathematical models the issue of population thresholds would become irrelevant.

Tom Downs: I had hoped so, too. I might add that in a paper by Prof. Cornfield, he dealt with the issue of no observable effect levels. A no observable effect level is primarily a funtion of the sample size used. You would have to have a sample of size one-thousand to be reasonably sure of detecting something which affects a one-threehundredth or one out of three hundred of the population. The no observable effect level is fine for diseases other than cancer, I would say.

Brock Neely: How does a drug company deal with the use of developing a new drug and establishing a dose for humans? It seems to me, that boasts to what a threshold is. That is, somehow or other, establish that a certain dose is going to have an effect or a certain dose will not have an adverse effect. Do they deal with that statistically?

Tom Downs: I know they try it out on animals first. I'm no expert on that. I'd rather pass that question to somebody else.

Leon Golberg: Would anybody in the audience like to commment on that question of thresholds and decisions on drug use in man. If not, we will pass on to a question for Dr. Neely. Dole and Peto estimate that about 5 percent of cancers are due to "the environment" such as air and water. Assuming that this estimate is approximatley correct, to what extent should environmental regulatory agencies impose new requirements or establish elaborate toxicology programs for this purpose. For the purpose of dealing with this 5 percent of cancers due to environment.

Brock Neely: It strikes me that if we are really serious about wanting to control the level of cancer we should institute a very active program to cut down the frequency of smoking. Until we really get at that problem I don't think we are going to change the statistics of cancer very much.

William Gaffey: One brief comment, if I'm not mistaken the figure is not 5 percent. I think their point estimate is 2 and the range is one to five. So the problem, although there isn't that much difference between two and five, is perhaps not even as big as has been suggested.

Leon Golberg: I have here another question that indirectly deals with threshold, but I think it is just a conceptual one. The recent advances in molecular biology concerning oncogenes have been astounding. Has there been any formal attempt within the field of toxicology to see if these concepts can be used on a theoretical or practical level in risk assessment and testing? Relevant concerns would be the contribution of these ideas to the possibility of establishing a threshold and the shape of the dose reponse curve at low doses. As Dr. Butterworth knows we tried to set up a meeting dealing with oncogenes and their potential contribution to present day toxicology. But, we really didn't think the time was right to be able to deal with that effectively.

I have another question here which poses an experimental situation in which a Compound A was found to produce cancer in rats. It was found to be metabolized to three metabolites X, Y and Z, of which metabolite X binds to DNA. How do we assess the risk to humans of compound A under those conditions?

Robert Lutz: I guess the answer, again, given my perspective on the problem would be in the extrapolation question again. To determine in the human being how much compound X is manufactured by the humans based on a given doses of the initial Compound A whatever it was. That can be done in a quantitative sense if you have some ideas of some of the rates of metabolism. That is a quantitative answer in the sense that it could tell you how much of compound X exists in the human but whether that same quantity is going to be effective as a carcinogen in the human involves a lot of biochemistry that I am afraid I cannot answer.

William Gaffey: I think one of the other things one would almost have to do is to see if there is a group of people with exposure to the substance and actually look at them. Even if you don't find anything I think you are obligated to look if the possibility exists for that kind of observation.

Leon Golberg: Perhaps look for the metabolite X by some of these sophisticated means we have been talking about.

William Gaffey: That would also be a possibility, yes.

Leon Golberg: I'd like to ask a question of Dr. Anderson. This has to do with the latest IRDC study on saccharin. In the course of which, it was re-established that saccharin at high doses produces a very beautiful dose-reponse relationship with regard to bladder cancer in rats. But among the experimental groups there was one in which the saccharin exposure was begun immediately postnatally by giving the saccharin to the mother and then as the pups began to consume food giving them the saccharin at high doses. An interesting thing was that in the final outcome those results were indistinguishable from the cancers produced starting by in-utero exposure. I wonder to what extent that might be found to be a more general phenonmenon, if one did enough detail work of this sort, so that one might ultimately avoid the in-utero exposure in testing. That is the way that the FDA expects you to do in food additives.

Lucy Anderson: Your question is whether immediate post-natal exposure could replace in-utero exposure for risk assessment tests.

Leon Golberg: We are talking now about food additives not necessarily alkylating agents like ethylnitrosourea.

Lucy Anderson: I understand. This idea has been proposed by others as well. It seems to me personally, and this is a personal opinion and not one which necessarily reflects any NCI policies, this is a rather good idea in some circumstances. It is not always practical to do a total life exposure study, even though I recommended it yesterday, starting with preconception and moving through gestation and so forth. There are a lot of problems with this, statistical as well as biological. There may be situations where because of the economics of it, the numbers of chemicals that need to be dealt with, so on and so forth, that beginning with birth will be a pretty good substitute. The perinatal or immediate postnatal animal is probably just as sensitive, and perhaps more so in some cases, because it doesn't have the benefits of maternal and placental protection from the chemical that it did in-utero and there are examples that can be given for this. I think it is a possibility that ought to be considered but it would need to be validated with additional experimentation of a sort that you have just described for saccharin.

Leon Golberg: I believe Dr. Homberger has a question for us.

Freddie Homberger: I wondered whether any of you believe that in the foreseeable future, let's say one or two generations, the establishment of safety of chemicals can ever be done by means of *in vitro* short term tests along. If you do not believe so, how do you think that the current unsatisfactory *in vivo* bioassays could be improved.

William Gaffey: It might be easy for me to answer because I don't really know what I'm talking about. It seems to me that our biggest problem is to improve the generalizability of the classical *in vivo* toxicology study and that probably the more we learn about metabolic pathways of different things the better off we'll be. The weaknesses of our generalizations now are simply weaknesses in our ability to determine what a real dose response relationship is because we don't know enough to characterize the true dose. People are beginning to learn now about all the interesting things that really go on in living organism. That can be, I think, a tremendously complicated series of jobs for all the possible substances one could think of. I think that is the way to make toxicology more generalizable. I think that may well happen. It will make people like me suitably modest when I talk about toxicologists next time.

Leon Golberg: I feel very strongly that the long term tests have a long way to go before they are perfected. The process is going on and there is a special committee been appointed by Dr. Rall to look into all this. If we can apply some of the principles of pharmacokinetics and metabolism that are available, I think the tests can be greatly improved. I feel we should not give up at this point, but press on and try to bring about these major improvements as soon as possible. In order that the money used in the bioassays is well applied and fruitfully employed.

Tom Downs: With regard to the bioassays, I would like to add that NCI is considering re-designing these assays perhaps with different numbers of animals in the various dose groups. Currently, they have the same number in each group. I would like to see it where besides the maximum tolerated dose (MTD) and a half or a fourth of it they were to use, that middle dose group with a much smaller dose, maybe one-tenth the MTD be used. I think preferably the choice should be guided by pharmacokinetic considerations and to check with data from the bioassay of what you think is going on pharmacokinetically.

Brock Neely: It seems to me we should be able to learn more from the drug agency because they have a wealth of experience in extrapolating from animal data to human. We can some how or other make some generalizations about chemical structure that is used for all these drugs and how they are metabolized in humans. I don't know if there is any work going on in that area or not.

Leon Goldberg: Does anyone feel capable of responding to that? Is there no one from the drug industry here?

Freddie Homberger: If nobody responds, I would like to make a comment because I really asked the question hoping that it would bring out some uncertain tests and uncertain parameters. I do believe that we need to improve not only our knowledge of the pharmacokinetics and metabolism, but also our ability to detect the induced-tumors, earlier by markers: chemical markers, as well as by imaging techniques. We should also subject species other than mouse, hamster and rat to studies of metabolic mechanisms for standard groups of compounds. I don't see or I couldn't find among the other potential species, such as gerbils, chipmunks, squirrels and numerous other possible animals that the classic organisms and so forth, models that could fit much better. Human metabolic processes are now available in my laboratory.

Brock Neely: That is why we use the monkey. They are supposed to simulate man pretty well.

Freddie Homberger: You have some limitations of course with the very offensive animals such as monkeys, dogs, horses, so forth. I don't believe we have exploited a regular approach with the potential of the other scale of animals.

Brock Neely: The field of comparative biochemistry is going to become more and more important.

Freddie Homberger: I gain more and more respect for it every day.

Brock Neely: You do have a problem of scale-up.

David Schaeffer: I have a question to anybody. Is there any sort of good data base of toxicologic dose response information related to human beings? Any endpoint? When you want to do extrapolation from species to species what do you use to appropriately measure human beings?

Leon Goldberg: There have been dose response curves for smoking and numbers of cigarettes. Dr. Bridges published a paper with regard to puyar therapy using soralun and ultraviolet light. There isn't a great deal.

Brock Neely: Radiation I would suspect would be one.

Tom Downs: There is a lot of haggling about the doses that the people in Japan have been exposed to as a result of the atomic bombs. One of our students is the statistician for that and he is re-doing all of what were the previous estimated doses. This is all going to be redone, so that is by no means clear cut. As with most epidemilogic data, actual doses are a real problem.

Leon Golberg: I had a question for Dr. Boyd, but unfortunately he is not with us, but I will mention it just the same. I've been struck by the increasing amount of information and evidence of damage to the olfactory epithelium that is being produced with a wide variety of compounds. At one time one was conscious that hexamethylphosphoramide and a few other things could do severe damage to the olfactory epithelium and go on to produce tumors. I at least was not conscious of the fact that severe damage can occur with a great many compounds such as dimethylamine, methacrylates of various sorts and so on. Is anyone in the audience able to comment on this? Is it just that we've never looked hard enough at the olfactory neuroepithelium and gone into it in sufficient detail. The sort of damage that is being seen is pretty gross and is being picked up in matter of hours after exposure. Of course, in the past, people haven't looked there in any considerable detail.

(Reponse to this question could not be heard - William Ribelin was talking.)

Leon Golberg: Of course that is one problem. One can't do human biopsies up there. One can do biopsies of the respiratory epithelium fairly readily and these have been done, of course, in many instances. However, olfactory epithelium is a little more difficult.

Leon Golberg: Dr. Butterworth, you know I am a great supporter of what you have been doing but I haven't noticed it being taken up with any great avidity by the rest of the genotoxicity community. Do you think this is just conservatism or is it actually being taken up and we're just not aware of it?

Byron Butterworth: A few people have. But like they said yesterday, in many instances, for various reasons the Ames test is the only thing that ever gets around. Often times if you are voluntarily testing something and you get a negative in the Ames tests, that's it, you don't go any further than that. I think that the more advanced laboratories, those that are really concerned, are beinning to do it. We get inquiries all the time. I know the people here at Monsanto and those at DuPont are starting it up. I think there is just a little lag time between development and actually getting it applied.

Leon Golberg: Talking of the Ames test, I was absolutely staggered by some people who have got the computer program from Joyce McCann that tells you whether your Ames test results are significant or not. I have always thought that rule of thumb of twice the number of revertants was a pretty sound way of judging, but this computer program comes out with positive results that baffle the imagination. The differences are so small. I wondered whether anyone has had experience of trying to judge the results of Ames tests by that or other computer programs. Maybe it wasn't functioning properly.

Larry Kier: We have used a number of statistical programs to analyze Salmonella results. I think we have to distinguish between biological significance and statistical significance. If you get enough data you can get a response which is reproducible and much less than two-fold background. We have done that. However, the original two-fold rule, I believe, was intended to indicate biological significance.

Leon Golberg: Probably the same as the rule that you never do Ames tests on Thursday.

Larry Kier: We do at Monsanto because I occasionally come in on weekends.

Steven Lewis: I'm struck by the lack of notice or lack of attention given to one more dimension of uncertainty in all of these considerations, particularly as it relates to metabolism and pharmacokinetics. That is, there are some of us who are unlucky enough to work with materials that are complex mixtures. I offer you unleaded gasoline, Dr. Goldberg, as an example. Where the relevance of molecular mechanisms of action and pharmacokinetics begin to take on rather bizzare, arcane and most of the time irrelevant reference. Do any of you believe there is opportunity to apply metabolism studies and pharmacokinetics in the toxicologic profile for complex mixtures?

Brock Neely: It seems to me that you have the same problem there that people have had with the PCBs being a complex mixture. You almost have to look at it piece by piece to look at the different homologs. When you do that you begin to notice major differences between the various isomers. I suspect it would be the same thing with gasoline. I don't see how you can treat it as a entity. You have to break it down.

Al Li: I have worked with complex mixtures. There are thousands of chemicals in, for instance, diesel exhaust emission. I don't think it is practical to test every single component of such a complex mixture.

Leon Golberg: The alternative is to decide on a particular compound which may not even be part of that mixture as being sufficiently representative. I think perhaps decoline, in the case that you referred to might be regarded as a prototype in the case of the renal toxicity. Of course studies on that compound are going on right now. I have a similar problem that might be given some thought. Are we ever going to make progress in some of these difficult issues in toxicology that have been with us for half a century? This one refers to the question of the relationship of bladder stones and bladder cancer. Of course we have been over that. There has been some brilliant work involving putting glass beads into the bladder and getting bladder cancer in the rat. The fact is that melamine was studied by the NTP. Great masses of melamine stones were found in the bladder, as well as bladder cancer. The conclusion of the NTP was that you couldn't completely exclude the possibility that the melamine contributed to the bladder cancer quite separately and distinctly from any effect that the bladder stones may have had. It was pronounced a carcinogen. It so happens that Ciba-Geigy has a larvicide that is fed to chickens and produces melamine in the feces and thereby enables the intensive culture of chickens without an accompanying mass of flies. I think that is a very valuable product from a social-economc point of view. That has now been banned by the FDA, under the Delaney clause, because melamine is a carcinogen. This merely goes to indicate how the ramifications, for what I think is a fundamentally wrong decision, just keep on and have such decisions in the past. They have been upheld by the courts, and yet there seems to be this very distinct relationship between stones and bladder cancer in the rat. I think most of the scientific community accept that, but in any given instance, there is that element of uncertainty as to whether we can totally ignore those bladder cancers just because a mass of stones was present. I don't know if anyone would like to comment on that, but I find it rather sad in that toxicologists simply cannot get over a hurdle like that.

Jim Stevens: I work for Ciba-Geigy. First of all, it is not banned by the FDA. It is controlled and regulated under the EPA and essentially the action taken was the suspension of Section 18 which is emergency use of the product before it is registered. It is under consideration at the EPA, as to whether it is a real problem and the registration of this product will be considered. Risk extrapolation was done for melamine as a metabolites of Larvade and the highest level risk obtained was 1 in 10 million. Numbers in the order of Avogradro's number were higher were also seen with different models. We have applied the standard risk assessment model and have not seen a problem.

Leon Golberg: It raises the question why the Delaney clause should be invoked. If there is a trace of melamine detectable in the flesh of the chickens, then the Delaney clause would apply irrespective of what numbers your risk assessment arrived at.

Jim Stevens: That is correct and that is the issue we have to deal with, significant risk or not, as long as the Delaney clause stands there is potential for a ban as well. It is still under regulatory action as to whether melamine should be completely banned or eliminated. The FDA position on melamine is that it is not a carcinogen and they are as my understanding in opposition to the NTP.

Richard Albertini: Furthermore it is negative in short term tests.

Leon Goldberg: That point needs to be stressed that it is not genotoxic.

Jim Stevens: There is more data available at lower doses which do not show an oncogenic response.

Leon Golberg: I know that American Cyanamide sponsored a study using a technique that was developed by Dr. Heck at CIIT in connection with thilthalic acid. The material was fed immediately post-natally and within the matter of a few weeks the bladders of the neonates were absolutely solidly packed with stones. In the case of melamine it was really dramatic what happened. Material that has that propensity surely cannot be regarded as constituting a hazard at these very very low environmental levels.

Brock Neely: I have a question I would like to ask Dr. Heath. With a little fear and intrepidation I do. I can't let a guy from CDC leave without asking about agent orange and dioxin. Does he has any comments on agent orange and the massive studies that are going on with the Viet Nam veterans.

Clark Heath: Basically I do not have any comments. But you're right there is a massive study going on. There are actually two studies. One much more massive than the other. The more massive one hasn't yet started. There is a large case control study being carried out with respect to reproductive outcomes. Looking at babies with birth defects and babies without born in the Atlanta area, with respect to father's service in Viet Nam. This is a unique study from a epidemiologists stand point because it utilizes many more cases than controls so such is the sample size. That study is partly directed to the question of agent orange, but since the question of the dose that men might have received in Viet Nam is difficult to approach, the study realistically approaches rather the question of service in Viet Nam or not. The larger study is the one which the veteran's administration had been developing over the last several years with the help of outside advice. It was to be in some form a follow-up of some large group of veterans in a comparison manner. The structure of that study is not yet clear but it would have to be a very large and highly expensive study. I can't really comment on where that stands. All of this of course is very much in the public eye and is a very complex social issue. It may be an unapproachable scientific issues.

Leon Golberg: I'd like to ask Dr. Julian Preston to give us his views on the use of SCEs as an index of genotoxicity. There is alot of loose talk whenever a controversial issue arises about a particular compound. If it is known that it is capable of producing SCEs that is immediately jumped on as evidence that it is genotoxic. What is your view about extrapolation to health effects as distinct from simply an indicator of exposure?

Julian Preston: There are several parts to the question. As I indicated yesterday, just to identify an increase in sister chromatid exchanges, if you have done the experiment correctly and you have only one real variable in a group of control individuals or unexposed individuals and exposed individuals, if the only variable is the agent you're interested in and you can show an increase in sister chromatid exchanges you can declare there has probably been an exposure to that agent. The dose response curve, if you could get such a dose response curve, for which there are some indications with ethylene oxide there might be a dose response curve in humans, but the dose ranges for any individual are rather large and the SCE frequency is very rounded. There is an indication of a dose response curve. If you can get a dose response curve it is not directly related to the exposure. As I pointed out it will be indirectly related to the exposure because of the timing of the production of the sister chromatid exchanges. The time of sampling of individuals after an exposure, if it is an acute exposure, or even for chronic exposures will influence the dose response curve. Then we get the problem what do you do with those data. The thing is there is no known effect, other biological effect, associated directly with increases in sister chromatid exchanges. There are implied relationships between increases in SCE's and increases in mutations, specifically locus mutations to work with. Carrano and others at Livermore indicated a relationship. They found straight line relationships if you plot SCE's on one axis against mutations on the other axis. The thing is you almost inevitably will get straight lines because SCE dose response curves are linear and mutation dose response curves are linear so if you plot one against the other you are going to get linear relationships. It is the question of where the position of the relationship is. For some agents you get no increases in SCE but increases in mutation. Radiation is the classic case. In others you can get increases in mutation and no increases in sister chromatid exchange. Neocarcinostatin is a classic example of that. There are unusual relationships. There might be a relationship. It's not been established, so in terms of an increase in SCEs and subsequent adverse health effects there is no relationship at this point so you cannot use the data. At this point you can use SCE data for indicating on a group level, not an individual level, whether or not there has been an exposure. Not the size of that and no subsequent adverse health effects.

Leon Golberg: Thank you. That is valuable clarification.

David Schaffer: Would someone care to comment about experiments which seem to indicate protective effects. For example, Salsberg has been publishing several papers where he has re-analyzed the National Cancer Institute studies and his belief is that several of those studies which suggest that the animals that were exposed had higher survivability than the animals that we used as controls. Thereby, indicating a protective effect. Would anyone care to comment on how toxicology should handle such data?

Leon Golberg: Some statistican (I can't remember who it was) has suggested that these are more apparent than real.

David Schaffer: The dilema is that we are willing to take a 5 percent if it goes in the direction that we believe it should go, then it should show an effect. What about the 5 percent in the other direction showing better condition of the treated versus the untreated.

Leon Golberg: Sometimes they are far more dramatic than that.

Tom Downs: There was a recent article, I forget the exact journal right now, he had looked at some 25 recent studies, NCI bioassays, and for half of them I think there were significant lowering of spontaneous (tumor) rates on some sites and significant raising of spontaneous (tumor) rates on other sites. This author also pointed out that there was an increase in longevity in the dosed groups in some cases. Maybe you should look at the other side of the coin and select the most favorable site for the most favorable sex and for the most favorable species and you might see things differently. There is a problem with the statistical analysis that when you do this, the sample sizes are a limiting factor in the quality and sophistication of the statistical analysis. It is certainly worthwhile and I'd like to see more things done in that area.

David Schaffer: I think that the subjective bias of the statistician introduces is that generally they use one-sided tests and it is always the upper one-sided test.

Tom Downs: That is another bone of contention of mine, too. It would help if you did it this way, look at the most favorable site, as well as the worst one. This would tend to get rid of such biases. You would be forced to use two-sided tests then. I think this is appropriate. If that bothers you, then you can raise the alpha level.

David Schaffer: The comment referred to specific animal tests. If the same sort of comment is likely to be true with some of the genetic screening tests, that is that you can observe protective effects and maybe these need to be accounted for.

Leon Golberg: Anti-mutagens have been described of course by a number of authors, but I don't know that we have incorporated that into our thinking. There was a striking example of antagonism of this sort published by Culter and Walkeny in which they used ethylnitrosourea as transplacentally producing brain tumors in rats. They found if they gave methy-S-oxy methanol immediately before the ethylnitrosourea they virtually wiped out the neurogenic tumors that results. While methy-S-oxy methanol by itself produces a substantial yield of neurogenic tumors. Would Dr. Anderson like to comment on that?

Lucy Anderson: Actually I would like to comment on several of these points. With regard to the reduction in tumor rate in the animals. First the investigator would look at the food consumption and the weight gain. If these had been suppressed the chemicals then you suspect that there is a general effect which is not particularly related to the chemical of interest and you can sort of write if off. If that hasn't occurred, then the compound seems to be of interest as a protective agent and ought to be pursued further in that regard for a quite a different reason than you started with nevertheless of great interest. With regard to Dr. Down's point about the sensitive animals I take some flack about this from time to time because I use the mouse lung tumor a lot. I think the point could be made, at least for purposes of argument, that the people that get the cancers are the ones that are the most sensitive to whatever the causative agent is. The organ in which they get it is the organ that is the most sensitive to this causative agent. There is a reason to use these sensitive models that nature has provided for us that they may be quite relevant to the human causation process.

Leon Golberg: There may also be factors determining localization. There was a beautiful experiment published from a dental school in Science not long ago in which they gave ethyl nitrosourea parenterally and then applied a piece of sharp wire around various teeth. Wherever the wire caused local damage to the buccal mucosa that is where the cancer resulted from the ethyl nitrosourea.

Freddie Homberger: I'd like to add to the discussion of long survival in treated animals. In our experience every lifetime feeding study that we have conducted with the Syrian hamster regardless of the nature of the compound, treated animals had significantly increased survival times. About a dozen of these studies have been done.

Leon Golberg: There certainly are occasions when the compound obviously has protective action against bacteria, for example with the benzylacetate study. The benzyl alcohol formed, protected against intercurrent disease and all kinds of things like that and caused much better survival.

Subject Index

Subject Index

A

AAF, *see* 2-Acetylaminofluorene
Abnormal pregnancy, environmental risk assessment and, 254–256
2-Acetylaminofluorene, 35
Adaptive repair, in kinetic models, 232
AFP, *see* α-Fetoprotein
Alkylated derivatives, in hemoglobin and urine, 8
Alkylation, and repair of intracellular macromolecules, 6–7
Ames test, 33–34
Anchorage independence, 28,29,99
Anchorage independent transformed human fibroblasts, 27
Antigen distribution, monocyte-macrophage phagocytosis and, 173–174
1-β-D-Arabinofuranosylcytosine, 135,136; *see also* Cytosine arabinoside
Arene oxide, 115
Atopy, 6

B

BaP, *see* Benzo(a)pyrene
Benzene, in Unit World model, 241
Benzo(a)pyrene
 in antibody response, 168
 in DTH response, 171
 in transplacental carcinogenesis, 186,190,191
3,4-Benzopyrene, metabolic cooperation and, 83
Betapropiolactone, in DCB test, 94–95
BHT, *see* Butylated hydroxytoluene
Biological model, in quantitative risk assessment, 129
Biotransformation of chemicals, 105–107
Bladder stones and bladder cancer, 268–269
Blood flow, time-scaling of, 138–141
Blood flow limitation, 136–137
BP, *see* 3,4-Benzopyrene
BPDE, *see* 7,8-Diol-9,10-epoxide of benzo(a)pyrene
Butylated hydroxytoluene, 81–82

C

Cancer
 bladder stones and bladder cancer, 268–269
 environmental risk assessment and, 263–264
 pharmacokinetic models in risk assessment and, 145–146
Carbon tetrachloride, 100
Carcinoembryonic antigen, 68
Carcinogen-metabolizing enzymes, and tumorigenesis, 186
Carcinogenesis, as problem of local intercellular communication, 80
Carcinogenetic chemicals, and formalin-treated cells, 93–96
Carcinogenicity determination, human cells in, 17–29
Carcinogens; *see also* Environmental carcinogens
 cytotoxic effect of, 18–21
 mutagenic effect of, 21–24
4-CBP, *see* 4-Chlorobiphenyl
Cell free homogenate preparations, validity of, 160
Cell-mediated immunocompetence, assessment of, 169
Chemical-induced immunomodulation, 213–220
 DEM in, 216
 DES in, 216,220
 DMN in, 219,220
 host resistance assays, 214–215
 immune function assays, 215
Chemically-induced DNA repair, 35–38
 in human bronchial epithelium, 37
 in human hepatocytes, 36
 in rat alveolar macrophages, 38
 in rat hepatocytes, 35–36
 in rat nasal epithelium, 37
 in rat spermatocytes, 38
 in rat tracheal epithelium, 36–37
Chemicals, establishing safety of, 265
Childhood cancer, and transplacental carcinogenesis, 181
Chlordecone, *see* Kepone
Chlorine, in hexachlorobiphenyls, 107
Chlorobenzene inhalation pharmacokinetics, 151–157
 analysis of variance in, 152
 dose dependent decrease and, 147
 elimination kinetics in, 155,156
 excretion in, 153–154,156,157
 multiple versus single exposure regimen and, 157
 tissue burdens in, 153,156,157
 urinary metabolites and, 155–157
4-Chlorobiphenyl, 84
Chlorodeoxyuridine, 48

SUBJECT INDEX

Chloroform, 100
Clonal efficiencies, 56–58
Cloned T-lymphocytes, 59–61
Comparative biochemistry, 266
Complex mixtures, toxicologic profile for, 267–268
Covalent binding
  metabolic activation and, 120–121
  of PCB-equivalents, 112
  of radioactive material, 121
Cryopreservation, 55
Cysteine, 159
Cytochrome P450, 159, 208
Cytogenic endpoints, in human lymphocytes, 41–48; see also Lymphocyte assays
Cytolytic killer cell activity, assessment of, 171–172
Cytosine arabinoside, 47–48

D

DCB, see DNA-cell binding assay
4-DCB, see 4,4'-Dichlorobiphenyl
DEHP, see Di(2-ethylhexyl) phthalate
Delaney clause, 268
Delayed-type hypersensitivity, 169
  measurement of, 170–171
DES, see Diethylstilbestrol
Desmethylminsonidazole, pharmacokinetic model of, 137–138
Di(2-ethylhexyl) phthalate, 100
  metabolic cooperation and, 84
4,4'-Dichlorobiphenyl
  HPLC analysis of, 111
  metabolism of, in vitro versus in vivo results in, 113, 115
  metabolites of, 111
  as model for metabolism of PCBs, 109–110
Diethylstilbestrol
  in antibody response, 168
  in chemical-induced immunomodulation, 216, 220
  transplacental carcinogenic effect of, 180
  vaginal carcinoma and, 179–180
Dihydrofolate reductase, 134
7,12-Dimethyl-benz(a)anthracene, 70
  in transplacental carcinogenesis, 183, 186, 189, 191
1,2-Dimethylhydrazine, 70
Dimethylnitrosamine, 35, 171
  in antibody response, 168
  in chemical-induced immunomodulation, 219, 220
  in transplacental carcinogenesis, 182, 188, 190
Dimethylsulfoxide, metabolic cooperation and, 84–85
1,6-Dinitropyrene, 36
7,8-Diol-9,10-epoxide of benzo(a)pyrene, 21, 22
Diphtheria toxin, resistance to, 21
Diphtheria toxin resistant human T-lymphocytes, 59
Diploid human cells, neoplastic transformation of, 17
Diploid human fibroblasts, neoplastic transformation and, 26–27
Direct mutagenicity testing, definition of, 51
DMBA, see 7,12-Dimethyl-benz(a)anthracene
DMH, see 1,2-Dimethylhydrazine
DMN, see Dimethylnitrosamine
DMSO, see Dimethylsulfoxide
DNA
  neoplastic transformation and, 27–29
  UV-induced damage to, 18
DNA adducts, detecting, 9
DNA-cell binding assay, 93–96
DNA excision repair, 18
DNA methylation, 6–7
DNA repair, chemically-induced, see Chemically-induced DNA repair
DNA synthesis, 24–26, 29
DNP, see 1,6-Dinitropyrene
Dose-response models, 227–232, 235
  common dose-response models, 228–230
  dose units, 227–228
  kinetic models, 230–232
Dose-response risk assessment model, 129–130
Dose-response test sensitivities, 61
Drug metabolizing enzyme systems, 119–126
Drug-metabolizing enzymes, metabolic activation and, 120
DT, see Diphtheria toxin
DTH, see Delayed-type hypersensitivity

E

Endogenous N-nitrosation, measurement of, 7–8
ENU, see Ethylnitrosourea
Environmental carcinogens, 67–75
  retrogenetic expression by animals with cancer, 69–74
  retrogenetic expression by humans with cancer, 74
  retrogenetic expression of, 68–69
Environmental distribution and fate, 235–244
  models for estimating, 237–244
Environmental risk assessment, 253–260
  abnormal pregnancy and, 254–256
  cancer and, 263–264
  cytogenic observations in, 257–259
  factors complicating direct assessment of human health risk in, 253–254
  no observable effect level in, 263
Epidemiology versus toxicology, 247–250
  before the fact versus after the fact, 247–248
  dose versus response, 249
  experimental versus observational studies in, 248–249
  generalizability, 249

SUBJECT INDEX

E

Ethanol
  hepatic blood flow in clearance of, 137
  metabolic cooperation and, 84
Ethoxybenzamide
  binding studies of, 134
  Vmax and Michaelis constants for, 137
Ethylnitrosourea, 21,22
  in transplacental carcinogenesis, 182–185,190
Exogenous metabolic activation systems, 99
Exposure assessment, 235

F

Fetal protein, cell-mediated immunity and, 73
α-Fetoprotein, 68–70
Flow-limited tissues, pharmacokinetic effects in, 142
N-2-Fluorenylacetamide, in transplacental carcinogenesis, 186
Formaldehyde, inhalation of, 5
Formalin-treated cells, in DNA-cell-binding assay, 93–96
Furan derivatives, 122

G

Gehring-Blau model, 230–231
Genetic toxicology, 33–38
  genotoxicity assays in, 34
  in regulatory process, 34–35
  short-term tests in, 33–34
Genotoxic chemicals, 93–96
Genotoxicity, SCEs as index of, 269–270
Glutathione conjugation, 151
  3MF and, 123–124

H

Haber's law, 5
Hazard identification, 235
HCB, see Hexachlorobiphenyls
236-HCB, see Hexachlorobiphenyls
245-HCB, see Hexachlorobiphenyls
Helper T lymphocytes, 100
Hemoglobin, alkylated derivatives in, 8
Hexachlorobiphenyls, 106–107, 115
  HPLC analysis of, 110–111
  in vitro and in vivo results in, 113–115
  metabolites of, 110–111
  as model for metabolism of PCBs, 109–110
Host susceptibility, toxicological risk and, 5–6
HPRT, see Hypoxanthine-guanine phosphoribosyltransferase
Human cells, cytotoxic effect of carcinogens in, 18–21
Human direct mutagenicity test results
  and health outcomes of individuals tested, 62
  interpreting, 61
Human lymphocytes, cytogenetic endpoints in, 41–48

Human risk assessment, pharmacokinetic model and, 129–146
Human T-lymphocytes, 51–63; see also Lymphocyte entries; T-lymphocytes; 6-Thioguanine resistant; T-lymphocyte system
Hypoxanthine-guanine phosphoribosyltransferase
  deficiency in, 53
  in TG^r T-lymphocyte system, 52

I

Immune system
  assessing human risk to, using mouse model system, 176
  cellular components of, 166
  chemicals in, effects of, 165–176
  as target organ, 165–167
Immunologic alteration(s), 167–175
  antibody response to thymic-dependent antigen in, 168–169
  antigen distribution and monocyte-macrophage phagocytosis, 173–174
  cytolytic killer cell activity in, 171–172
  delayed hypersensitivity in, 170–171
  lymphocyte proliferation in response to mitogens, 172–173
  mechanisms of, dissecting, 174
  mixed lymphocyte response in, 171
  serum immunoglobulin and complement levels in, 174
  tier system of immunological assessment in, 174–175
Immunomodulation, see Chemical-induced immunomodulation
In-utero testing, avoiding, 264–265
Intracellular macromolecules, alkylation and repair of, 6–7
4-Ipomeanol, 159

K

K-hit model, 229,230
Kepone
  enteric model for transport of, 143–144
  tissue-to-blood distribution coefficients for, 134
Kinetic models, 230–232

L

Lesch-Nylan mutation, 52
Liver function tests, in environmental risk assessment, 256–257
LN mutation/LN syndrome, see Lesch-Nylan mutation
Log-normal model, 230
Logistic model, 230
Lymphocyte assays, 42–48
  chemical-induced aberrations and estimates of exposure in, 44–46

SUBJECT INDEX

Lymphocyte assays *(contd.)*
  chromosome aberrations and, 43
  increasing sensitivity of, 47–48
  methods of culture, 42–43
  radiation induced aberrations and estimates of exposure in, 43–44
  S-phase in, 45
  SCE and, 46–47
Lymphocyte proliferation, in response to mitogens, 172–173

M

Melamine, bladder stones and, 268–269
Membrane-limited tissues, pharmacokinetic effects in, 142
Metabolic activation, toxicity and, 120–122
Metabolic cooperation *in vitro*, 79–85
  cell growth regulation and, 80
  chalones or chalone-like substances and, 80
  hypothesis of, 79–80
  selected carcinogens and, 83–84
  solvents and, 84–85
  structurally diverse chemicals in, 82
  tumor promoters and, 81–83
  V79/HGPRT mutation assay and, 80–81
Metabolism, *in vitro–in vivo* correlation and, 136
Metabolizing enzymes, in teratogenicity testing, 208
Methotrexate, plasma half life of, 135
3-Methylfuran, 119–120,122–125
  background, 122–123
  carcinogenicity of, 160
  in environmentally polluted area, 159–160
  human risk assessment and, 125
  metabolic activation *in vitro*, 123–124
  nasal olfactory damage due to, 159
  target tissue toxicity, 124–125
O^6-Methylguanine-DNA methyltransferase, 7
Methylnitrosourea, in transplacental carcinogenesis, 185,190
3-MF, *see* 3-Methylfuran
Misonidazole, pharmacokinetic model of, 137
Mixed lymphocyte response, 169,171
MNNG, *see* N-methyl-N'-nitro-N-nitrosoguanidine
MNU, *see* Methylnitrosourea
Monocyte-macrophage, 166
Monocyte-macrophage phagocytosis, antigen distribution and, 173–174
Multi-hit model, 229,230
Multi-stage model, 229,230
Murine tumors, AFP in, 69–70
Mutagenicity, human cells in, 17–29
Mutant TG^r T-lymphocytes, 56–58
  method, 56–57
  results, 58
Mutational transformation, 99–100
Mutations
  excision before DNA synthesis and, 24–26
  thioguanine resistance and, 99

N

N-acetoxy-2-acetylaminofluorene, 21,22
N-acetoxy-4-acetylaminostilbene, 21
N-acetylcysteine, 159
N-methyl-N-nitro-N'-nitrosoguanidine, 22,70
Nasal epithelium, 3-MF and, 125
Natural killer cells, 166
Neoplastic transformation
  diploid human fibroblasts and, 26–27
  DNA damage and genetic changes in, 27–29
  measuring frequency of, 17
  mutagenesis and, similarities between, 27
  mutations in, 17–18
Nitrilotriacetic acid, metabolic cooperation and, 84
No observable effect level, 263

O

Olfactory epithelium, damage to, 266–267
OMDM, *see* O^6-Methylguanine-DNA methyltransferase
Oncofetal protein, 70–71
Oncofetal substances, 68
Oncogenes, and toxicology, 264
One-hit model, 228–229,230

P

PCB(s)
  compartmental flow diagram for, 132
  metabolic cooperation and, 84
  metabolism of, 106–107,115
    in vitro versus *in vivo* results in, 113–115
    rates of, 113
  metabolized, 136
PCB congeners
  blood distribution coefficients for, 133
  body weight and, 136
  pharmacokinetic model of distribution of, 131,132
  potential health risks associated with, 256–257
  in site specific modeling, 244
  species differences in elimination of, 108
  structures of, 109
PCB-equivalents, 112
PCB hydroxylation, 115
PCB metabolites, HPLC analysis of, 110–112
Perfusion rates, in tissue uptake, 138–139
Permeability-gut surface area product, 144
pha, *see* Phytohemagglutinin
Pharmacokinetic model(s), 129–146
  anatomical similitude among, 132–133
  in cancer risk assessment, 145–146
  of PCB distribution, 131,132
  physiological parameters of, 134–138
  purpose of, 131
  route of administration in, 143–145
  thermodynamic parameters of, 133–134
  transport in, 138–143
  for vapor inhalation, 144
Pharmacokinetics, in risk assessment, 145–146

SUBJECT INDEX

Phenol and phenol metabolites, 82–83
Phenytoin, clearances and half lives of, 137
Phorbol-12,13-dibutyrate, 81
Phorbol-12-myristate-13-acetate, 80
    DMSO and, 84–85
Physiological models, bias toward, 161
Physiological pharmacokinetics, *see*
    Pharmacokinetic model(s)
Phytohemagglutinin, 41,53,54
Plasma perfusion rate, 139
PMA, *see* Phorbol-12-myristate-13-acetate
Polychlorinated biphenyls, *see* PCB *entries*
Polymorphonuclear leukocyte, 166
Probit model, 230

Q

Quantitative risk assessment, 129–130

R

Radioactive material, covalent binding of, 121
Reactive electrophilic intermediates, 122
Replication, 100
Retrodifferentiation, 68
Risk assessment; *see also* Environmental risk
    assessment; Epidemiology and toxicology
    considerations in, 235
    defining, 235
    environmental distribution and fate in, 235–244
    exposure assessment in, 236–237
    metabolism studies in, 105–116
    models for estimating environmental
        distribution and fate in, 237
    pharmacokinetics in, 145–146
    threshold in, 263
Risk assessment model, 129
Risk characterization, 235
rRNA, hypomethylation of, 7

S

S-phase, lymphocyte assays and, 45
Saccharin, 264
Saturable membrane transport, 142
SCE, *see* Sister chromatid exchanges
SCM, *see* Sodium cyclamate
Semicarbazide, 123–124
Serum immunoglobulin and complement levels, 174
Sister chromatid exchanges, 46–47
    analysis of, 42,46
    as genotoxicity index, 269–270
Site specific modeling, 241–244
Site specific parameters associated with a
    river, 241–244
    alachlor and atrazine in Rathburn reservoir, 242
    chlorinated solvents in, 242–244
    chlorpyrifos applied to fish pond, 241–242
    PCBs in, 244
Sodium cyclamate, 82
Somatic cell biomonitoring systems, 60

T

T killer cells, 172
    function of, 169
T lymphocytes, 165,166; *see also* Cloned
    lymphocytes
    in DTH, 169
    immunoselection and, 59
    in MLR, 169
TAFA, *see* Tumor-associated fetal antigens
Technical grade dinitrotoluene, 36
Teratogenic risk, criteria for ideal test system
    for, 203–204
Teratogenicity testing, 203–210
    cell culture in, 205–206
    mammalian *in vitro* test culture system, 204,205
    metabolizing enzymes in, 208–209
    organ culture in, 206
    whole embryo culture, 206–208
TG, *see* 6-Thioguanine
TG^r T-lymphocyte system, *see* 6-Thioguanine
    resistant T-lymphocyte system
Thioguanine resistance, 99
6-Thioguanine, resistance to, 21
6-Thioguanine resistant T-lymphocyte system,
    52–58; *see also* Cloned T-lymphocytes;
    Mutant TG^r T-lymphocytes
    autoradiographic assay for, 53–56
    method, 53–54
    phenocopies, 54–55
    recent results, 56
    control labeling index formula for, 53
    mutants versus mutations, 61–62
    rationale for method, 52–53
    variant frequency formula for, 54
Thymic-dependent antigen, 168–169
Tissue-to-blood distribution coefficients, 134
Tissue-to-blood partition coefficients, 140
Toxic chemical agents, time course of tissue
    uptake of, 138
Toxic chemicals, dermal uptake of, 144–145
Toxicity
    metabolic activation and, 120–122
    route of administration of chemical in, 143–145
Toxicity testing, metabolism studies in, 105–116
Toxicological risk evaluation, 3–9
    alkylation and repair of intracellular
        macromolecules, 6–7
    host susceptibility and, 5–6
    human biological monitoring in, 7–9
    progress in, 3–4
    significant advances in, 4–5
Toxicology; *see also* Epidemiology versus
    toxicology
    complex mixtures and, 267–268
    dose response information related to human
        beings, 266
    oncogenes and, 264
    progress in, 268

Toxicology *(contd.)*
　protective effects for data in, 270
　statistical analysis in, 270–271
Transplacental carcinogenesis, 179–192
　BaP in, 186,190,191
　brain tumors and, 180
　cancer and, 180–181
　cellular determinants of risk in, 185–187
　childhood cancer and, 180–181
　DEN and, 182,183,188,189
　direct evidence in, 179–182
　DMBA in, 183,186,189,191
　DMN and, 182,188,190
　ENU and, 182–185,190
　N-2-fluorenylacetamide and, 186
　and human cancers of middle and old age, 181
　identification of, 187–191
　　assay systems, 187
　　in vivo assays, 187–189
　　short *in vitro* tests, 187
　indirect evidence from animal models, 181–182
　MNU in, 185,190
　modulating factors in, 182–187
　postnatal effects in, 184–185
　species effects in, 183–184
　target organs in, 183–184
　time-specific effects in, 183–184

Tumor-associated fetal antigens, 69–70
Tumorigenesis, carcinogen-metabolizing enzymes and, 186
Tumors, multi-stepped process in development of, 17

U

UDS, *see* Unscheduled DNA synthesis
Unit World model, 237–241
　data requirements in, 238–239
　processes operating in, 238
　proper ties required for operating, 240
　results from using, 240
Unscheduled DNA synthesis, 35
Urine, alkylated derivatives in, 8

V

Vaginal carcinoma, DES in, 179–180
Vinyl chloride dose-response curve, 231

W

Weibull dose-response model, 229,230

X

X-ray induced small bowel adenocarcinoma, 73

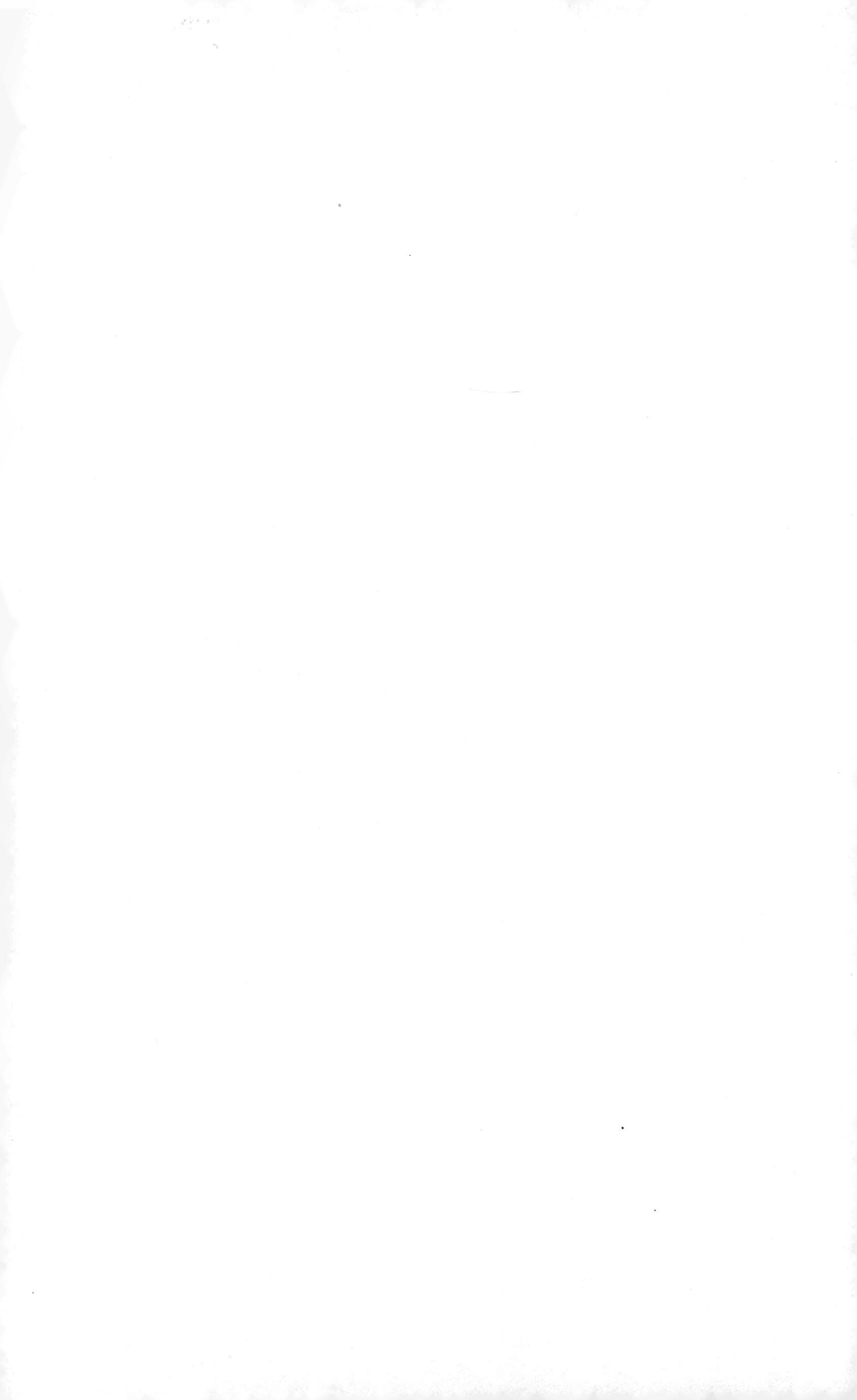